Mental Health Effects of COVID-19

Mental Health Effects of COVID-19

Edited by

Ahmed A. Moustafa
Department of Psychiatry, Wroclaw Medical University, Wroclaw, Poland

School of Psychology & Marcs Institute for Brain and Behaviour, Western Sydney University, Sydney, NSW, Australia

ELSEVIER

ACADEMIC PRESS

An imprint of Elsevier

Academic Press is an imprint of Elsevier
125 London Wall, London EC2Y 5AS, United Kingdom
525 B Street, Suite 1650, San Diego, CA 92101, United States
50 Hampshire Street, 5th Floor, Cambridge, MA 02139, United States
The Boulevard, Langford Lane, Kidlington, Oxford OX5 1GB, United Kingdom

Library of Congress Cataloging-in-Publication Data
A catalog record for this book is available from the Library of Congress

British Library Cataloguing-in-Publication Data
A catalogue record for this book is available from the British Library

ISBN 978-0-12-824289-6

For information on all Academic Press publications
visit our website at https://www.elsevier.com/books-and-journals

Publisher: Nikki Levy
Acquisitions Editor: Joslyn Chaiprasert-Paguio
Editorial Project Manager: Barbara Makinster
Production Project Manager: Omer Mukthar
Cover Designer: Mark Rogers

Typeset by SPi Global, India

Dedication

This book is dedicated to all people around the globe who have suffered from COVID-19.

Contents

Contributors xv
Preface xix
Acknowledgment xxi

Part I
Impact of COVID-19 on mental health

1. **COVID-19 and the impact on gambling, sex, and pornography use and addictions**
Anastasia Hronis and Patrick Dixon

Introduction 3
The impact of COVID-19 on gambling behaviors and addiction 4
Gambling and gambling disorder 4
Vulnerability to gambling disorder 5
The impact of COVID-19 on gambling use and gambling disorder 7
The impact of COVID-19 on sexual behaviors and addictions 10
Sexual behaviors and sex addiction 10
The impact of COVID-19 on sexual behaviors and addictions 11
The impact of COVID-19 on pornography use and addiction 12
Pornography use and addiction 12
The impact of COVID-19 on pornography use and addiction 13
Conclusion 14
References 14

2. **Care leavers' experiences of COVID-19 in Uganda and Ghana: Implications for their mental health and psychosocial wellbeing**
Paul Bukuluki, Kwabena Frimpong-Manso, and Francis Kato

Introduction 19
Methodology 21
Data analysis 23
Results 23
The effects of COVID-19 26
Employment and livelihood-related issues 26

Strained relationships and disrupted social support systems 27
Fear and anxiety 28
Coping mechanisms 29
Religion, faith, and prayer 29
Changing or holding on the known 30
Maintaining an optimistic position and accepting change 31
Connectedness to informal support systems 32
Discussion 32
Conclusion 34
References 34

3. The impact of COVID-19 on mental health of frontline health workers in Ghana and Uganda

Simon Peter Katongole, Peter Yaro, and Paul Bukuluki

Introduction 37
Methods 40
Results 41
Mental health and psychosocial challenges faced by the frontline health workers 41
Emotional effects of COVID-19 to frontline health workers 41
Psychosocial factors affecting frontline health workers engaged in COVID-19 services provision 48
Behavioral mental health challenges faced by frontline health workers 51
The coping mechanisms to overcome mental health and psychosocial challenges among frontline health workers during COVID-19 52
Interpersonal problem solving mechanisms 53
Selection of the health workers to be part of the response team 53
Appropriate scheduling of duties 53
Developing mutual support among the response team members 54
Good healthcare system leadership 55
Interpersonal emotional building mechanisms 55
Morale boosting from workmates 56
Family support 57
The intrapersonal coping strategies employed by frontline health workers in COVID-19 57
Adherence to infection prevention control and standard operating procedures 57
Staying away from family when one has been exposed 58
The sense of calling to serve patients 58
Developed positive thinking 59
Feeling of making a special contribution to the pandemic 60
Spirituality 60
Believing that COVID-19 in the hospitals is less severe than earlier thought about 60
Bearing in mind that one has no underlying medical condition that would put them at risk 61

Adequate training and preparedness 61
Taking COVID-19 as an opportunity to learn 62
Discussion 62
Conclusion 64
References 65

4. The psychosocial effect of COVID-19 on urban refugees: Narratives from Congolese refugees living in Kampala

Paul Bukuluki, Hadijah Mwenyango, Francis Kato, Agnes Kyamulabi, and Alex Bagabo

Introduction 69
Methodology 71
Design 71
Sample 71
Procedures 72
Results 73
Key findings: Psychosocial impact of COVID-19 on urban refugees 73
Fear of COVID-19 75
Anger/irritability 75
Financial distress 76
Anxiety 76
Sleep disorders 77
Social and physical isolation 78
Loss of social support 79
Social malfunction 80
Resilience and personal coping mechanisms 80
Discussion 81
Social role limitations and lost identity 82
Ruptured lives 83
Loss of personal control 83
Resilience and coping mechanisms 84
Do refugees need psychosocial support? 84
Conclusion 85
References 86

5. Psychological distress, social support, and psychological flexibility during COVID-19

Richard Tindle and Ahmed A. Moustafa

Psychological distress during COVID-19 90
Social support 92
Psychological flexibility 94
Conclusions 96
References 97

6. The impact of COVID-19 social restrictions on culture and psychosocial well-being: The Ghanaian experience

Alfred Dickson Dai-Kosi, Victoria Akuorkor Acquaye, Kingsley Kwadwo Asare Pereko, Paa-Kwesi Blankson, and Christian Ackom

Introduction 103
COVID-19 lockdowns and restrictions 104
COVID-19 and sociocultural challenges of Ghanaians 105
Influence of restrictions and lockdowns on individuals 107
Conceptualization of health problems and COVID-19 compliance 109
Conclusion 113
References 113

7. "Alone, but not lonely": The impact of COVID-19 on older persons and the role of technology in staying connected

Ceylan Okan, Gabrielle Weidemann, and Phoebe E. Bailey

Introduction 117
Chapter overview 117
Loneliness in older age and mental health implications 118
Loneliness and mental health impacts during the coronavirus pandemic 120
Alternative ways to socialize? Online communication and social media use by older adults 123
Older adults and online communication during the coronavirus pandemic 126
Conclusion 127
References 127

8. Social isolation as a laboratory model of depression

Gunes Unal

Introduction: Social isolation as a laboratory model of depression 133
Sociality and the meaning of isolation 134
Defining social isolation 136
Self-imposed/voluntary vs. enforced isolation 137
The behavioral effects of social isolation 138
The physiological effects of social isolation 140
Conclusion: The uniquely human aspect of social isolation 142
References 143

9. **Increased hallucinations in patients with Alzheimer's disease during the Covid-19 lockdown: A presentation of two cases**

Mohamad El Haj and Frank Larøi

The two cases	154
Hallucination assessment and results	155
Discussion	155
References	157

10. **Eating disorders during a coronavirus pandemic**

Samantha Hayes and Evelyn Smith

Introduction	159
Eating disorders	160
Clinical implications	165
Conclusion	169
References	169

11. **Obsessive-compulsive disorder during and after Covid-19 pandemic**

Anıl Şafak Kaçar

Introduction	171
Obsessive-compulsive disorder	171
How to decide excessive behavior during the Covid-19 pandemic?	174
Effect of Covid-19 pandemic on OCD patients	175
Expected increase in OCD prevalence	179
Conclusions	181
Acknowledgments	182
References	182

Part II
Recent topics on impact of COVID-19 on health

12. **The role of nutrition in respiratory disease and COVID-19 management**

Kingsley Kwadwo Asare Pereko, Enock Dugbatey Mensah, Victoria Akuorkor Acquaye, Christiana Nsiah-Asamoah, Flora Chadare, Freda Dzifa Intiful, Jacob Setorglo, Nancy Innocentia Ebu, and Alfred Dickson Dai-Kosi

Introduction	187
Background	188
Nutrition and immunity	188
Nutrition infection cycle	192

Nutrition and infectivity 193
Nutrition and disease recovery 194
Nutrition and respiratory illness 195
Nutrition and respiratory infectivity 195
Nutrition and immunity against respiratory illness 196
Nutrition and recovery from respiratory illness 198
Nutrition and COVID-19 199
Contemporary evidence on nutrition and COVID-19 199
Nutrition and immune development in COVID-19 200
Nutrition and COVID-19 infectivity 200
Nutrition and recoveries from COVID-19 201
Nutrition for optimal mental health during COVID-19 202
Nutrition in management of COVID-19 204
Conclusion 205
References 206

13. Physical activity as a counteracting measure to mitigate the harmful effects of COVID-19 lockdowns: Special focus on healthy children, adolescents, adults, elderly, athletes, and people with Down syndrome

Monoem Haddad, Zied Abbes, Amine Ghram, Germina Cosma, and Karim Chamari,

Introduction 215
Preventing COVID-19 spread 217
Consequences of COVID-19 on health 217
Sedentary behavior, bed rest, and physical inactivity during COVID-19 lockdown 218
Why are physical activity and sports important for health? 219
Physical activity and sports in healthy adults 219
Physical activity and sports in elderly 220
Physical activity and sports in children and adolescents 222
Physical activity and sports in athletes 223
Physical activity in individuals with Down syndrome 224
Conclusion 226
References 227

14. Parenting through the COVID-19 pandemic

Natalie M.V. Morrison and Ben. W. Morrison

Introduction 235
The changing landscape of parenting 236
Relational models of the parent-child dynamic 238
COVID-19 parental stressors 240
Health anxiety 241
Role collision and navigation 242
Financial burden 246

Sleep deprivation 246
Family separation 247
Parental burnout 247
Family violence 249
Parental coping through COVID-19 250
Parent-led posttraumatic growth 253
Conclusion 254
References 255

15. Compliance with health-protective behaviors in relation to COVID-19: The roles of health-related misinformation, perceived vulnerability, and personality traits

Zahir Vally

Introduction 263
Health-related misinformation 265
The propagation of health-related misinformation on social media 266
Factors associated with the sharing of COVID-19 misinformation 267
Evidence of the association between belief in conspiracy theories and COVID-19 health-protective behaviors 269
Perceived risk and health-protective behaviors 271
The role of personality traits in the adoption of health-protective behaviors 273
Summary and conclusion 275
References 276

16. Social media use, experiences of social connectedness and wellbeing during COVID-19

Jacqui Taylor-Jackson, Imogen Abba, Alessandra Baradel, Jeremy Lay, Jasmin Herewini, and Amber Taylor

Literature review 283
Social connectedness and psychological wellbeing 285
Social media and social connectedness 285
Social media and negative impacts on psychological wellbeing 287
Methodological limitations of research relating to social media use and wellbeing 287
Rationale 288
Method 288
Results 289
Quantitative data analysis 289
Qualitative data analysis 289
Discussion 295
Conclusions and further research 297
References 297

17. Cognitive behavior therapy for COVID-19 related distress

Karen Moses and Bethany M. Wootton

COVID-19 and distress 301
Assessment of COVID-19 related distress 302
Cognitive behavior therapy for COVID-19 related distress 304
Individualized case formulation 304
Psychoeducation 305
Situation selection 305
Cognitive restructuring 305
In vivo exposure 306
Imaginal exposure 307
Eliminating safety behaviors 308
Structured problem solving 308
Physiological arousal and stress reduction 309
Activity scheduling 309
Sleep hygiene 310
Crisis support 310
Remote CBT 311
Conclusion 312
References 312

Index 319

Contributors

Numbers in parentheses indicate the pages on which the author's contributions begin.

Imogen Abba (283), School of Psychology, Western Sydney University, Sydney, NSW, Australia

Zied Abbes (215), Department of Physical Education, College of Education, Qatar University, Doha, Qatar

Christian Ackom (103), Department of Psychological Medicine and Mental Health, School of Medical Sciences, College of Health and Allied Sciences, University of Cape Coast, Cape Coast, Ghana

Victoria Akuorkor Acquaye (103, 187), Department of Psychological Medicine and Mental Health, School of Medical Sciences, College of Health and Allied Sciences, University of Cape Coast, Cape Coast, Ghana

Alex Bagabo (69), Department of Social Work and Social Administration, Makerere University, Kampala, Uganda

Phoebe E. Bailey (117), School of Psychology, Western Sydney University, Sydney, NSW, Australia

Alessandra Baradel (283), School of Psychology, Western Sydney University, Sydney, NSW, Australia

Paa-Kwesi Blankson (103), Department of Oral and Maxillofacial Surgery, Korle-Bu Teaching Hospital, Accra, Ghana

Paul Bukuluki (19, 37, 69), Department of Social Work and Social Administration, Makerere University, Kampala, Uganda

Flora Chadare (187), Laboratoire de Sciences et Technologie des Aliments et Bioressources et de Nutrition Humaine, Université Nationale d'Agriculture, Ketou, Benin

Karim Chamari (215), Aspetar, Qatar Orthopaedic and Sports Medicine Hospital, Doha, Qatar

Germina Cosma (215), Department of Theory and Methodology of Motor Activities, University of Craiova, Craiova, Romania

Alfred Dickson Dai-Kosi (103, 187), Department of Community and Preventive Dentistry, School of Medicine and Dentistry, University of Ghana, Legon, Ghana

Patrick Dixon (3), Graduate School of Health, University of Technology Sydney, Ultimo, NSW, Australia

Nancy Innocentia Ebu (187), School of Mursing and Midwifery, College of Health and Allied Sciences, University of Cape Coast, Cape Coast, Ghana

Mohamad El Haj (153), Laboratoire de Psychologie des Pays de la Loire (LPPL–EA 4638), Nantes Université, University of Angers, Nantes; Unité de Gériatrie, Centre Hospitalier de Tourcoing, Tourcoing; Institut Universitaire de France, Paris, France

Kwabena Frimpong-Manso (19), Department of Social Work, University of Ghana, Accra, Ghana

Amine Ghram (215), Department of Exercise Physiology, Faculty of Physical Education and Sport Sciences, University of Tehran; Department of Cardiac Rehabilitation, Tehran Heart Center, Tehran University of Medical Sciences, Tehran, Iran

Monoem Haddad (215), Department of Physical Education, College of Education, Qatar University, Doha, Qatar

Samantha Hayes (159), School of Psychology, Western Sydney University, Penrith, NSW, Australia

Jasmin Herewini (283), School of Psychology, Western Sydney University, Sydney, NSW, Australia

Anastasia Hronis (3), Graduate School of Health, University of Technology Sydney, Ultimo, NSW, Australia

Freda Dzifa Intiful (187), Department of Dietetics, School of Biomedical and Allied Health Sciences, College of Health Sciences, University of Ghana, Korle-Bu, Ghana

Anıl Şafak Kaçar (171), Graduate School of Health Sciences, Koç University; Koc University Research Center for Translational Medicine (KUTTAM), Istanbul, Turkey

Francis Kato (19, 69), Department of Social Work and Social Administration, Makerere University, Kampala, Uganda

Simon Peter Katongole (37), Uganda Martyrs University, Faculty of Health Sciences, Nkozi, Uganda

Agnes Kyamulabi (69), Department of Social Work and Social Administration, Makerere University, Kampala, Uganda

Frank Larøi (153), Department of Biological and Medical Psychology, University of Bergen, Bergen, Norway; Norwegian Center of Excellence for Mental Disorders Research, University of Oslo, Oslo, Norway; Psychology and Neuroscience of Cognition Research Unit, University of Liège, Liège, Belgium

Jeremy Lay (283), School of Psychology, Western Sydney University, Sydney, NSW, Australia

Enock Dugbatey Mensah (187), Department of Biochemistry, School of Biological Sciences, College of Agricultural and Natural Sciences, University of Cape Coast, Cape Coast, Ghana

Ben. W. Morrison (235), Department of Psychology, Macquarie University, Macquarie Park, NSW, Australia

Natalie M.V. Morrison (235), School of Medicine; Translational Health Research Institute, Western Sydney University, Penrith, NSW, Australia

Karen Moses (301), School of Psychology, Western Sydney University, Sydney, NSW, Australia

Ahmed A. Moustafa (89), Department of Psychiatry, Wroclaw Medical University, Wroclaw, Poland; School of Psychology & Marcs Institute for Brain and Behaviour, Western Sydney University, Sydney, NSW, Australia

Hadijah Mwenyango (69), Department of Social Work and Social Administration, Makerere University, Kampala, Uganda

Christiana Nsiah-Asamoah (187), Department of Clinical Nutrition and Dietetics, School of Allied Health, College of Health and Allied Sciences, University of Cape Coast, Cape Coast, Ghana

Ceylan Okan (117), School of Psychology, Western Sydney University, Sydney, NSW, Australia

Kingsley Kwadwo Asare Pereko (103, 187), Department of Community Medicine, School of Medical Sciences, College of Health and Allied Sciences, University of Cape Coast, Cape Coast, Ghana

Jacob Setorglo (187), Department of Medical Biochemistry, School of Medical Sciences, College of Health and Allied Sciences, University of Cape Coast, Cape Coast, Ghana

Evelyn Smith (159), School of Psychology, Western Sydney University, Penrith, NSW, Australia

Amber Taylor (283), Division of Psychology and Language Science, University College London, London, United Kingdom

Jacqui Taylor-Jackson (283), School of Psychology, Western Sydney University, Sydney, NSW, Australia

Richard Tindle (89), Faculty of Business, Justice and Behavioural Sciences, School of Psychology, Charles Sturt University, Port Macquarie, NSW; School of Health and Behavioural Sciences, Discipline of Psychology, University of the Sunshine Coast, Sippy Downs, QLD, Australia

Gunes Unal (133), Behavioral Neuroscience Laboratory, Department of Psychology, Boğaziçi University, Istanbul, Turkey

Zahir Vally (263), Department of Clinical Psychology, United Arab Emirates University, Al Ain, United Arab Emirates; Nuffield Department of Population Health, University of Oxford, Oxford, United Kingdom

Gabrielle Weidemann (117), School of Psychology, Western Sydney University, Sydney, NSW, Australia

Bethany M. Wootton (301), Graduate School of Health, University of Technology Sydney, Sydney, NSW, Australia

Peter Yaro (37), Basic Needs Ghana, Accra, Ghana

Preface

The COVID-19 pandemic is most likely transmitted to the human population in December 2019. The movement of people from Wuhan resulted in massive spread nationally and internationally where people travelled during the holidays. The World Health Organization (WHO) declared COVID-19 as a pandemic on 11th March 2020 by the time it has already spread to about 114 countries with 118,000 cases and it killed 4291 people around the globe. According to WHO "If countries detect, test, treat, isolate, trace, and mobilize their people in the response, those with a handful of cases can prevent those cases becoming clusters, and those clusters becoming community transmission".

Mental health is one of the biggest problems which needs to be addressed post-COVID-19 pandemic as this crisis has generated tremendous stress to the public. Lockdowns, the spread of fake news, and poor understanding of the seriousness have contributed to several mental, as well as physical, health problems. Moreover, ethical dilemma in treating patients with health problems added more burdens on medical professionals due to COVID-19, which we also discuss in this book. This book provides several chapters on how the COVID-19 pandemic could endanger the mental well-being of millions of individuals causing depression, anxiety, insomnia, distress, and even suicidal attempts. In conclusion, an immediate measure should be taken to assess and provide mental and psychosocial support services to vulnerable people as well as healthcare workers during and following the COVID-19 pandemic.

In this book, we also provide a comprehensive analysis of mental health problems due to COVID-19, including eating disorders, depression, problematic gambling, suicidal thoughts and attempts, trauma and obsessive-compulsive disorder (OCD) symptoms, among others. We further explain the impact of COVID-19 on the family's well-being, parenting, and society dynamics. We further provide chapters to explain how physical activity and social connectedness can help mitigate the impact of COVID-19 on mental health. We end up with a chapter to explain how cognitive behavioral therapy (CBT) methods can be used to reduce mental health problems due to COVID-19.

Acknowledgment

I would like to thank all chapter authors and contributors, including, but not limited to Anastasia Hronis, Paul Bukuluki, Victoria Acquaye, Ceylan Okan, Gunes Unal, Mohamad El Haj, Evelyn Smith, Anil Kacar, Kingsley Kwadwo Asare Pereko, Monoem Haddad, Natalie Morrison, Zahir Vally, Jacqui Taylor-Jackson, and Karen Moses. I also like to thank all coauthors as well for their efforts.

Part I

Impact of COVID-19 on mental health

Chapter 1

COVID-19 and the impact on gambling, sex, and pornography use and addictions

Anastasia Hronis and Patrick Dixon
Graduate School of Health, University of Technology Sydney, Ultimo, NSW, Australia

Introduction

COVID-19 has had a far-reaching impact on people throughout the world and has resulted in hardships that have cultivated a vulnerability to mental health difficulties. The mental health repercussions of COVID-19 on the global population have been estimated to be catastrophic if additional funding and supports are not put in place (Mucci, Mucci, & Diolaiuti, 2020). As of early 2020, it was indicated that mental health has been negatively impacted on a global scale due to COVID-19, with a rise in unemployment, financial uncertainty, and mental health disorders (Ahmed et al., 2020; Galea, Merchant, & Lurie, 2020; Mukhtar, 2020; Torales, O'Higgins, Castaldelli-Maia, & Ventriglio, 2020). Furthermore, rates of domestic violence have increased, placing those affected at further risk of mental health disorders (Bradbury-Jones & Isham, 2020; Mukhtar, 2020). With life as we once knew it being affected in plethora of domains, psychological harm has been predicted to continue to grow, with examples of adjustment disorder, acute stress, depression, and anxiety among some of the growing number of mental health concerns predicted to increase over time (Ahmed et al., 2020; Torales et al., 2020). Furthermore, the effects on mental health, due to COVID-19, are predicted to proceed long after the peak of the pandemic (Mukhtar, 2020). These delayed effects on mental health could last years after the peak and manifest in a diverse range of unhealthy internal and external psychosocial experiences.

COVID-19 has created particular vulnerability for those with preexisting addiction disorders and has increased risk for those with moderate- or high-risk behaviors. Moreover, many addictive behaviors often develop gradually, meaning that the full extent of new or resurfaced addictive behaviors may not fully emerge until the weeks and months following the pandemic. In addition to a potential increase in people developing problematic behaviors or experiencing lapses and relapses within addiction, there has also been a restriction of some service provisions available to those struggling. For example, social distancing

Mental Health Effects of COVID-19. https://doi.org/10.1016/B978-0-12-824289-6.00016-7

restrictions have meant that fewer people are able to access inpatient, outpatient, and rehabilitation facilities. In addition, most support groups such as 12 Step Recovery programs and SMART Recovery groups were required to stop face-to-face meetings and move to online sessions, creating barriers for those without the ability to access the online meetings.

The current chapter explores the impact of COVID-19 on gambling, sex, and pornography use, with a specific focus on problematic behavioral addictions, including gambling disorder, sex addiction, and pornography addiction.

The impact of COVID-19 on gambling behaviors and addiction

Gambling and gambling disorder

Problem gambling is a multifaceted mental health issue and is categorized in the Diagnostic and Statistical Manual of Mental Disorders (5th ed., DSM 5; American Psychiatric Association, 2013) as an addictive disorder. Gambling disorder is the experience of persistent and recurrent problematic gambling behavior leading to significant impairment or distress over a 12-month period (American Psychiatric Association, 2013). An individual may experience symptoms such as requiring increasing amounts of money to gamble in order to achieve the desired excitement, restlessness or irritability when attempting to cut down or stop gambling, repeated unsuccessful efforts to control or stop gambling, a preoccupation with gambling in an individual's thought patterns, gambling to relieve emotional distress, chasing one's losses, relying on others to provide money, lying to conceal the extent of gambling, and gambling despite consequences to relationships, education, or career opportunities (American Psychiatric Association, 2013; Binde, 2013).

Gambling behaviors are not uncommon, with approximately 70%–80% of Australians participating in a gambling activity at least one time per year (Delfabbro & King, 2012). However, approximately 1% of the population have significant problems with gambling, with a further 1.4%–2.1% considered at risk of developing gambling disorder (Productivity Commission, 2010). These figures may in fact underestimate the number of gamblers who suffer problematic consequences, as these figures are based on screening tools used in community telephone surveys (Delfabbro & King, 2012), with a recent systematic review indicating that up to 12% of the population may have a gambling problem (Calado, Alexandre, & Griffiths, 2017). In 2015 it was estimated that 1.39 million Australian adults had experienced one or more gambling-related problems (Armstrong & Carroll, 2017; Dowling et al., 2016). This rate has continued to increase, with the number of betting platforms increasing, as well as betting companies and websites (Armstrong & Carroll, 2017). In comparison to twenty years ago, gambling has become more accessible and more common in Australia (Armstrong & Carroll, 2017). The gambling industry has had a catastrophic effect on Australia, with 18 billion AUD being spent on gambling in 2015, and approximately 24 billion AUD spent on gambling in 2017–18, which is more per capita than any other country in the world (Armstrong & Carroll, 2017; Australian Gambling Statistic, 2019).

There are many forms of gambling, including card games (e.g., poker, blackjack, baccarat), electronic gaming machines (i.e., poker machines), sports betting, lottery, and traditional casino games (e.g., roulette, craps). Poker machines or "pokies" are the main platform of gambling in Australia (Armstrong & Carroll, 2017; Dowling et al., 2016). Australians are among the highest gamblers in the world as demonstrated by the fact that Australians spend on average 15 billion AUD per year on poker machines (Armstrong & Carroll, 2017). In addition to these, more common forms of gambling, betting platforms have continued to add a variety of topics people can gamble on, from reality television to clothing items of the prime minister of Australia. The internet has provided a platform for a magnitude of new forms of gambling, making gambling now more accessible and more prominent than ever before (Gainsbury et al., 2014). Online gambling has made gambling more accessible, increasing chances for regular gamblers to acquire gambling disorder (Gainsbury et al., 2014). Furthermore, people who gamble using offshore gambling websites are more likely to experience problematic gambling in comparison with those who gamble using legal platforms (Gainsbury et al., 2014).

Vulnerability to gambling disorder

There are a number of factors which have been identified as contributing to the development of a gambling disorder. Factors which place an individual at risk of developing a gambling disorder include psychological distress, interpersonal difficulties, isolation, boredom, avoidance, mood modification, and filling feelings of emptiness (Barrault & Varescon, 2013; Ledgerwood & Petry, 2006; Wood & Griffiths, 2007). In addition, being male, demonstrating higher levels of aggression, and experiencing a higher number of depressed symptoms have been linked with problematic gambling (Sagoe et al., 2017). Specifically, adolescent males with higher levels of aggression (both verbal and physical) and greater symptoms of anxiety and depression have been shown to be at high risk of transitioning to problematic gambling from adolescents to adulthood (Sagoe et al., 2017). Stress in particular has been found to be a significant predictor of gambling behaviors and problem gambling with those who are under stress whether financial, health, social, family, professional, being more vulnerable to develop pathological gambling problems (Olason, Hayer, Brosowski, & Meyer, 2015).

Multiple pathways to developing a pathological gambling disorder have been identified. In Blaszczynski and Nower's (2002) seminal paper, the Pathways Model was proposed, integrating empirical and clinical knowledge linking biological, personality, developmental, cognitive, and environmental factors associated with problem gambling into one framework. Three specific pathways to the development of problem gambling are as follows: the behaviorally conditioned problem gamblers, the emotionally vulnerable problem gamblers, and the antisocial impulsivist problem gamblers. While ecological determinants, conditioning processes, and cognitive schemas are present in all pathways, problem gamblers with emotional vulnerabilities often present with premorbid anxiety or depression, poor coping and problem solving skills, and negative life experiences. The emotionally vulnerable gambler is in large motivated to engage in gambling in order to modulate affective states and meet specific psychological needs (Blaszczynski & Nower, 2002). Low mood reduces the tendency to gamble for enjoyment but increases the tendency to gamble in order to regulate emotional states, suggesting that gambling while depressed may be driven by the desire to modulate dysphoric or depressed states (Lloyd et al., 2010).

Regarding the neuroscience of gambling, dopamine, a key component within the brain's reward system, is a central reason as to why gambling can be so addictive (Clark et al., 2013; Love, Laier, Brand, Hatch, & Hajela, 2015). When the brain experiences reward, the neurotransmitter dopamine gets released to activate the feeling of pleasure and euphoria, leading to a continuous desired effect. Due to the sense of euphoria and the ease of access to gambling, gambling is reinforced as a positive experience, thus continuing the cycle of gambling (Clark et al., 2013). Over repeated use, desensitization occurs, that is, the euphoria release is not experienced at the same level as it was initially, which increases the urge to gamble more in order to strive for that same euphoric sensation (Clark et al., 2013). Throughout this process, dependence to gambling occurs, meaning that a person gambles to feel stability rather than the euphoria that was once experienced (Clark et al., 2013; Love et al., 2015). The neurological processes which occur with gambling are similar to those with other addictions (Linnet, Møller, Peterson, Gjedde, & Doudet, 2011; Love et al., 2015).

Problem gambling has been shown to have negative effects on personal, professional, social, and psychological aspects of the people involved and those associated with them. Problem gambling affects more people than just the individual participating in the gambling, with studies estimating that at least six people in addition to the individual gambling are negatively impacted (Goodwin, Browne, Rockloff, & Rose, 2017). Gambling can also have negative consequences on an individual's overall mental health and well-being. People with a gambling disorder are up to 20 times more likely to display psychological distress, approximately 2.5 times more likely to be depressed, and just under 50% of people with gambling disorder experience anxiety (Victorian Department of Justice, 2009). They also experience high rates of drug and alcohol use (Armstrong & Carroll, 2017). Problematic gambling can also induce feelings of guilt and shame from dishonesty with self and loved ones, lessened sense of self-worth due to difficulty ceasing gambling habits, financial difficulties including loss of assets, borrowing money, and dependence on welfare, and potential increase in criminal activity like petty theft to fuel problem gambling. These behaviors can result in an incongruence between one's ideal self and their current self, further diminishing self-esteem and facing reality, which manifests into further avoidance of reality and leads to urges to gamble to avoid (Brown, Oldenhof, Allen, & Dowling, 2016).

The impact of COVID-19 on gambling use and gambling disorder

On March 23, 2020, COVID-19 lockdown measures were imposed in Australia and as a result, many Australians were forced to stay longer times at home. As part of the lockdown, pubs, clubs, and casinos were all closed, meaning that Australia's 194,000 poker machines were no longer accessible to the 15%–25% of the population who access them (Australian Gambling Statistics, 2019). Furthermore, COVID-19 has ravished the world with uncertainty that has manifested in an increase in stress across a range of critical domains. The rates of unemployment have dramatically increased since COVID-19 as the financial stability of once prosperous industries has diminished, resulting in financial stress for many individuals (Baker, Bloom, Davis, & Terry, 2020). Furthermore, the stress of the uncertainty of physical health associated with the threat of COVID-19 has multiplied the rate and intensity of mental health concerns across the country (Fiorillo & Gorwood, 2020). These stressors, as identified earlier, are factors which create an increased vulnerability for people to develop problematic gambling behaviors. Psychosocial stress is a key driver of high risk and addictive gambling, and there are few situations more stressful, and at the same time boring, than what COVID-19 and the lockdown restrictions have brought about. In addition, the Australian government has allowed people to withdraw up to $20,000 from their superannuation accounts, which for individuals at risk of problem gambling or with a gambling disorder, could prove to be very dangerous.

During COVID-19, an increase in online gambling was noticed. From Jun 2019 to June 2020 (the time of writing this chapter), the average monthly amount of money spent on online gambling in Australia has fluctuated until March 2020, whereby it started to increase each month. Spending on online gambling in Australia increased by 67% during the first week of April (Alphabeta, 2020). Australian gamblers spent 90% more on gambling during June 2020 than in June 2019. These Australians spent $802 each on average in June 2020, while the average spend in June 2019 was $421. The number of gambling transactions per person also more than doubled in June 2020 compared to June 2019, with a 140% increase. Spending on online gambling in June 2020 exceeded spending on online gambling in May 2020 by 32%. In June 2020 the amount spent on gambling per gambler averaged at $802 which was $194 higher than May 2020 ($608), resulting in June 2020 having the highest average spend per person on gambling in the past 12 months. The average amount spent per transaction increased by $12 from $66 in May 2020 to $78 in June 2020, and the average number of online gambling transactions per gambler also saw a 12% rise. Research on the numbers of online gambling transactions found results that indicated there had been a 142% increase in transactions from March 2020 to the beginning of May (Alphabeta, 2020). Furthermore, people who gamble using offshore gambling websites are more likely to experience problematic gambling in comparison with those who gamble using legal platforms (Gainsbury et al., 2014). With the closing of pubs and clubs around Australia and the world, the lure for online offshore gambling is also predicted to increase (Gainsbury et al., 2014).

A study conducted in Sweden compared gambling rates before and during the COVID-19 pandemic (Håkansson, 2020). The research was conducted using participants from the general population, with 9% of the total number of participants reporting either a moderate to high risk of problematic gambling behaviors (Håkansson, 2020). The results suggested that the majority of participants had not increased their gambling since the pandemic; however, those who had reported prior to COVID-19 a gambling problem increased in their gambling as well as increased their alcohol intake (Håkansson, 2020). Furthermore, participants that identified that they had increased other forms of online gambling (i.e., online casino) due to sports cancellations were more likely to have gambling problems than those that did not (Håkansson, 2020), transitioning their gambling from one form to another. The results from this study suggest that the general population may be less likely to increase their gambling due to COVID-19; however, those people with preexisting gambling problems are more likely to increase their gambling habits and alcohol consumption since the onset of COVID-19 (Håkansson, 2020).

An Australian study has found similar preliminary results, showing that during COVID-19 lockdown, almost three in four respondents in a self-selected sample reported spending less time gambling during the shutdown, with reported monthly gambling spend reducing from AUD $450 on average pre-lockdown, to $200 during lockdown (Gainsbury, Swanton, Burgess, & Blaszczynski, 2020). Of the people who reported an increase in gambling behaviors, over half were identified as having gambling problems or engaging in moderate risk gambling. Higher psychological distress and COVID-19 related financial difficulties appear to be linked with increases in gambling expenditure, but not increases in gambling frequency. Most participants reported expecting to resume their normal gambling patterns post-shutdown. Similar findings have been noted in the UK, with a survey of people who gamble regularly in the UK indicating that approximately two-thirds of participants had either continued to gamble the same as before or had increased their gambling behaviors since the onset of COVID-19 and the associated restrictions (Survation, 2020).

For some, COVID-19 and the lockdown produced positive benefits. A study which specifically looked at sports betting via an online casino found evidence to suggest that frequent gamblers continued to gamble at a similar rate, whereas infrequent gamblers reduced or even stopped online gambling (Auer, Malischnig, & Griffiths, 2020). The study focused on people who gambled on sporting competitions online and the change in online casino gambling when sports stopped due to COVID-19. Sports bettors did not switch to playing more online casino games and that there was also a significant reduction in playing online casino games among sports bettors. It is also estimated that with pubs and clubs with poker machines in Australia closing due to COVID-19 restrictions, an estimated 1.5 billion AUD has been saved (Gambling Reform, 2020). The closing of casinos across Australia has shown a further 500 million AUD saved on gambling losses (Gambling Reform, 2020).

While COVID-19 led to the restriction of access to traditional land casinos, pubs, and clubs, novel ways to gamble were developed. During the COVID-19 pandemic, gamblers could wager on how often President Donald Trump used his "favorite" words and phrases during his daily COVID-19 task force briefings. "Return to action" markets were also offered on major international sporting events where punters could bet on whether the next game would be played before June, July, or August 2020. The rise of online gambling is further dangerous due to targeted advertising. People who are using gambling websites during the pandemic will likely continue to see advertisements for these online services for many months after use, with constant reminders potentially making it harder to stop using these sites through retargeting advertising strategies.

Volatility in the stock market during the first half of 2020 is linked to a significant increase in Australians trading on the stock market. In May 2020 Australian Securities and Investments Commission (ASIC) reported that more than 140,000 new investors signed up to brokers between 24 February and 3 April, an average of 4575 new accounts per day (Australian Securities and Investments Commision, 2020). This is an increase of approximately 3.4 times compared to the previous six months, with new investors accounting for approximately 21% of all existing accounts. The search on Google for the term "how to buy shares" in Australia spiked at the start of March after global stock markets plunged. While some may see this as an opportunity to enter the market at a low point, others may be out of work and searching to buy and sell shares on short time frames as a source of income. It is important, however, that this also be considered an alternative to gambling, posing the same risks as sports betting, casinos, or poker machines.

Unfortunately, COVID-19 has also brought about restrictions in the ways people can now access treatments and supports for gambling problems. Multidisciplinary inpatient and community outpatient health and mental health services have become in high demand for people with addictive behaviors due to the increased demand caused by COVID-19, leaving people at higher risk than before of relapse, increased problematic behavior, and less essential immediate support (Dubey et al., 2020). Furthermore, restrictions due to social distancing and quarantine guidelines have meant people with addictive disorders including gambling have less exposure to group therapy, and therefore, are more likely to either relapse or increase their addictive behavior in the context of COVID-19 (Columb, Hussain, & O'Gara, 2020). Furthermore, hospitals that treat addiction disorders including gambling have reported that since COVID-19, the topic of therapy has shifted from relapse prevention and addiction management strategies to anxiety and stress management in the context of the uncertainty and life difficulties that have come from the impact of COVID-19 (Columb et al., 2020). Many group therapy approaches to treating gambling addiction reduced or changed, with the 12 Step Fellowship Gambler's Anonymous (GA) stopping face-to-face sessions and some moving to online meetings.

Government responses to COVID-19 have been promising. It was proposed that governments consider banning or reducing access to online gambling in the context of COVID-19 given the predicted increases in problem gambling rates and predicted high severity of impact that COVID-19 may have on people with problem gambling and gambling disorder (Columb et al., 2020). The Latvian government implemented a ban on online gambling since COVID-19 (Columb et al., 2020), while the UK stopped television and radio advertisements during the COVID-19 lockdown to try to reduce problem gambling (Skentelbery, 2020). Within Australia, the Australian Communications and Media Authority provided information on the risks of online gambling, illegal gambling, and provided a platform in which to make complaints against illegal online gambling platforms. Online mental health supports and access to overall mental health and addiction services were increased and expanded.

The impact of COVID-19 on sexual behaviors and addictions

Sexual behaviors and sex addiction

Sex addiction is defined by repetitive compulsive urges, thoughts, and acts, surrounding sex that impairs functioning and intimacy (Hall, 2011, 2014). Sex addiction is not recognized in the DSM–V; however, it is recognized in part in the ICD-11 as Compulsive Sexual Behavior Disorder. Compulsive Sexual Behavior Disorder falls into the Impulse Control Disorder section of the ICD-11 (World Health Organization, 2018). It is further characterized by a persistent pattern of failure to control intense, repetitive sexual impulses or urges resulting in repetitive sexual behavior. An individual with Compulsive Sexual Behavior Disorder may experience sexual activities becoming a central focus of the person's life at the expense of health, other interests, activities, and responsibilities. Other symptoms may include unsuccessful efforts to significantly reduce repetitive sexual behaviors, and continued repetitive sexual behaviors despite adverse consequences or deriving little or no satisfaction from it.

Sex addiction has been formulated to become a problem for an individual for a range of biopsychosocial reasons. Biologically speaking, it has been theorized with empirical backing that like other addictive behaviors, genetic predisposition to risk-taking behavior, emotion dysregulation, and impulsivity can create a higher vulnerability to become addicted to sex (Hall, 2011, 2014; Rosenberg, Carnes, & O'Connor, 2014). In terms of psychological components that contribute to sex addiction, mental health concerns such as personality disorders, anxiety, depression, and bipolar disorder have been linked with higher sexual promiscuity and sex addiction (Hall, 2011; Phillips, Hajela, & Hilton Jr, 2015). Furthermore, sex addiction has been linked with other addictions like drug and alcohol abuse (Hall, 2011; Phillips et al., 2015; Zapf, Greiner, & Carroll, 2008). For many, sex addiction is described as bringing about feelings of shame, inadequacy, and guilt due to an incongruence between the moral compass of the individual and the urges and behaviors associated with sex addiction (Hall, 2011).

The impact of COVID-19 on sexual behaviors and addictions

There is limited research at present, indicating the impact of COVID-19 on sexual behaviors and sex addiction. During the COVID-19 lockdown it was recommended that people avoid physical proximity with people outside of their households, to avoid spreading the virus, which has the potential to significantly impact the sexual activity of a person currently not in a relationship, or in a relationship living apart from their partner (Luria & Nesher, 2020). A study conducted by Li, Li, Xin, Wang, and Yang (2020) found among a self-selected sample of responders that 44% of participants reported a decrease in the number of sexual partners they engaged with, and approximately 37% reported a decrease in sexual frequency. There was an overall reduction in risky sexual behaviors, with only 5% of people within the study reporting an increase in risky sexualized behaviors since the start of COVID-19. There was also a reduction in sexual satisfaction with a partner, though it is unclear from the research as to why this may be the case Li et al. (2020). Additionally, 25% experienced a reduction in sexual desire, while only 18% of men and 8% of women reported an increase in sexual desire Li et al. (2020). Furthermore, both men and women reported a reduction in sexual satisfaction during COVID-19. It was however, noted, that 32% of men and 18% of women stated that they were inclined to increase the number of sexual partners and/or risky sexual behaviors once the pandemic came to an end. Within the UK, it was found that almost 40% were engaging in sexual activity at least once per week, and being male, younger age, married, consuming alcohol, and a higher number of days in isolation were all associated with greater sexual activity compared to their counterparts (Jacob et al., 2020). These findings correspond to the existing literature during nonpandemic times (Grabovac et al., 2020; Lee, Nazroo, O'Connor, Blake, & Pendleton, 2016; Smith et al., 2019).

It has been predicted that there will be a reduction in cases of sexually transmitted diseases (STDs) during the COVID-19 pandemic as a result of reduced sexual activity. A free service for the prevention and treatment of STDs recorded an average of approximately 70 daily outpatient visits in April 2019, compared to approximately 30 daily outpatient visits during COVID-19 (Gaspari et al., 2020). An Australian study surveyed men who have sex with men, and found that 87% stopped having casual sex during COVID-19, and 35.2% decreased their number of sexual partners (Chow et al., 2020). A survey of gay and bisexual American men during lockdown orders (April 10 and May 10, 2020), found that significant changes were made to sexual behavior in response to the pandemic (McKay et al., 2020). Nine out of ten men reported having either one sexual partner or no sexual partner during this period, which, for many, was a substantial decrease compared to before the pandemic. The men in the sample also reported making changes to the kinds of partners they had and their sexual activities with partners (e.g., more virtual sex), engaged in new strategies to reduce their risks of infection from partners, and expressed high levels of concern about how HIV may affect COVID-19 risk, treatment, and recovery. However, the percentage of men who disclosed that they had had COVID-19 symptoms to their sexual partner was low, at 40%. Thus targeted messaging around how to have conversations with partners about COVID-19 symptoms and how to better navigate the risks would be warranted (McKay et al., 2020).

It is also important to note, that as with gambling disorder treatments, many group therapy approaches to treating sex addictions were subject to restrictions due to lockdowns and social distancing. Many of the 12 Step Fellowships, including Sex and Love Addicts Anonymous (SLA), moved to online only meetings, meaning those with limited access to technologies and internet may have been at a disadvantage. Overall, it seems that COVID-19 has resulted in a decrease in sexual behaviors and risky sexual behaviors; however this is based on extremely limited research. It cannot at this point be predicted if and how these patterns may change over time.

The impact of COVID-19 on pornography use and addiction

Pornography use and addiction

Pornography use is a worldwide phenomenon, with people in countries around the world increasingly accessing pornography in recent years (Luscombe, 2016; Mestre-Bach, Blycker, & Potenza, 2020). The increased ease of access to the internet and its accessibility across multiple digital devices, including smart phones, has provided a plethora of opportunity for people to access pornography more than ever before (Luscombe, 2016). The World Health Organization has declared that pornography will often be part of the sexual education learned by adolescents (World Health Organization, 2018).

Pornography addiction, also referred to as Problematic Pornography Use (PPU), or Self-Perceived Pornography Addiction (SPPA), has been defined in a number of different ways within the research literature focusing on pornography use (Duffy, Dawson, & Das Nair, 2016). The difficulty in reaching a consensus for a definition for pornography addiction has led to some inconsistencies with research findings (Duffy et al., 2016). Despite this, common features of the definitions of pornography addiction are the continued watching of pornography on an increased level over time, despite efforts to stop, and the amount of time spent watching pornography is more than desired to the detriment of the individuals functioning (Brand, Blycker, & Potenza, 2019). Pornography addiction, although not currently included in the DSM-5, has been shown to have similar psychological and neurological effects as substance disorders and gambling disorder, and is therefore been largely recognized as a behavioral addiction as opposed to just a compulsive sexual behavior (Brand et al., 2019; Love et al., 2015).

Much like other behavioral addictions and substance addictions, pornography addiction can start as a result of the suppression of uncomfortable emotions including loneliness, fear, shame, boredom, and sadness (Young, 2008). The initial use of pornography can begin from curiosity, and the instant gratification and release of dopamine can reinforce its use as a means to feel better when faced with difficult emotions (Love et al., 2015; Young, 2008). Research indicates that pornography use results in or contributes to relationship difficulties, a decline in sexual satisfaction and libido, increased masturbation, and lower self-esteem and confidence (Campbell & Kohut, 2017). Furthermore, pornography addiction can become problematic for other aspects of life such as social, professional, and financial (Campbell & Kohut, 2017). Pornography addiction can cause functional impairment, emotional avoidance, and psychopathology (Mestre-Bach et al., 2020).

A number of psychosocial risk factors have been associated with pornography use and addiction, with depression, anxiety, and substance use disorders commonly occurring in people with people with pornography addiction (Brand et al., 2019). Research has indicated that men tend to view pornography more than women (Hald, 2006). Specifically, factors that were linked with pornography use were being male, younger age of first exposure to pornography, and higher frequency of masturbation (Hald, 2006).

The impact of COVID-19 on pornography use and addiction

COVID-19 has led to uncertainty and increased psychological distress across the world (Torales et al., 2020). Furthermore, isolation, limited contact with others outside of the household, has heightened the stress and limited access to previous coping strategies such as socializing with friends and family, exercising at gyms and health clubs, and working (Hwang, Rabheru, Peisah, Reichman, & Ikeda, 2020; Torales et al., 2020). Stress and uncertainty, which has increased due to the repercussions of COVID-19, have cultivated a situation where addictive behaviors such as pornography use become more tempting (Mestre-Bach et al., 2020).

Preliminary research shows that the use of the internet, particularly websites relating to pornography and video gaming, has markedly increased during the period of lockdown (Király et al., 2020). An increase in distress, loneliness, and boredom, as well as limited access to face-to-face support groups for addiction are potential influential factors associated with the increased rate of pornography use in the context of COVID-19 (Mestre-Bach et al., 2020). In 2019 one of the largest pornography websites, Pornhub, reported to have had 42 billion visits to the website (Pornhub, 2019, 2020). Pornhub reported an increase of 11.6% worldwide in visits to their website as of March 17 with the increased impact of COVID-19, and an increase of 24.4% on March 25 after it offered free access to its premium site to encourage people to stay indoors and distance themselves socially (Pornhub, 2020). Furthermore, in regions where Pornhub promoted a free premium trial, rates of pornography use increased from 38% to 61% (Pornhub, 2020).

Conclusion

Overall, COVID-19 has changed the patterns of engagement with gambling, sex, and pornography. While online gambling statistics indicate that more people were gambling online during the pandemic, self-reported measures indicate that many people maintained or reduced gambling, while those who are at moderate risk or have a gambling problem increased their use. There appears to be an overall decrease in sexual activity, though for those with higher rates of sexual engagement and sex addiction prior to COVID-19, an increase in sexual behaviors is noted. Finally, access to online pornography appears to have increased during the COVID-19 lockdown period. Due to limited preliminary research, and the constant changes that the pandemic brings, it is difficult to say whether these changes to gambling, sex, and pornography will be maintained, or if people will return to their usual patterns after the pandemic.

References

Ahmed, M. Z., Ahmed, O., Aibao, Z., Hanbin, S., Siyu, L., & Ahmad, A. (2020). Epidemic of COVID-19 in China and associated psychological problems. *Asian Journal of Psychiatry, 51*(1). https://doi.org/10.1016/j.ajp.2020.102092.

Alphabeta. (2020). *COVID-19 economic impact: Real time tracking*. Retrieved June 30, 2020, from https://www.alphabeta.com/illiontracking.

American Psychiatric Association. (2013). *Diagnostic and statistical manual of mental disorders* (5th ed.). Arlington, VA: American Psychiatric Association.

Armstrong, A., & Carroll, M. (2017). *Gambling activity in Australia*. Melbourne, Australia: Australian Gambling Research Centre, Australian Institute of Family Studies.

Auer, M., Malischnig, D., & Griffiths, M. D. (2020). Gambling before and during the COVID-19 pandemic among European regular sports bettors: An empirical study using behavioral tracking data. *International Journal of Mental Health and Addiction*, 1–8. https://doi.org/10.1007/s11469-020-00327-8.

Australian Gambling Statistics. (2019). *Australian gambling statistics*. Retrieved 30 June, 2020, from https://www.qgso.qld.gov.au/issues/2646/australian-gambling-statistics-35th-edn-1992-93-2017-18.pdf.

Australian Securities & Investments Commision. (May, 2020). *Retail investor trading during COVID-19 volatility*. Retrieved June 30, 2020 from https://download.asic.gov.au/media/5584799/retail-investor-trading-during-covid-19-volatility-published-6-may-2020.pdf.

Baker, S. R., Bloom, N., Davis, S. J., & Terry, S. J. (2020). *Covid-induced economic uncertainty (No. w26983)*. National Bureau of Economic Research. Retrieved June 28, 2020, from https://www.nber.org/papers/w26983.

Barrault, S., & Varescon, I. (2013). Cognitive distortions, anxiety, and depression among regular and pathological gambling online poker players. *Cyberpsychology, Behavior and Social Networking*, *16*(3), 183–188. https://doi.org/10.1089/cyber.2012.0150.

Binde, P. (2013). Why people gamble: A model with five motivational dimensions. *International Gambling Studies*, *13*(1), 81–97. https://doi.org/10.1080/14459795.2012.712150.

Blaszczynski, A., & Nower, L. (2002). A pathways model of problem and pathological gambling. *Addiction*, *97*(5), 487–499.

Bradbury-Jones, C., & Isham, L. (2020). The pandemic paradox: The consequences of COVID-19 on domestic violence. *Journal of Clinical Nursing*, *29*(13–14), 2047–2049. https://doi.org/10.1111/jocn.15296.

Brand, M., Blycker, G. R., & Potenza, M. (2019). When pornography becomes a problem: Clinical insights. *Psychiatric Times*, *36*(12), 48–51.

Brown, M., Oldenhof, E., Allen, J. S., & Dowling, N. A. (2016). An empirical study of personality disorders among treatment-seeking problem gamblers. *Journal of Gambling Studies*, *32*(4), 1079–1100.

Calado, F., Alexandre, J., & Griffiths, M. D. (2017). Prevalence of adolescent problem gambling: A systematic review of recent research. *Journal of Gambling Studies*, *33*(2), 397–424. https://doi.org/10.1007/s10899-016-9627-5.

Campbell, L., & Kohut, T. (2017). The use and effects of pornography in romantic relationships. *Current Opinion in Psychology*, *13*, 6–10. https://doi.org/10.1016/j.copsyc.2016.03.004.

Chow, E. P., Hocking, J. S., Ong, J. J., Schmidt, T., Buchanan, A., Rodriguez, E., … Fairley, C. K. (2020, July). Changing the use of HIV pre-exposure prophylaxis among men who have sex with men during the COVID-19 pandemic in Melbourne, Australia. In *Open forum infectious diseases*. US: Oxford University Press. (Vol. 7, no. 7, p. ofaa275).

Clark, L., Averbeck, B., Payer, D., Sescousse, G., Winstanley, C. A., & Xue, G. (2013). Pathological choice: The neuroscience of gambling and gambling addiction. *Journal of Neuroscience*, *33*(45), 17617–17623. https://doi.org/10.1523/JNEUROSCI.3231-13.2013.

Columb, D., Hussain, R., & O'Gara, C. (2020). Addiction psychiatry and COVID-19: Impact on patients and service provision. *Irish Journal of Psychological Medicine*, *37*(3), 164–168. https://doi.org/10.1017/ipm.2020.47.

Delfabbro, P., & King, D. (2012). Gambling in Australia: Experiences, problems, research and policy. *Addiction*, *107*(9), 1556–1561. https://doi.org/10.1111/j.1360-0443.2012.03802.x.

Dowling, N. A., Youssef, G. J., Jackson, A. C., Pennay, D. W., Francis, K. L., Pennay, A., & Lubman, D. I. (2016). National estimates of Australian gambling prevalence: Findings from a dual-frame omnibus survey. *Addiction*, *111*(3), 420–435. https://doi.org/10.1111/add.13176.

Dubey, M. J., Ghosh, R., Chatterjee, S., Biswas, P., Chatterjee, S., & Dubey, S. (2020). COVID-19 and addiction. *Diabetes and Metabolic Syndrome: Clinical Research and Reviews*, *14*(5), 817–823. https://doi.org/10.1016/j.dsx.2020.06.008.

Duffy, A., Dawson, D. L., & Das Nair, R. (2016). Pornography addiction in adults: A systematic review of definitions and reported impact. *The Journal of Sexual Medicine*, *13*(5), 760–777. https://doi.org/10.1016/j.jsxm.2016.03.002.

Fiorillo, A., & Gorwood, P. (2020). The consequences of the COVID-19 pandemic on mental health and implications for clinical practice. *European Psychiatry*, *63*(1), E32. https://doi.org/10.1192/j.eurpsy.2020.35.

Gainsbury, S. M., Russell, A., Hing, N., Wood, R., Lubman, D. I., & Blaszczynski, A. (2014). The prevalence and determinants of problem gambling in Australia: Assessing the impact of interactive gambling and new technologies. *Psychology of Addictive Behaviors*, *28*(3), 769–779. https://doi.org/10.1037/a0036207.

Gainsbury, S., Swanton, T., Burgess, M., & Blaszczynski. (2020). *The impact of the COVID-19 shutdown on gambling in Australia Preliminary results from Wave 1 cross-sectional survey*. Gambling Treatment and Research Clinic, Brain & Mind Centre. https://www.sydney.edu.au/content/dam/corporate/documents/brain-and-mind-centre/usyd-covid-gambling-research-report-aug-2020.pdf.

Galea, S., Merchant, R. M., & Lurie, N. (2020). The mental health consequences of COVID-19 and physical distancing: The need for prevention and early intervention. *JAMA Internal Medicine*, *180*(6), 817–818. https://doi.org/10.1001/jamainternmed.2020.1562.

Gambling Reform (2020). Retrieved June 30, 2020 from https://www.pokiesplayyou.org.au/media_releases.

Gaspari, V., Orioni, G., Viviani, F., Raone, B., Lanzoni, A., & Bardazzi, F. (2020). Does COVID-19 influence sexual behaviors? *Dermatologic Therapy*, e14004. https://doi.org/10.1111/dth.14004.

Goodwin, B. C., Browne, M., Rockloff, M., & Rose, J. (2017). A typical problem gambler affects six others. *International Gambling Studies*, *17*(2), 276–289. https://doi.org/10.1080/14459795.2017.1331252.

Grabovac, I., Smith, L., Yang, L., Soysal, P., Veronese, N., Isik, A. T., … Jackson, S. (2020). The relationship between chronic diseases and number of sexual partners: An exploratory analysis. *BMJ Sexual & Reproductive Health*, *46*(2), 100–107.

Håkansson, A. (2020). Changes in gambling behavior during the COVID-19 pandemic—A web survey study in Sweden. *International Journal of Environmental Research and Public Health*, *17*(11), 4013. https://doi.org/10.3390/ijerph17114013.

Hald, G. M. (2006). Gender differences in pornography consumption among young heterosexual Danish adults. *Archives of Sexual Behavior*, *35*(5), 577–585. https://doi.org/10.1007/s10508-006-9064-0.

Hall, P. (2011). A biopsychosocial view of sex addiction. *Sexual and Relationship Therapy*, *26*(3), 217–228. https://doi.org/10.1080/14681994.2011.628310.

Hall, P. (2014). Sex addiction—an extraordinarily contentious problem. *Sexual and Relationship Therapy*, *29*(1), 68–75. https://doi.org/10.1080/14681994.2013.861898.

Hwang, T., Rabheru, K., Peisah, C., Reichman, W., & Ikeda, M. (2020). Loneliness and social isolation during the COVID-19 pandemic. *International Psychogeriatrics*, 1–4. https://doi.org/10.1017/S1041610220000988.

Jacob, L., Smith, L., Butler, L., Barnett, Y., Grabovac, I., McDermott, D., … Tully, M. A. (2020). Challenges in the practice of sexual medicine in the time of COVID-19 in the United Kingdom. *The Journal of Sexual Medicine*, *17*(7), 1229–1236.

Király, O., Potenza, M. N., Stein, D. J., King, D. L., Hodgins, D. C., Saunders, J. B., … Abbott, M. W. (2020). Preventing problematic internet use during the COVID-19 pandemic: Consensus guidance. *Comprehensive Psychiatry*, 152180.

Ledgerwood, D. M., & Petry, N. M. (2006). Psychological experience of gambling and subtypes of pathological gamblers. *Psychiatry Research, 144*(1), 17–27. https://doi.org/10.1016/j.psychres.2005.08.017.

Lee, D. M., Nazroo, J., O'Connor, D. B., Blake, M., & Pendleton, N. (2016). Sexual health and well-being among older men and women in England: Findings from the English longitudinal study of ageing. *Archives of Sexual Behavior, 45*(1), 133–144.

Li, W., Li, G., Xin, C., Wang, Y., & Yang, S. (2020). Challenges in the practice of sexual medicine in the time of COVID-19 in China. *The Journal of Sexual Medicine, 17*(7), 1225–1228. https://doi.org/10.1016/j.jsxm.2020.04.380.

Linnet, J., Møller, A., Peterson, E., Gjedde, A., & Doudet, D. (2011). Dopamine release in ventral striatum during Iowa gambling task performance is associated with increased excitement levels in pathological gambling. *Addiction, 106*(2), 383–390. https://doi.org/10.1111/j.1360-0443.2010.03126.x.

Lloyd, J., Doll, H., Hawton, K., Dutton, W. H., Geddes, J. R., Goodwin, G. M., & Rogers, R. D. (2010). Internet gamblers: A latent class analysis of their behaviours and health experiences. *Journal of Gambling Studies, 26*(3), 387–399.

Love, T., Laier, C., Brand, M., Hatch, L., & Hajela, R. (2015). Neuroscience of internet pornography addiction: A review and update. *Behavioral Science, 5*(3), 388–433. https://doi.org/10.3390/bs5030388.

Luria, M., & Nesher, S. P. (2020). Challenges in the practice of sexual medicine in the time of COVID-19 in Israel. *The Journal of Sexual Medicine, 17*(7), 1209–1211.

Luscombe, B. (2016). Porn and the threat to virility. *Time, 187*, 4047.

McKay, T., Henne, J., Gonzales, G., Quarles, R., Gavulic, K. A., & Garcia Gallegos, S. (2020). *The COVID-19 Pandemic and Sexual Behavior among Gay and Bisexual Men in the United States*. Available at SSRN 3614113.

Mestre-Bach, G., Blycker, G. R., & Potenza, M. N. (2020). Pornography use in the setting of the COVID-19 pandemic. *Journal of Behavioral Addictions, 9*(2), 181–183.

Mucci, F., Mucci, N., & Diolaiuti, F. (2020). Lockdown and isolation: Psychological aspects of COVID-19 pandemic in the general population. *Clinical Neuropsychiatry: Journal of Treatment Evaluation, 17*(2), 63–64.

Mukhtar, S. (2020). Psychological health during the coronavirus disease 2019 pandemic outbreak. *The International Journal of Social Psychiatry*. https://doi.org/10.1177/0020764020925835.

Olason, D. T., Hayer, T., Brosowski, T., & Meyer, G. (2015). Gambling in the mist of economic crisis: Results from three national prevalence studies from Iceland. *Journal of Gambling Studies, 31*(3), 759–774.

Phillips, B., Hajela, R., & Hilton, D. L., Jr. (2015). Sex addiction as a disease: Evidence for assessment, diagnosis, and response to critics. *Sexual Addiction & Compulsivity, 22*(2), 167–192. https://doi.org/10.1080/10720162.2015.1036184.

Pornhub. (2019). *The 2019 Year in review*. Retrieved June 20, 2020, from https://www.pornhub.com/insights/2019-year-in-review.

Pornhub. (2020). *Coronavirus insights*. Retrieved June 25, 2020, from https://www.pornhub.com/insights/corona-virus.

Productivity Commission. (2010). *Gambling. Productivity Commission draft report*. Canberra: Productivity Commission.

Rosenberg, K. P., Carnes, P., & O'Connor, S. (2014). Evaluation and treatment of sex addiction. *Journal of Sex & Marital Therapy, 40*(2), 77–91. https://doi.org/10.1080/0092623X.2012.701268.

Sagoe, D., Pallesen, S., Hanss, D., Leino, T., Molde, H., Mentzoni, R. A., & Torsheim, T. (2017). The relationships between mental health symptoms and gambling behavior in the transition from adolescence to emerging adulthood. *Frontiers in Psychology, 8*, 478. https://doi.org/10.3389/fpsyg.2017.00478.

Skentelbery, G. (2020). *UK gambling firms stop advertising during the COVID—19 lockdown.* Retrieved June 30, 2020, from https://www.warrington-worldwide.co.uk/2020/05/04/uk-gambling-firms-stop-advertising-during-the-covid-19-lockdown/.

Smith, L., Yang, L., Veronese, N., Soysal, P., Stubbs, B., & Jackson, S. E. (2019). Sexual activity is associated with greater enjoyment of life in older adults. *Sexual Medicine*, *7*(1), 11–18.

Survation. (2020). *Survation Clean Up Gambling Online Survey Data Tables (1) [Data file].* Retrieved on June 29, 2020, from https://www.survation.com/covid-19-survation-survey-for-clean-up-gambling-campaign-points-to-addiction-concerns-during-coronavirus-lockdown/.

Torales, J., O'Higgins, M., Castaldelli-Maia, J. M., & Ventriglio, A. (2020). The outbreak of COVID-19 coronavirus and its impact on global mental health. *International Journal of Social Psychiatry*, *66*(4), 317–320. https://doi.org/10.1177/0020764020915212.

Victorian Department of Justice. (2009). Retrieved on 30 June, 2020, from. In *Gambling*. https://www.justice.vic.gov.au/safer-communities/gambling.

Wood, R. T., & Griffiths, M. D. (2007). A qualitative investigation of problem gambling as an escape-based coping strategy. *Psychology and Psychotherapy: Theory, Research and Practice*, *80*(1), 107–125.

World Health Organization. (2018). *International classification of diseases for mortality and morbidity statistics (11th Revision).* Retrieved June 30, 2020, from https://icd.who.int/browse11/l-m/en.

Young, K. S. (2008). Internet sex addiction: Risk factors, stages of development, and treatment. *American Behavioral Scientist*, *52*(1), 21–37. https://doi.org/10.1177/0002764208321339.

Zapf, J. L., Greiner, J., & Carroll, J. (2008). Attachment styles and male sex addiction. *Sexual Addiction & Compulsivity*, *15*(2), 158–175. https://doi.org/10.1080/10720160802035832.

Chapter 2

Care leavers' experiences of COVID-19 in Uganda and Ghana: Implications for their mental health and psychosocial wellbeing

Paul Bukuluki[a], Kwabena Frimpong-Manso[b], and Francis Kato[a]
[a]*Department of Social Work and Social Administration, Makerere University, Kampala, Uganda,*
[b]*Department of Social Work, University of Ghana, Accra, Ghana*

Introduction

In Ghana and Uganda, two low-income sub-Saharan African countries, an increasing number of young people leave residential care each year to begin life on their own in the wider society. The increase in young people making their transitions to adulthood from care contexts is because, in both countries, many children live outside without parental care because of a complex and interrelated set of socioeconomic factors, consisting of poverty, orphanhood, abandonment, and detrimental cultural practices (Casey, 2011; Ministry of Gender, Labour and Social Development, and UNICEF Uganda, 2015). In Ghana, children under 18 make up 45% of the population of 25,904,600. Despite economic growth and peaceful political environment, a third of the populace live below the poverty line and food insecurity, with Ghana ranked 142/189 on the United Nations Human Development Index (Better Care Network & UNICEF, 2015). Uganda is ranked 161/186 in the United Nations Human Development Index and is among the countries with the fastest growing populations in Africa, with an annual population growth rate of 3.2% (UBOS and ICF, 2018). Youth (aged 12–30) constitute almost 80% of Uganda's 34.6 million citizens (UBOS & ICF, 2018). Uganda is among the countries that experienced high prevalence of HIV and AIDS and armed conflict. It is estimated that because of these and other factors including poverty, Uganda has about 2 million orphans (Wylde, Ssewankambo, & Baryabanoha, 2012).

Most orphan and vulnerable children (OVC) live in informal foster care provided by extended family members (Milligan, Withington, Connelly, & Gale, 2017). However, for some OVCs, these informal care arrangements are

Mental Health Effects of COVID-19. https://doi.org/10.1016/B978-0-12-824289-6.00018-0

either unsuitable or unavailable. For such children, the State, through the 2004 Children's Act Cap 59 (Uganda) and 1998 Children's Act 560 (Ghana), assumes responsibility for their care and protection. Despite reforms to reduce the institutionalization, residential care remains the main formal alternative care option, due to the unavailability of foster care, domestic adoption, and family support services (Frimpong-Manso, 2014; Mutenyo, Machingaidze, Okello, Otai, & Asekenye, 2019). In Uganda, recent estimates show that almost 50,000 children, 80% of who have one or both parents alive, live in 800 residential care facilities, the majority of them private orphanages (Koenderink, 2019). In 2013, 4332 Ghanaian children were living in residential care in Ghana (Better Care Network & UNICEF, 2015).

While in both countries residential care is a temporary arrangement, the evidence suggests that some children spend their entire childhood in these facilities (Frimpong-Manso, Deliege, Wilson, & Norman, 2019; Walakira, Dumba-Nyanzi, & Bukenya, 2015). As a result, several children, once they turn 18 years, the age of majority in both countries, have to leave residential care to live independently in the community. The scant research from Ghana and Uganda (Ddumba-Nyanzi, Fricke, Hong Max, Nambooze, & Riley, 2019; Frimpong-Manso, 2018; Luboyera, 2014) and other African countries (e.g., Diraditsile & Nyadza, 2018; Pryce et al., 2015; Sekibo, 2019) suggests that many young people who leave care experience several challenges.

Unemployment is high among care leavers, and those working often doing temporary, low-paying informal sector self-employment (Pouw, Hodgkinson, Le Mat, & van Dam, 2017). Several African studies report that the limited job opportunities result in many care leavers experiencing exploitation, intimidation, and sexual abuse from employers (Dziro & Rufurwokuda, 2013; Pouw et al., 2017; Pryce et al., 2015). The care leavers struggle to find jobs because they usually have limited social connections to tell them about jobs or provide references that employers require (Pryce et al., 2015). Pouw and her colleagues highlight that though the policy of many residential facilities is to provide young people with vocational training and entrepreneurship, many care leavers lack the capital or support to start their own businesses. The care leaver's inability to secure jobs makes it difficult for many care leavers to access and maintain housing, healthcare, and further their education (Sekibo, 2019). Many care leavers also experience stigma and discrimination due to their care or orphan identity. Several studies (e.g., Dziro & Rufurwokuda, 2013; Luboyera, 2014; Pryce et al., 2015) report that they struggle to get accepted in their families and communities and denied housing and jobs as they are seen as deviant youth who do not share in the cultural norms and practices of the wider society. The experiences of stigma and social exclusion result in low self-esteem and reduction of social capital.

A major reason for the challenges faced by care leavers is the lack of statutory policy and mandated services for young people during and after their transition from care (Bond, 2018). Much of what exists depends on the policies of individual care facilities, but they provide this in an ad hoc fashion because of the lack of resources (Mhongera & Lombard, 2016). Preparatory programs have been found to be effective in equipping youth leaving with the socioemotional, psychological, and economic resources to cope with and adjust to life after care (Tanur, 2012). For example, work readiness programs are effective in facilitating self-reliance of care-experienced youth through employment in the formal sector and self-employment (Bukuluki, Kamya, Kasirye, & Nabulya, 2019). There is the lack of after-care support from the residential facility for care leavers in most African countries (Frimpong-Manso, 2012; Gwenzi, 2018). Young people who leave care cannot count on or receive support from their families and communities because they often lose contact with these informal networks while in care and also lack the social skills to build relationships to access support from these support systems. The purpose of the assessment on which this chapter is based was to appreciate the mental health and psychosocial experiences, challenges, and coping mechanisms of young adults who left residential care that can be attributed to the COVID-19 pandemic. The information generated would help inform policy and programming for care leavers in the context of COVID-19 and other pandemics.

Methodology

We employed a qualitative approach and followed a phenomenological design to gain an in-depth understanding of the lived experiences of participants (Groenewald, 2004; Hycner, 1999). Given the study sort to understand the lived experiences of the participants, phenomenology was an appropriate design (Kvale, 1996; Welman & Kruger, 1999). The essence of qualitative research is the focus on a person's own perspective, views, and experiences (Curtin & Fossey, 2007; Qu & Dumay, 2011) about a phenomenon.

Purposive sampling was used to select care leavers who meet the following criteria: had been in residential care and left care in less than a year. The research team, working closely with practitioners in residential care facilities, identified and nominated care leavers who met the inclusion criteria. In addition, recruited participants were to provide information about their potential peers who would take part in the study. Overall, 11 care leavers consented and participated in the study. Six of the care leavers had left the care of SOS children village in Uganda while five had left care in SOS children's Village in Ghana. Care leavers from the SOS Children's Village were purposively selected because of its presence in the two countries and similar approaches to care across the two countries. We contacted three of the 11 participants through a snowball process. The participants had all left residential care within a period ranging from 11 months to 2 months before the interviews and were facing the COVID-19 pandemic as care leavers. All the participants we interacted with have been in residential care with SOS children Villages either Uganda (6) or Ghana (5). Given the risks that the COVID-19 pandemic presented and considering the PH&S measures, such as the Lockdown, stay at home orders, social distancing, and restriction on both private and public means of transport, we deemed telephone inquiry proper for interviewing the participants Table 1.

TABLE 1 Summary of social demographic data of the care leavers who participated in the study.

Pseudo Name	Gender		Civil status	Age	Employment	When left care	Education	Country of residence
	F	M						
Phiona	X		Cohabiting	25	Student	July 2020	University	Uganda
Moses		X	Cohabiting	25	Employed	December 2019	University	Uganda
Hillary		X	Cohabiting	26	Employed	December 2019	University	Uganda
Joan	X		Single	23	Teacher	December 2019	University	Uganda
peter		X	single	21	Employed	December 2019	Technical institute	Uganda
Evelyn	X		Single	23	Volunteer	July 2019	University	Uganda
Brian		X	Single	24	Self-employed	August 2019	Technical College	Ghana
Joan	X		Single	22	Employed	November 2019	University	Ghana
David		X	Cohabiting	24	Working	August 2019	Higher National Diploma	Ghana
Gerald		X	Single	23	Self-employed	October 2019	Senior High School	Ghana
Adrian		X	Single	22	Employed	October 2019	University	Ghana

We interviewed the participants between May and June 2020. An unstructured interview guide was used to facilitate the interactions (interviews) with the care leavers (Knox & Burkard, 2009). We prepared the guide with (substantive) questions aligned to the study objectives (Knox & Burkard, 2009; Taylor, Bogdan, & DeVault, 2015). The key domains covered in the guide included experiences in relation to social networks/relationships, social support, resilience, and personal coping mechanisms, socioeconomic and psychosocial status, and family dynamics. The intention was to facilitate an understanding of these domains from the experiences and viewpoint of the care leavers (Vaismoradi, Jones, Turunen, & Snelgrove, 2016). Before the interview, the researchers called each participant to explain the purpose of the study, the time needed, possible risks, and benefits. They emphasized voluntary participation and the right to withdraw. Permission to audio-record the interview was requested, and each participant was also encouraged to appoint schedules convenient to them for the interview to take place. As we did the interviews through telephone calls, it was not possible to make visual observations of the nonverbal cues of the participants. This could have provided additional data that could have possibly offered different dimensions to further enrich the study's findings (Lechuga, 2012). We conducted all interviews in English, which was the preferred language by the participants.

Data analysis

Thematic analysis was used to organize the data into meaningful themes and subthemes. Following each interview, the researchers listened to the audio recordings generated to familiarize and make sense of the views presented. The audios were then transcribed and processed into Microsoft Word document to support further familiarity and reflection on the content, and support the extraction of codes, subthemes, and themes (Vaismoradi & Snelgrove, 2019. Manual analysis was conducted using a matrix with codes, themes, and subthemes (Vaismoradi et al., 2016). We illustrate an example in Table 2.

It is from such a matrix that the researchers were able to transform the voices of the participants into themes and subthemes and arguments on experiences of study participants with of the COVID-19 pandemic and the related MHPSS effects.

Results

The themes generated from the data transcripts illuminate the challenges these young people faced and how they dealt with them. We divided results into two sections, the first section focusing on the care leavers' psychosocial and mental health.[a] In the second part, we look at the different ways the young adults approached the challenges, paying attention to the resource systems both intrapersonal and connected to external systems of support and their role in coping.

---

a. The term young adults in the current chapter will be used synonymously with care leavers to reflect our target population.

TABLE 2 Matrix illustrating the output from the data explication process.

Main theme	Subtheme	Relevant extract	Extract Source	Additional notes
Coping	**Faith, religion, and prayer**	*Our head pastor has been just be supportive, and he calls, he calls us, to check on us how we are doing and he just pray with us, assuring us it will be well and we will get back to our normal times, we should just believe in God and have faith in God and it will soon pass away....*	Gerald, Ghana	
	Financial discipline	*I had savings that's what was saving me in the start yeah and I had to just cut my budget short and later I got some kids to coach you know so I can be there*	Joan, Uganda	Being mindful of one's consumption patterns
	Social Support (family and Friends)	*Oh yeah, I think it could be because sometimes I sit down to think if I didn't have a foster family, (Someone speaking at the background) what would I have done? Because now I'm out of work, I'm not working.*	Adrian, Ghana	Difference in experience comparing those with and without known families
		I think they have gone through the worst and at some point yes I think so because at least they don't have anyone, they don't expect any help from anyone at least me am lucky if I don't have food I can get from home but I think they experiences it in a hard way for them to go through a hard situation us	Evelyn, Uganda	

Resilience	**Optimism and accepting change**	*I stay positive because I know that these things will not last, these are challenges that come and go, I watch TV, movies and all that just to keep myself occupied busy and talk to neighbors.*	Phiona, Uganda	
		In the start I was losing concentration but right now am kind of even getting used to the situation, am kind of getting used to everything so I no longer lose concentration that much.	Joan, Uganda	
	Constant fear of COVID-19 infection at work place	*Well, for me I have been stressed, I feel stressed Because I still go to work […] the people even if you go privately in your own ride or something okay, is still not safe, you interact with people in their offices, I mean, yeah, for me is still usual. I mean, nothing really has changed, probably quality, in terms of running shift in office, and you feeling insecure about your new customers that come your way, when there is […] maybe a face to face or in person meet up okay, interactions outside the virtual ones, well that's all I have to say.*	David, Ghana	
		Okay, during this period, I feel unusual because recently within our area where I live, we heard that there were some cases, some cases within our locality, so, they have to come and pick up those patients who have and it was a bit scary for me personally and so I had to tread very cautiously with my family anytime I am going out for any essential need.	Gerald, Ghana	

The effects of COVID-19

The participants reported several experiences that reflected the psychosocial and mental health issues and challenges attributed to or associated with the situation at hand. The related issues and challenges are further described as follows.

Employment and livelihood-related issues

There were several employment issues with psychosocial and mental health implications. The young adults we interacted with had distinct realities in terms of employment. Some had lost their jobs, which was producing stressful outcomes for them. Even those who kept their positions and continued working reported feeling insecure because of sustained fear of contracting COVID-19 through their interactions with clients/customers at the workplace. Others felt frustrated about losing additional income streams besides their formal employment:

> *Well, for me I have been stressed, because I still go to work and I feel unsafe. You interact with people in their offices, I mean, yeah, for me is still usual. I mean, nothing really has changed, probably in terms of running shift in office, yes it and has. You feel insecure about new customers that come when there is [...] maybe a face to face or in person meet up.*
>
> (Brian, Ghana).

> *Because I am into IT, I would get gigs that you would get me some money. But here I have to stay home and depend only on my salary. It is frustrating because how am I going to deal with things like my rent when I am only relying on my salary.*
>
> (Moses, Uganda).

Those who lost their jobs expressed a sense of hopelessness and stress as it often led to the total loss of livelihoods. Not being able to work put the young adults in situations of idleness and constrained their capacity to deal with negative thoughts, especially around livelihoods which having a job helped to confront. Consequently, several of them, especially those who in single-headed households, reported the presence of depression.

> *I was chef but for the past three months I have been in the house due to COVID. Right now, a lot of staff have been laid off so, things have been...bad for me because it has made my business come down*
>
> (Adrian, Ghana).

> *COVID means stress... the mere fact that you aren't receiving any money from anyone and yet you don't have a source of income, not being able to buy what you want like. I don't know like having nothing to rely on even if 20k or 10k. So, it's kind of depressing, especially if you are not working and on top of it, you won't be getting what you have been getting*
>
> (Evelyn, Uganda).

No particularly my job no—I don't think they will resume this year because even the way the president speaks about it there is no hope for schools don't think they will resume this year because even the way the president speaks about it there is no hope for schools

(Joan, Uganda).

Strained relationships and disrupted social support systems

The young adults reported difficulties managing their social relations including interactions with their immediate families and intimate partners, during the lockdown. They explained that the difficulties were as a result of the burden of providing economically for themselves and their others they were living, without their inability to travel and communicate with friends and relatives due to the existing public health and social measures:

COVID-19 has affected my relationship with my siblings, my two (2) little sisters. When they closed down the Universities, she asked me to allow her to come to my place. I am somehow [...] for example if I want something, it should be like that, more so when it is at my place. So, my sister came. I don't know maybe if I was..... She wants a nice phone, chicken, meat, ice-cream, pizza and those things. So, I would shop for food, for example 50,000 Ugandan shillings and it would literally get done in a week, and she is alone at home. She was staying at my place alone so it would really puzzle me and whenever I would talk to her, and she would get pissed.

(Hillary, Uganda).

Visiting family and friends is difficult because of the lockdown. We sometimes talk on phone and WhatsApp or chat on Facebook, but because I am not working, I don't have money to buy internet or airtime

(Adrian, Ghana).

Some of the young adults reported that they experienced limited access to needed support during the COVID-19 period, especially difficulty accessing advice and other emotional support to deal with their challenges. This was because the networks they tried to reach out to cited COVID-19 and the corresponding public health and social measures as contributing to their inability to offer help.

Like there something's that happen and you would feel I wish I can talk to someone but because [...] you can't talk to them about the same issue to be much easier unless you are talking face to face about it yes it stresses

(Peter, Uganda).

There is a challenge in accessing advice and other help. When you are in trouble and you try to reach out for advice or help, people tell you they can't assist now—during this COVID time

(Moses, Uganda).

Fear and anxiety

The pandemic and related controls have created concern for the young adults because it introduced anxiety and fear about their survival during and after the pandemic, especially as they had no help from former carer (SOS children's villages). The findings also indicated that the fear and anxiety exhibited by some of the young adults was related to the lack of 'biological family' who they could rely on for support.

> *Yeah, what makes me worried is one—am always worried about my tomorrow like how is my tomorrow going to look like. This what am worried about […] I don't have any connection or anyone close to. You don't have anyone you can run to. You don't have anyone you can cry to. Because personally if I had someone I can run to or someone I can cry on. Am worried as the way Uganda is right now everything is about who knows you, the connection […] people don't have time of listening to yourself so it is a big worry and I feel like I don't really know how my tomorrow will be, I really don't know how life will be like if you aren't so close*
>
> (Peter, Uganda).

> *It [COVID-19] is stressed me. That was the time my medications [for mental health issues] were also not working and the drugs I taking were not working. It was because of the stress, being locked down and the uncertainty around the whole virus things and no one to talk to….*
>
> (Brain, Ghana).

For other young adults, the anxiety resulted from the fact that they had used up their savings, uncertainty about the prospects of keeping their jobs, or being able to revive their small businesses after the lockdown. This kept the young adults wondering about what would happen to them next.

> *What worries me most is that the year is going to end when am just at home, my savings I have now used them up like there is nothing I totally have, this is a school that has just started this was its third year so being that she is not earning am worried and she was already speaking of closing it up and starting something else, am like by the time we resume will it still be there*
>
> (Joan, Uganda).

> *Yeah… right now I've felt terrible and worried because one… I was working, but because of the COVID, I have been in the house for the past three months. I'm doing some errands and stuff to get something to at least get some money to feed myself…*
>
> (David, Ghana).

Because of the anxiety and fear related to the uncertainties resulting from the pandemic, several of the young adults reported irregular sleep patterns; sleeping for only a few hours. They slept late and still woke up early because they felt stressed by the challenging situations they found themselves as illustrated by Evelyn from Uganda and David from Ghana.

You just wake up in the middle of the night. You lack sleep because maybe you sleep at midnight and wake up at 3 am. It has been happening during this period [COVID-19], like sleeping only to wake up, check and its still 3 or 4 am. I may go back to sleep around 6 am, but when you wake up you are tired.

(Evelyn, Ghana).

A not eating well and sleeping at all too. I am always tired. I go to bed tired, wake up tired, and I spend fewer hours in bed. It is like I go to bed I cannot sleep I get like two, four hours of sleep. And I wake up I am still tired.

(David, Ghana).

Coping mechanisms

The narratives from the young adults depicted several ways in which they coped with the psychosocial and mental health issues or challenges they were experiencing, including the use of intrapersonal resources and the others associated with connectedness to support systems.

Religion, faith, and prayer

A number of young adults pointed out the important role of faith and prayer to their ability to cope with the challenges caused by the pandemic. Those who belonged to a faith group found their networks of support very useful as they received encouragement from their religious leaders through constant follow-ups, praying together, and reassurance that things would be well. The participants noted that having these support instilled a sense of hope.

Our head pastor has been just be supportive. He calls, he calls us, to check on us how we are doing and he just pray with us, assuring us that it will be well and we will get back to our normal times. That we should just believe in God and have faith in God and it will soon pass away, because it is said that, it said in the Bible that, everything shall pass away but except the word of God, so we are, we are having faith and we are believing having hope that surely it will come to a time where by it will be there no more and we will turn to our normal times.

(Gerald, Ghana).

I wouldn't say am so much of the church person, but at least somehow it has made me more committed to God. I pray a little more and actually spend more time with the pastor. Yeah because they aren't allowing gatherings in churches so I have this pastor [priest belonging to Pentecostal Christian Churches] this side, he is actually a missionary so we normally at gather at his home about 10 people and we pray from there so I would say that somehow to me it has brought me closer to God

(Hillary, Uganda).

Changing or holding on the known

The narratives of the participants suggested that they made several adjustments to their lifestyle to fit with the wider changes brought about by COVID-19. Several mentioned that they changed their eating patterns by cutting down on the number of meals they had daily.

> *You have to reduce some expenses. Yeah, there are some things I had to do away with. One was eating the normal course meal, that is the three meals—morning, afternoon and supper. I now either eat breakfast and supper, or you eat breakfast, lunch and leave supper.*
>
> (Moses, Uganda).

The young adults also mentioned a reasonable level of financial discipline through forethought consumption decisions in the study. Having accessed information about the lockdown, they stocked up essential items in anticipation of the lockdown imposed to combat COVID-19.

> *I prepared myself well enough, yeah, by God's grace I got the stuff I needed. I made sure that my internet was intact and working so I wouldn't have to step out of the house [often during the lockdown]. I prepared because I was already following the news from other countries, lockdown is the same so you should speculate that it is possible this could happen to us*
>
> (Brian, Ghana).

Others made adjustments to their budgets as Joan from Uganda illustrated, "I had savings that's what was saving me in the start yeah and I had to just cut my budget short and later I got some kids to coach you know so that I can be there."

The results showed that practicing adherence or nonadherence to some measures to combat COVID-19 was considered by the participants as ways to cope with the challenges of the time. Some of the young adults seemed relaxed on the vigilance to social distancing where they were involved in interaction with friends, in part due to the desire to maintain the friendship and avoiding hurting it. This was despite the recognition of the risk of transmission of the virus.

> *It should be easy to comply. But let me say you are talking to a friend or a person you are used to, you will forget about COVID-19. You will move closer, something like that. I won't lie, I haven't practiced social distancing, maybe isolating myself....*
>
> (Evelyn, Uganda).

Faced with a sense of dwindling hope and rising anxiety, some young adults complied with the instituted guidelines as matter of finding reassurance against the constant fear of contracting COVID-19.

> *You have to be very cautious and also looking at you with your family and moreover too I was bereaved, my wife.... My in-law passed on so it was a blow to us,*

we had to go to a private funeral in May and looking at the COVID – 19 situation; we were scared going for the private funeral. We had to take care of precautions like the measures: wear our nose mask, and using our sanitizer...

(Gerald, Ghana).

However, it [COVID] has also increased in one way or the other my personal hygiene because I'm always cautious of washing my hand like every time, I'm very careful of who I touch, I don't just go out anyhow. I'm... like I'm mostly indoors and very reserved.

(Joan, Ghana).

Maintaining an optimistic position and accepting change

The interactions we had with the young adults showed that when the COVID-19 events unfolded, there was a loss of concentration, a panic mode that anyone one can experience when faced with a situation of the magnitude of a global pandemic. However, as time went on, some became more optimistic and developed plans to deal with COVID-19 and it is ensuing challenges. For instance, Phiona shared:

I stay positive because I know that these things will not last, these are challenges that come and go. I watch TV, movies, and all that just to keep myself occupied busy and talk to neighbors

(Phiona, Uganda).

Yes, one of the things, just like you take long to see a friend, psychologically, you miss each other, we are not going to do things like the way we have been doing, changes are going to come in where few people will participate and others will not. Then you find that some people within that same click that you would want to interact with so psychologically it brought in the change of I would say missing someone

(Moses, Uganda).

A number of the young adults reported starting up business ventures, for example rearing of chicken with the view not only surviving in the lockdown but basing on these ventures as a plan for the post-COVID-19 period. There were also those who turned to expanding on their skills. At the time of collecting the data that informed the current chapter, countries such as Ghana had lifted the lockdown, and some young adults felt disappointed that they could not accomplish the skills training they started during lockdown.

Is been a bit positive right...I got occupied during the lockdown, I find myself.... I study, catch up, learn new stuff, you know, perfect my skills and all those things in the house. So when the lockdown was lifted, I was actually disappointed because I couldn't cover everything.

(Joan, Ghana).

Connectedness to informal support systems

Narratives from the young adults who we interviewed showed that they recognize the importance of support from family and friends. The support from their informal social networks came in different forms—both material and emotional (e.g., offering advice or showing concern during the pandemic). To some extent, the participants who received such support wondered what the situation would have been like if it was unavailable. This can be observed in the following excerpts:

> *Sometimes I sit down to think if I didn't have a foster family, what I would have done [in this situation] because, [right] now I'm out of work, I'm not working.*
>
> (David, Ghana).

> *... My grandfather calls me and they ask me how am I the sickness...so am I going to work ...yes...they really care about me so they will call me and find out... because they know that the sickness is dominating in Accra so they are also afraid for me, My grandfather says don't go out—make sure you take your sanitizer, your protective things when you are going out. If I'm not going to do anything, I should stay at home...he advises me. So, I took the advice and it has really helped me.*
>
> (Gerald, Ghana).

Discussion

Care leavers are generally vulnerable and marginalized young adults who have received residential care in institutions and transitioned out of care (Kelly et al., 2020). Our study revealed that common mental health and psychosocial challenges facing young people transitioning out-of-care in Ghana and Uganda, in the context of the COVID-19 pandemic, include loss of employment and livelihoods, disrupted and reduced social support, and stress resulting from the fear and anxiety of the unknown. These experiences have also been documented by Bukuluki, Mwenyango, Katongole, Sidhva, and Palattiyil (2020) in their article on urban refugees in Uganda.

While the loss of jobs within this period is not peculiar to care-experienced young adults and impact several other people, the consequence for them is dire and more severe, especially as many care leavers in Africa, without these extra hardships, are already struggling to find stability and lack a strong support system, on which they can fall on (Frimpong-Manso, 2015; Mhongera & Lombard, 2016; Ddumba-Nyanzi et al., 2019). The care leavers in this study have heightened stress levels that could cause mental health issues or exacerbate existing ones such as the case of the Ghanaian care leaver because of the limited social support. This study has also demonstrated limited awareness and access to mental health and psychosocial support services among the care leavers. In many cases, availability of mental health and psychosocial support services is limited or even nonexistent, aggravated by the public health measures and presidential directives in response to COVID-19 that limited mobility of people, and in many communities these services were not considered among the essential services (Bukuluki et al., 2020).

Generally those who had employment or a source of livelihood coped better and were more resilient compared to their counterparts with no stable employment opportunities (also see Bukuluki et al., 2019). However, this is happening in the context where globally, and particularly in developing countries like Uganda and Ghana, COVID-19 has led to the reduction in incomes or no earnings, especially for those working in the informal economy (Daily Monitor, 2020a, 2020b). These effects of the lockdown were mostly felt in the services sector, informal trade sector, domestic transport, and retailers among others. These are activities that employ most of the care leavers and young people in Africa (Pouw et al., 2017).

Regarding social protection, this study revealed that most of the care leavers interviewed in this study had not benefited from social assistance programs from the state or nongovernment organizations, possibly because in both countries care leavers were not prioritized and categorized as part of the vulnerable and marginalized groups who could be hardest hit by the COVID-19 pandemic. Care leavers felt abandoned by the government and the care institutions they had come to their rescue, contributing to the further weakening of their social support system and rendering them vulnerable to negative coping strategies, highlighting the need for policies in both countries that guarantee statutory support for care leavers during this period of crisis and also beyond it.

The study also reveals a combination of positive and negative coping mechanisms. The positive coping mechanisms included relying on spirituality through prayer and faith-based networks and adapting to challenges, factors, that other studies have also found as vital to the resilience of care leavers (Frimpong-Manso, 2018; Refaeli, 2017). However, some care leavers engaged in less resilient coping strategies which included reducing spending by cutting down on the number of meals they had and social isolation through withdrawal from networks (Bukuluki et al., 2020). Some, particularly the female care leavers, were forced to make compromises and move with their boyfriends earlier than they had planned because they could not live independently. Less resilient coping or maladaptive coping strategies were common among those who lacked employment and sources of livelihoods that did not have strong linkages to families and other forms of social support (also see Kelly et al., 2020). This too is similar to findings by Frimpong-Manso (2018) that the care leavers were experiencing challenges with employment, housing, and social integration. He noted that risk factors for lack of resilience included having inadequate social and cultural skills and leaving care without employment.

Therefore such effects combined with lack of strong and systematic social protection responses for young people, particularly care leavers, have driven some of them to engage in negative coping strategies, such as cutting down on consumption to the bear minimum. There is need for care to prioritize vulnerable young people especially care leavers in providing social protection, mental health, and psychosocial support services to further build their resilience to cope with the impact of the COVID-19 pandemic. In terms of preparing children to leave care, this study points to the need to strengthen focus on employable skills, building social networks, and strengthening linkages to the families (Kelly et al., 2020). Care leavers who had these opportunities and resources shared experiences of resilience, and the reverse was true for their counterparts without these resources.

Conclusion

In spite of the limitation of having a small sample of care leavers from one care institutions, this study has highlighted the challenges care leavers in Uganda and Ghana are experiencing during the COVID-19 pandemic. It has shown that care leavers have a limited fallback mechanism, unlike their peers with no care experience, to deal with the loss of jobs and social isolation imposed by the public health restrictions, which pose a serious risk to their mental health. While care leavers are ingenious in drawing on their internal resources such as their spirituality and adjusting their lifestyle to adapt to their challenges and utilizing the limited social resources, they need more formal support as this pandemic is exacerbating existing challenges that they encounter on their own as independent adults. The findings raise policy questions as the child welfare systems in both countries have ignored issues pertaining to this group of young adults whom the state has been their 'parent.' We need further research using mixed methods (quantitative and qualitative) and a big sample to further enhance our understanding of the situations of young people during pandemics like COVID-19 and how they cope with them.

References

Better Care Network & UNICEF. (2015). *Country care profile*. Ghana: UNICEF. Retrieved from: http://bettercarenet/work.org/bcn-in-action/technical-guidance/country-careprofiles/country-care-profile-ghana.

Bond, S. (2018). Care-leaving in South Africa: An international and social justice perspective. *Journal of International and Comparative Social Policy*, *34*(1), 76–90.

Bukuluki, P., Kamya, S., Kasirye, R., & Nabulya, A. (2019). Facilitating the transition of adolescents and emerging adults from care into employment in Kampala, Uganda: A case study of Uganda youth development link. *Emerging Adulthood*, 1–10. https://doi.org/10.1177/2167696819833592.

Bukuluki, P., Mwenyango, H., Katongole, S. P., Sidhva, D., & Palattiyil, G. (2020). The socio-economic and psychosocial impact of Covid-19 pandemic on urban refugees in Uganda. *Social Sciences & Humanities Open*, *2*(1). https://doi.org/10.1016/j.ssaho.2020.100045, 100045.

Casey, S. (2011). *Report of the mapping and analysis of Ghana's child protection system*. Kowloon: Child Frontiers.

Curtin, M., & Fossey, E. (2007). Appraising the trustworthiness of qualitative studies: Guidelines for occupational therapists: guidelines for occupational therapists. *Australian Occupational Therapy Journal*, *54*(2), 88–94. https://doi.org/10.1111/j.1440-1630.2007.00661.x.

Daily Monitor (August 28, 2020a). National News: More than 80% households report decline in incomes. This report cited a speech by the Director Uganda Bureau of Statistics providing highlights of a household survey carried out during the COVID-19 Pandemic. Available at: www.monitor.co.ug.

Daily Monitor (May 21, 2020b). Economy suffers major revenue losses. Available at: https://www.monitor.co.ug/News/National/Economy-suffers-major-revenue-losses/688334-5559328-4rh161/index.html.

Ddumba-Nyanzi, I., Fricke, M., Hong Max, A., Nambooze, M., & Riley, M. (2019). *The care leaver experience: A report on children and young people's experiences in and after leaving residential care in Uganda*. Ugandan Care Leavers.

Diraditsile, K., & Nyadza, M. (2018). Life after institutional care: Implications for research and practice. *Child & Family Social Work*, *23*(3), 451–457.

Dziro, C., & Rufurwokuda, A. (2013). Post-institutional integration challenges faced by children who were raised in children's homes in Zimbabwe: The case of "ex-girl" programme for one children's home in Harare, Zimbabwe. *Greener Journal of Social Sciences*, *3*(5), 268–277.

Frimpong-Manso, K. (2012). Preparation for young people leaving care: The case of SOS Children's village, Ghana. *Child Care in Practice*, *18*(4), 341–356.

Frimpong-Manso, K. (2014). From walls to homes: Child care reform and deinstitutionalisation in Ghana. *International Journal of Social Welfare*, *23*(4), 402–409.

Frimpong-Manso, K. (2015). The social support networks of care leavers from a children's village in Ghana: Formal and informal supports. *Child & Family Social Work*, *22*(1), 195–202.

Frimpong-Manso, K. (2018). Building and utilising resilience: The challenges and coping mechanisms of care leavers in Ghana. *Children and Youth Services Review*, *87*, 52–59.

Frimpong-Manso, K., Deliege, A., Wilson, T., & Norman, Y. (2019). Residential childcare in Ghana: Analysing current trends and drivers. *Scottish Journal of Residential Child Care*, *18*(2), 1–13.

Groenewald, T. (2004). A phenomenological research design illustrated. *International Journal for Qualitative Methods*. Available at: https://journals.sagepub.com/doi/pdf/10.1177/160940690400300104.

Gwenzi, G. (2018). The transition from institutional care to adulthood and independence: A social services professional and institutional caregiver perspective in Harare, Zimbabwe. *Child Care in Practice*, *25*(3), 248–262.

Hycner, R. H. (1999). Some guidelines for the phenomenological analysis of interview data. In A. Bryman, & R. G. Burgess (Eds.), *Qualitative research* (Vol. 3, pp. 143–164). London: Sage.

Kelly, B., et al. (2020). *Building positive futures: A pilot study on leaving care in Africa. Easy Read Summary*. Queens University Belfast, United Kingdom.

Knox, S., & Burkard, A. W. (2009). Qualitative research interviews. *Psychotherapy Research*, *19*(4–5), 566–575.

Koenderink, F. (2019). *Alternative care for children around the globe: A desk review of the child welfare situation in all cobbuntries in the world*. Retrieved from: http://socialserviceworkforce.org/resources/alternative-care-children-around-globe-desk-review-child-welfare-situation-all-countries.

Kvale, S. (1996). *Interviews: An introduction to qualitative research interviewing*. CA: Sage Thousand Oaks.

Lechuga, V. M. (2012). Exploring culture from a distance: The utility of telephone interviews in qualitative research. *International Journal of Qualitative Studies in Education*, *25*(3), 251–268.

Luboyera, F. (2014). *Unsettled youth: Examining the life experiences of resettled youth raised under institutional care in Uganda (Unpublished Master's Thesis)*. The Netherlands: University in The Hague.

Mhongera, P., & Lombard, A. (2016). Who is there for me? Evaluating the social support received by adolescent girls transitioning from institutional care in Zimbabwe. *Practice*, *29*(1), 19–35.

Milligan, I., Withington, R., Connelly, G., & Gale, C. (2017). *Alternative child care and deinstitutionalisation in sub-Saharan Africa: Findings of a desk review*. CELCIS, European Commission and SOS Children's Villages International.

Ministry of Gender, Labour and Social Development & UNICEF Uganda. (2015). *Situation analysis of children in Uganda*. UNICEF.

Mutenyo, F., Machingaidze, S., Okello, W., Otai, M., & Asekenye, M. (2019). Multistage processes of identifying children at risk or out of family care: A case of DOVCU project methods in Uganda. *Global Social Welfare*. https://doi.org/10.1007/s40609-019-00140-9.

Pouw, N., Hodgkinson, K., Le Mat, M., & van Dam, K. (2017). *The social exclusion of vulnerable youth synthesis report: Côte d'Ivoire, Guatemala, Indonesia, Kenya, Malawi and the Netherlands*. SOS Children's Villages International & University of Amsterdam.

Pryce, J., Jones, S., Wildman, A., Thomas, A., Okrzesik, K., & Kaufka-Walts, K. (2015). Aging out of care in Ethiopia: Challenges and implications facing orphans and vulnerable youth. *Emerging Adulthood*, *4*(2), 119–130.

Qu, S. Q., & Dumay, J. (2011). The qualitative research interview. *Qualitative Research in Accounting & Management*, *8*(3), 238–264.

Refaeli, T. (2017). Narratives of care leavers: What promotes resilience in transitions to independent lives? *Children and Youth Services Review*, *79*, 1–9. https://doi.org/10.1016/j.childyouth.2017.05.023.

Sekibo, B. (2019). Experiences of young people early in the transition from residential care in Lagos State, Nigeria. *Emerging Adulthood*, *8*(1), 92–100.

Tanur, C. (2012). Project Lungisela: Supporting young people leaving state care in South Africa. *Child Care in Practice*, *18*(4), 325–340.

Taylor, S. J., Bogdan, R., & DeVault, M. (2015). *Introduction to qualitative research methods: A guidebook and resource*. John Wiley & Sons.

UBOS & ICF. (2018). *Uganda demographic and health survey* (2016). Uganda; Rockville, MD: Kampala.

Vaismoradi, M., Jones, J., Turunen, H., & Snelgrove, S. (2016). Theme development in qualitative content analysis and thematic analysis. *Journal of Nursing Education and Practice*, *6*(5), 100–110. https://doi.org/10.5430/jnep.v6n5p100.

Vaismoradi, M., & Snelgrove, S. (2019). Theme in qualitative content analysis and thematic analysis. *Forum Qualitative Sozialforschung/Forum: Qualitative Social Research*, *20*(3), 23. https://doi.org/10.17169/fqs-20.3.3376.

Walakira, E. J., Dumba-Nyanzi, I., & Bukenya, B. (2015). *Child care institutions in selected districts in Uganda and the situation of children in care: A baseline survey report for the strong beginnings project*. http://www.anppcanug.org/wp-content/uploads/research_reports/2015/Baseline_Survey_Report_Full.PDF.

Welman, J. C., & Kruger, S. J. (1999). *Research methodology for the business and administrative sciences*. Johannesburg: International Thompson.

Wylde, E., Ssewankambo, E., & Baryabanoha, W. (2012). *Uganda social protection public expenditure review*. Kampala, Uganda: Expanding Social Protection Programme, Ministry of Gender Labour and Social Development.

Chapter 3

The impact of COVID-19 on mental health of frontline health workers in Ghana and Uganda

Simon Peter Katongole[a], Peter Yaro[b], and Paul Bukuluki[c]
[a]*Uganda Martyrs University, Faculty of Health Sciences, Nkozi, Uganda,* [b]*Basic Needs Ghana, Accra, Ghana,* [c]*Department of Social Work and Social Administration, Makerere University, Kampala, Uganda*

Introduction

The Corona Virus disease 2019 (COVID-19) has evolved as one of the crises that has hit the world in recent times affecting all kinds of people and regions in different ways (Adhikari et al., 2020). The pandemic in Africa arrived at later stages compared to other continents. The first case of COVID-19 was reported on 21 March 2020 which was an imported case from Dubai. On the other hand, Ghana had its first COVID-19 reported cases on 12 March 2020 (Lone & Ahmad, 2020). These were two cases of infected returnees from Europe one from Norway and the other from Turkey. As of August 24, 2020, Uganda had 2362 cases (Ministry of Health, 2020a). Twenty-two COVID-19 deaths had been registered in Uganda by 24th August 2020(Ministry of Health, 2020a). This makes it one of the countries with the least deaths due to the pandemic among the counties reporting (Ministry of Health, 2020b). The first death reported was of a health worker, a support staff in one of the primary health facilities in the Eastern region of the country (Ministry of Health, 2020c). As of August 24th, 2020, Ghana has had 43,622 confirmed cases among which are 263 deaths (Ghana Health Services, 2020). This makes Ghana the 9th ranking country in Africa with the highest death among the 40 countries out of the 53 that are reporting COVID-19 (World Health Organization Regional Offices for Africa, 2020). As of July 29, 2020, more than 10,000 healthcare workers in Africa have been infected with COVID-19—some of these also succumbing to the pandemic (WHO African Region, 2020). The numbers being reported though are from countries that have complied with the reporting mechanisms about the disease indicating that the burden of the disease among health workers could be much more than is orthodoxly reported.

Mental Health Effects of COVID-19. https://doi.org/10.1016/B978-0-12-824289-6.00014-3

Health workers at the forefront of the management of this pandemic may be classified as clinical (also called medical) and nonclinical health workers (also known as support staff or support services providers). From the clinical perspective, these include nurses, doctors, psychologists, psychiatrists, laboratory personnel, and midwives. The support staff in one way or another play various roles in the response to the pandemic and include the cleaners, drivers, mortuary attendants, guards, and hospital administrators. By virtue of their interactions with people who are being treated for COVID-19 and the roles they play, health workers are on an increased risk of getting infected with COVID-19 compared to other members of the population. The proportion of health worker infections among persons with COVID-19 in Uganda and Ghana stands at 2.6% and 4.8%, respectively, as of a 19th August 2020 WHO African Region report on COVID-19 situation in Africa (World Health Organization Regional Offices for Africa, 2020). With the COVID-19 cases escalating on the African continent, this is expected to have a toll on not only the healthcare delivery system of the African countries but also on the mental health and psychological wellbeing of the numerous health workers of various disciplines all over the continent (Olum & Bongomin, 2020).

Various biological, physiological, and psychological responses have been implemented as a way of combating the disease and its physical, physiological, mental, and psychosocial effects (Kaseje, 2020; Lone & Ahmad, 2020; WHO African Region, 2020). Similarities and differences exist in the two countries' approaches to COVID-19 management and more so in the two hospitals considered in this review. The similar approaches that the two countries have taken include border closure, specifically, with no more entry for passengers entering the countries by land and air except for cargo and apart from specially arranged repatriation of noncitizens and citizens of the specific countries. In both cases, returnees and those deemed to have been exposed to people who are being treated for COVID-19 are quarantined while people who are confirmed to have COVID-19 are isolated while receiving treatment in designated COVID-19 treatment hospitals. Both countries have also suspended public gatherings and decreed the wearing of face masks in public places. While Ghana imposed total lockdown in two cities, Kumasi and Accra that were most affected, Uganda imposed a total lockdown for close to 3 months (Agyeman-Manu, 2020; Olum & Bongomin, 2020). Both countries have introduced risk allowances for frontline health workers with that of Ghana being 50% salary allowance on basic salary and had tax relief for health workers for 4 months which was later extended for two more months (The Presidency of the Republic of Ghana, 2020). Uganda, on the other hand, pays its frontline health workers a risk allowance that ranges between 5.5$ and 21$ depending on the classification of risk to the frontline health worker (Wafula, 2020). These responses, however, have diverse effects on the mental and psychological effects of the health workers.

With its health systems having unique challenges, sub-Saharan Africa was bound to be impacted by the COVID-19 pandemic in a rather different way compared to other continents (Lone & Ahmad, 2020). The shortage of health workers, poor infrastructure, lack of adequate financing for health, poor information management, and inadequate responses to outbreaks have previously been mentioned as hindrances to outbreak management in the sub-Saharan African countries. This consequently affects the mental health of the human resources for health (Kaseje, 2020; Lone & Ahmad, 2020). Previous research on the Ebola outbreaks in Uganda and Sierra Leone has revealed that health workers are more likely to be infected and thus get impacted diversely compared to any other groups (Hewlett & Amolat, 2003; McMahon et al., 2016). Many other countries have reported mental health and psychosocial related effects of COVID-19 to health workers (Black Dog Institute, 2020; Dong & Bouey, 2020; El-Hage et al., 2020; Khanal, Devkota, Dahal, Paudel, & Joshi, 2020; Munawar & Choudhry, 2020). These range from anxiety, depression, fear, and stigma among others. These effects could either be as a result of the disease itself or due to the response strategies put in place to combat the spread of the pandemic (World Health Organization, 2020). The lessons learned elsewhere may not be deduced to the African context since the pandemic arrived at a later stage in Africa when health workers had observed how the pandemic was impacting in other countries. Moreover, the pandemic has taken a different trajectory altogether in the different health systems of the different countries (Kaseje, 2020). In addition, the approaches taken to respond to the pandemic in different countries may present unique manifestation of the mental health challenges as well as call for different coping mechanisms.

Much of the research on COVID-19 has majorly centered on the biological and physiological effects of the disease. Where attempts have been made to document the mental health effects of COVID-19, the focus has majorly been on the general population and some of the vulnerable populations. Little effort has been placed in studying the subject from the health workers' perspective. This could be because, hitherto, expression of mental health effects among health workers has been considered as a taboo (Barello & Graffigna, 2020). There is a dearth of current research on the effects of COVID-19 on the mental health of health workers in sub-Saharan African settings and how they have managed to cope in order to continue attending to the pandemic response services. Understanding the mental and psychosocial experiences of frontline health workers and the coping mechanisms they employ to overcome these experiences is crucial in strengthening the current response plans in both countries as well as in promoting the resilience of the health workers. The information also helps future planning of responses, especially from the mental health response plan for epidemics that may occur. Thus this chapter explores self-reported mental health and psychosocial effects of the pandemic on frontline health workers in hospitals located in sub-Saharan Africa and self-reported coping mechanisms.

Methods

A phenomenological approach was employed using in-depth interview techniques to establish experiences, beliefs, and perceptions on the mental health and psychosocial effects COVID-19 has had on frontline health workers treating people who are being treated for COVID-19 (Groenewald, 2004; Jodi, 1994). Questions were as well asked to draw out health workers' experiences, perceptions, and explanations on the coping mechanisms employed toward the challenges observed. The interviews were carried out between the months of May and July which was 2–3 months into the pandemic. This time was deemed so vital to examine the two countries' responses to the pandemic and how the responses and the course of the disease may have impacted on the health workers in the two countries. The health workers included four nurses, five doctors, one hygienist, one ambulance driver, and a hospital manager.

We interviewed frontline health workers from two hospitals, Seven in Entebbe Hospital and Six in Tamale Teaching Hospital. These two hospitals were taken as case studies because of their centeredness in the COVID-19 response in the two countries. Both hospitals are regional referral hospitals with Entebbe hospital serving as the regional referral hospital for the most populous district in Uganda, Wakiso district and its surroundings with over three million people altogether. Being nearer Entebbe airport, and with COVID-19 having been considered imported especially from Asia and the western world, Entebbe hospital was designated as COVID-19 treatment center with all other service to the general population thereof suspended. On the other hand, Tamale Teaching Hospital serves as the regional referral hospital for the Northern region of Ghana and has served as the testing hospital for Savannah, Upper West, Upper East, and North East regions (UNICEF GHANA, 2020). The hospital also receives people who are being treated for COVID-19 from some parts of Burkina Faso and Ivory Coast. In both cases, all COVID-19 cases managed free of charge.

Due to the stringent social distancing measures put in place by the government and the difficulty to access Entebbe hospital, all but one of the seven interviews in Uganda were conducted remotely by phone. All interviews conducted in Tamale Teaching Hospital were carried out face to face with the interviewer and interviewees ensuring that they observed the public health measures and using personal protective equipment. We sought permission from the hospital management of the respective hospitals to interview the health workers after which verbal consent from the interviewees was obtained prior to the interview. The interviews were audio recorded and transcribed based on the orthographic principles where a verbatim account of every word uttered was written down as explained by Braun and Clarke (2006). Analysis was conducted by all the three authors independently and included reading the transcripts multiple times to establish codes, subthemes, and major themes following the thematic analysis framework (Aronson, 1999; Vaismoradi, Jones, Turunen, & Snelgrove, 2016; Vaismoradi & Snelgrove, 2019). Any disagreements that arose were agreed upon after reaching consensus.

Results

Mental health and psychosocial challenges faced by the frontline health workers

The findings of the effects of mental health and psychological effects of COVID-19 to health workers have been categorized into three major themes, namely emotional, psychosocial, and behavioral effects. The emotional effects in this context are described as the thoughts and feelings that have manifested within the health workers by virtue of the services they are rendering to people who are being treated for COVID-19 and what significance the health workers have attached to them. Borrowing from the definition of (Upton, 2013), the psychosocial effects are described as the influences COVID-19 has impacted on the frontline health workers from the social perspective including relations with others, society, and family.

Emotional effects of COVID-19 to frontline health workers

The emotional health of the health workers while managing people who are being treated for COVID-19 is important as it helps health workers to be in control of their own relationships, feelings, thoughts, and how they behave and how they will cope with any challenges coming their way. The COVID-19 pandemic has emotionally impacted on the health workers in diverse ways. Expressions such as feeling of incompetence, stress, irritability, doubt, depression, expression of worry, mental fatigue, shock, blaming one's self, and psychological trauma were highlighted as emotional impacts of the pandemic to the health workers.

Fear has been the prominent human emotion that affected frontline health workers with some reporting that COVID-19 has been the most scaring moment in their lives. This fear manifested in several ways and at different course of the pandemic. Prior to the reporting of cases, the fear was mainly driven by the uncertainty surrounding the disease which was novel to the health workers, with no initial information on how to go about it. Additionally, unlike the hemorrhagic fevers where a patient is mainly infectious when symptomatic, it was quite different with COVID-19 given that most cases were asymptomatic at the time of disease detection. At that time, the international media reported infection rates and deaths occurring in other countries such as Italy, Spain, United States, and other countries in the West. Most health workers who had keenly followed the news were alarmed by the rate at which both the infections and deaths were occurring. These were developed countries assumed to have better health systems and were thus anticipated to be on top of the pandemic and yet people were dying at such a rate! It was thus assumed that a much worse situation would be observed in sub-Saharan Africa where the health systems are not as good as it is in the West. Accordingly, health workers became apprehensive of what might happen, especially should cases be reported in here. As the trend of the pandemic in the West was being reported, some health workers started posing questions to themselves, especially questioning which category of people they would fall into if they ever caught the virus. The thought of whether one would be in the category of people who are asymptomatic and end up getting fine or those who may develop mild symptoms or those who go to the extent of developing severe symptoms lingered on the minds of some health workers and caused a lot of panic.

When the first case was announced, the reality dawned to the health workers that what they had been dreading about all along and only seeing on TV in other countries had finally landed to them and they had to face it. Pre-COVID-19 health workers had kept attending to their routine work. However, the announcement of the index case was a game changer. Panic engulfed almost everyone including doctors, the laboratory personnel, cleaners, especially when they received information that they were being traced for having been contacts of the index case that had tested positive. They all thought that they were going to be infected and die. It was a rare pandemic people did not know what to do and there was no proper direction.

Initially, the hospital management of the Ugandan case study had called upon all those who wished to be part of the COVID-19 response team to register. However, just as many as 30 health workers out of the over 400 health workers in the hospital heeded to this call and remained to be trained for to be part of the response team. More so, most of those who remained were those who had had prior experience with managing Ebola and other hemorrhagic fevers such as Marburg, Crimean-Congo hemorrhagic fever, and yellow fever that had previously affected the country. Such health workers came with confidence and vigor that as they survived those diseases so it will be with COVID-19. The situation was not much different in the Ghanaian case study as the nursing response team attracted just as many as 25 nurses out of the over 1400 nurses in the teaching hospital, with only two being female. Attracting only those few willing health workers was attributed to the fear of acquiring the infection that they had already gotten scared about given the little experience and capability they had in managing it.

The fear among the health workers was further exacerbated when news of health workers acquiring the infection started trickling in. In Ghana, a high profile death at the University of Ghana Medical Centre (UGMC) of a former Rector of the Ghana College of Physicians and Surgeons, an academic and at the time a consultant physician at Komfo Anokye Teaching Hospital Kumasi, the second-largest hospital in Ghana in April 2020 sent waves of fear among health workers. In Uganda's case, some health workers who had slowly gained interest of joining the COVID-19 response teams again because of now the fear upon hearing of the admission of the first health worker admitted to the hospital abandoned the idea and started dodging entering the hospital. When health workers got sick and yet they had ostensibly used personal protective equipment (PPE) and adhered to the standard operating procedures (SOPs) laid down to prevent catching the disease, it became apparent that maybe just adhering to these was not enough. This further amplified the fear factor among some health workers and caused panic. It was thus adduced that even though protection was somewhat guaranteed at places of work while using personal protective equipment, one could still be infected outside their work place hence necessitating one to further keep protecting themselves at all times. Contemplating about the death of people who are being treated for COVID-19 who actually did not have any underlying conditions, especially those who were young was another of the drivers of fear.

Health workers who got involved in some surgical procedures such as those who assisted women with COVID-19 to deliver especially by cesarean section, the thought of having to get involved in such a procedure that was presumed to further increase the risk of exposure was very scaring. The fear of what may go wrong to the patient or to the surgeon lingered around some of those to be involved in the procedures. As the day for the operation drew closer, the fear level also rose higher more so the night before the operation. Relatedly, in the Ghanaian setting especially the thought of losing a patient who had come in for dialysis and now diagnosed with COVID-19 also brought in fear. When the fear got hold of such health workers, they started getting upsets and downs. In some of the health workers, the fear once in a while happened, especially when the hype in cases is reported. It is worsened if health workers are among the reported cases. To the health workers who had been exposed, the fear further deepened and persisted for as long as samples had been collected from them tested and fear only waned when they had received negative results.

Detecting a person who has COVID-19 in people who are being treated for COVID-19 originally admitted for other conditions became a catalyst of fear in the Ghanaian setting where the hospital continued operations in normal way in addition to hosting people who are being treated for COVID-19. This was worsened by the fact that the measures that had been taken in the hospital on the general wards were quite different from those in the COVID-19 isolation centers. Whereas with adequate personal protective equipment, health workers working in the COVID-19 Isolation Treatment Unit (ITU) felt a bit protected, their colleagues working at the general wards with only face masks and aprons as the only available personal protective equipment felt not adequately protected. As a matter of fact, the first case in the hospital was that of a patient who had initially been admitted for a kidney infection and needing dialysis but eventually was diagnosed with COVID-19. Most of the health workers had come into contact with this patient, later panicked due to the fear of having contracted the virus from this patient.

In the Ghanaian case study where health workers continued staying in their homes in the process interacting with their families, in addition to the fear at personal level carried with them the fear of contracting this disease and taking it back home. Most importantly, health workers had young children with whom it was extremely difficult to avoid interacting with in order to avoid infecting them in an event that health workers had been infected in the process of looking after people who are being treated for COVID-19. Similar sentiments were echoed by health workers in the Ugandan context who despite having been isolated from their families faced the challenge at the beginning of the response before the isolation had been initiated. Even when they had been permitted to visit families after undergoing testing, the fear of infecting the family members persisted especially with the belief that maybe in the process of waiting for the results and having interacted with people who are being treated for COVID-19 the night before, they had eventually acquired the infection.

In the early stages of the pandemic, especially with the announcement of the index case, the fear of infecting the family members after supposedly having been exposed to the case forced one of the frontline health worker in Uganda upon returning home to first undress and thoroughly bath from outside his house, in the process bathing three times until he was satisfied that he was noninfectious. In addition, he had to wait for all family members to sleep before he could take his sleep in the sitting room, wake up earlier than anybody else, clean all his clothes and beddings, and leave the house back to the hospital to start his quarantine. It thus was cited that the fear of infecting family members would only cease when no more cases are reported and health workers are swabbed at once and for all, with no more anticipated interactions with cases and the whole COVID-19 chapter is closed. Relatedly, the thought of having to undergo periodic swabbing for checkup brought fears of its own, especially with the discomfort that is associated with the procedure of swabbing.

The fear of acquiring COVID-19 from fellow health workers also engulfed most of the health workers. In this case, health workers have shunned getting closer to colleagues they presume are of increased risk, especially those who have attended to people who are being treated for COVID-19. Drivers of ambulances that drive people who are being treated for COVID-19 are shunned so are the nurses and doctors who come into contact with people who are being treated for COVID-19. Even colleagues who are quarantined are feared so much that health workers who end up attending to spend a little time with them when they are attending to them.

Many health workers attending to people who are being treated for COVID-19 in Ghana and Uganda reported feeling stressed during the time they have spent at the frontline of services provision to patients with COVID-19. Stress is much more pronounced in Uganda's case study contributed mainly by factors including having to live at the treatment centers away from home, daily interactions with people who are being treated for COVID-19, working for long hours leading to work overload, fatigue, and burn out. Some of the health workers mention that they are stressed because the family members they left home have no food, and that their children are getting sick as revealed by one health worker.

> *Even at the point I went to quarantine myself, and left my toddlers at home with just their dad, and nobody else to support him and one of them got ill while I was in quarantine, these are nights I cried and wished I would get out and be with my kids.*

The stress was majorly experienced in the first 3 weeks of the response more so before the mandatory isolation of the health workers was changed. For health workers retained at the place of work, staying in the same unit for a long time was stressing and led to mental fatigue. The introduction of occasional short home visits somehow relieved this stress. Initially, even the hospital management put a blind ear to the expressions of stress by the health workers as they had nothing to do about it. In both countries, the news of the increasing deaths of people who are being treated for COVID-19 in the western world also intensified the stress.

On the other hand, the hospital management has had its stress factors especially emanating from the lack of adequate logistics. For example, logistics to cater for the quarantined health workers, and contacts right away from the basic needs as clothes, slippers, toilet papers, and all the sundries the liability of the hospital management team for all the days they were quarantined. In the early stages of the pandemic the hospital management had to deal with the stress from the relatives of especially the first admitted COVID-19 people who are being treated for COVID-19 and those quarantined. The relatives constantly sought for information about the progress of their relatives. Providing such information to the relatives who were corroborating it with that being received from both the main and social media became difficult since in most cases the facts in it differed. The social media, for example, kept feeding the public with false information that relatives got to read about. Besides, having to adhere to the principles of confidentiality and providing information to the relatives to allay their fears became challenging and stressing. In some health workers, stress due to COVID-19 has been associated with irritability of the health workers.

In the early stages of the pandemic, health workers kept casting doubt on what would happen if the disease progressed to the levels being witnessed elsewhere in the western world. They voiced their lack of confidence of managing people who are being treated for COVID-19 who may advance to severe disease especially due to the lack of equipment and supplies. Take an example of a patient with kidney complications, if the dialysis machine is used on that patient it may not be used on another patient. If a respirator was to be used on a patient with airway complications, it may not be used on another patient because that respirator is deemed to already have the Corona virus.

Furthermore, when health workers were subjected to mandatory tests after being exposed, even when they received negative results, they kept doubting them not until they completed the 14 days of mandatory quarantining and ultimately tested negative as echoed by a health worker:

> *But as a person, when you think about what happened and that the incubation period of this disease is fourteen days, you say but now, when you have swabbed me today and I have not fished the fourteen days, it is like I have done nothing. So you start again thinking then now, after fourteen days, what will happen? Maybe we may turn positive because we suspect this virus may still be in incubation period.*

Some health workers were in denial of the existence of COVID-19. They also cast doubts on the severity of the disease especially by the time of interviews were undertaken in the two hospitals, no death had occurred in Uganda and only three deaths had been registered in Tamale Teaching Hospital. The belief that the disease was not as dangerous as originally portrayed strongly existed in some health workers. Because of this, others have actually thought that the whole story of COVID-19 is not real as mentioned by one of the health workers:

> *But there are days I do wake up and say, but this whole virus thing, it is just a scam. It is just a joke. It is a movie. We will wake and one day we will say it is nothing. You know!*

With a second thought, reality has gotten back to such health workers and get to believe the reality of the disease as observed again by the same health worker who cast doubt to the reality of COVID-19 in the hospital:

> *And then, the other side of it gets back, and I say I have to get serious, I have to be realistic and think about it. So, I have been there and there*

Closely related to doubt was skepticism in a way that some health workers had taken COVID-19 as a disease of the temperate regions. Hence, they questioned whether really COVID-19 would take the same course in Africa as it had done elsewhere. One nurse had made the following observation:

> *Being a nurse, I was wondering what this was all about. I was a bit skeptical as whether this will really strive with us, and so I had to block my mind thoughts that ok just a few cases, they will get fine and everything will go back to normal.*

After observing that indeed what has happened in the temperate regions can indeed occur in any other regions, all this skepticism has however disappeared.

Depression was also reported as another emotional consequence of COVID-19 mainly suffered by health workers who interacted with the first people who were being treated for COVID-19 to be diagnosed in the Ugandan case study. Whenever the health workers received news that someone they had interacted with had tested positive what would follow next was a feeling of pseudo symptoms such as loss of appetite, thoughts about deaths, being uncomfortable, shivering, and feeling uneasy. In some other cases, the people who are being treated for COVID-19 and people who may have COVID-19 did not cooperate and sometimes hid their identity when picked by the testing team. In one situation, a person was a contact of a person with COVID-19 concealed his identity when he was contacted for testing. He indicated that he was to direct the team tasked to pick him to where the person they were looking for was. As they arrived to pick him, he insisted in occupying the front seat of the ambulance as they were to drive him to where he wanted a request that was not accepted. Upon arrival at his home this is when he revealed that he was actually the contact being looked for. This shocked the contact team and left some depressed thereafter when tested positive.

The issue of constant worry has also been on the health workers' minds. This is mainly pointed out in the Ghanaian context where health workers are continuing to run normal ward duties. As news of new cases trickle in, the question that follows next is who is actually negative? One nurse thus remarked:

> *This person who comes into my ward and I am taking care of, is this person really negative or positive? You cannot tell whether this person is negative or positive. You wake up and then you know that, well, things might get out of hand. We hope it doesn't but we have to prepare for it.*

Consequently, this makes health workers to take more caution for themselves and for their colleagues. With the new faces of colleagues one has to work with, you have to take extra care for yourself to not pick this disease from a person you are not sure of or you infecting them and indirectly protect their family members.

The other dimension of worry is that of the possibility of losing patients that have been attending the chronic disease illnesses such as diabetes, people having uncontrolled hypertension or controlled on medication, kidney, people with congestive cardiac failure disease hovered over some of the health workers' minds especially physicians much more than it was for losing people who are being treated for COVID-19. The people with chronic conditions depended on coming for review either weekly, twice every other week, or monthly for survival so cutting that was going to put my patients in danger. Even after spending the whole day attending to people who are being treated for COVID-19, the minds of some physicians are on the people who have chronic conditions who have missed two or three times of review and whose life might deteriorate if they are not reviewed. However, on another thought, it was also worrying to let the same patients come for review and then expose them to the high risk of catching COVID-19 and yet if such patients got the COVID-19 their risk of dying is increased.

COVID-19 has led to a blame game where countries, societies, and sometimes individuals blame each other for having been responsible for transmitting the disease. However, in the perspective of the frontline health workers, self-blame was the issue. Some blamed themselves for having accepted to partake in the response team. They considered that joining the response team was perhaps a mistake especially because it was then becoming a danger to their families and loved ones. Others even regretted having joined the health profession which was putting them at such a risk. Feelings such as:

> *[…] you are there for some time and that ask that why should I get myself in this or why should I involve' myself in this.*

Another lamented that

> *I kept blaming myself, my dear that may be I made a mistake. I was thinking a lot. Thinking about my young kids, and people are dying, you know, aah!*

Another one had this to say:

> *[…] with every human being feeling nervous, I do not understand what probably brought me into this job. If I had known, I would have taken a different or gone for a different career.*

Health workers have also reported feeling psychologically tortured because of their participation in the COVID-19 response. In the Ugandan case study, upon receiving the first people who may have had COVID-19 where one tested positive, all health workers that had come into contact with this person felt psychologically traumatized. The news came as a surprise since none of the people who may have COVID-19 had shown any suspicion of being infected. This was a time the picture of the disease in Uganda had been known and the thoughts on health workers' minds were how he/she should be managed especially if he/she ever develops severe disease. As more people who may have COVID-19 eventually tested positive for COVID-19 yet they had no cardinal signs and symptoms of the disease, health workers became more psychologically traumatized. From that time, the stigma subjected to health workers upon knowing that one works in a COVID-19 treating hospital is casing psychological trauma to health workers. What is more traumatizing is when a fellow health worker you meet anywhere else pulls on a mask the moment they get cognizance of your place of occupation being a COVID-19 treatment center and the pull out masks for protection.

Psychosocial factors affecting frontline health workers engaged in COVID-19 services provision

Stigmatizing health workers attending to people who are being treated for COVID-19 has been a common feature during this pandemic. Manifested in numerous ways, it has had a toll on the lives of these health workers For example, in Uganda, some doctors working with the government do dual practice in other clinics and hospitals when not on duty to supplement their incomes. However, during the COVID-19 pandemic, most of these were rejected, so because they were coming to Entebbe. Working in the COVID-19 treatment hospital had health workers being tagged as having COVID-19. An example is given in this quote from a one of the managers:

> *One morning I picked some of my staff from Kampala. But whenever we were stopped and asked where we were going, whenever we responded that we were staffs of Entebbe hospital going for work, they would say "Oh, you people go, you have COVID-19."*

The least place where this stigmatization would be expected is at the Ministry of Health. However, a visit by a health worker to any office at the Ministry of Health headquarters in Kampala would prompt workers to pull out a mask and put it on if they were not doing so as well as ensuring social distancing even beyond the required distance since all workers from the COVID-19 treatment hospital are considered to be contacts of people who are being treated for COVID-19. Any business conducted thereafter will have to done hurriedly to reduce the contact hours. This reaction is exaggerated especially with health workers and managers who are very well known to workers at the Ministry of Health. The story is not much different even in the hospital premises itself more so in the early stages where health workers who received and attended to the first case admitted in the hospital were for some time shunned by colleagues with the conviction that they had been infected in the process of attending to the first case. One health worker during the interviews noted that:

Actually up then, it was a bit like a challenge to them to interact with us. Even mere coming to you they would fear and say, that one is the one who received the first case, so they keep fearing even entering inside rooms where we were quarantined. Someone enters inside spends one second and finds excuse to not stay longer, saying I am not going to enter.

Stigma in the Ghanaian case study has manifested in a different way to that in Uganda because of the different approaches in the way the human resources for health responding to COVID-19 were handled. Stigma in this case has mainly occurred within the community. For example, in the communities, upon setting eyes on a health worker employed at Tamale Teaching Hospital and who is part of the response team, parents residing with such a health worker will gather their children and prevent them from interacting with the health worker. An example of such practice is noted by one of the health workers:

I was on duty, when I got home, some tenants had children who previously when I get home and they see me coming, they would run to me. But that day when I got home, I realized that everybody had taken their child out. So I felt a bit bad but since then, that didn't deter me from getting away from the children.

As is the case in Uganda, health workers attending to people who are being treated for COVID-19 have also been stigmatized by their colleagues working on the general wards. Since the health workers in the COVID-19 response team also continued attending with their previous duties, their colleagues on the general wards try to avoid them and isolate themselves from them when they report to the general wards. Similarly, the health workers who had contact with cases and got quarantined are stigmatized by their workmates with stereotypes such as "quarantinos" as noted by a health worker:

So when you are in that quarantine or if you have been quarantined everybody calls you "quarantino", "quarantinos". It's not easy coping up if you have been quarantined because you have a small parameter to move around.

For the health workers who are stigmatized, this problem could be much worse than the COVID-19. The worst scenario is that the stigmatization is pushed beyond the health worker to their family members especially in their neighborhood as noted in the quote that "*It goes along side not for you per but your whole family line will be stigmatized. Your children cannot go out to play freely.*"

Upon hearing that some of their tenants are part of the pandemic response team, some landlords responded by evicting such health workers even when their rent money was still due. This practice came as a result of the landlords being pressurized by some tenants who complained that they cannot live with people who are attending to people who are being treated for COVID-19. And if such a health worker is alone among many tenants, he or she will be sacrificed by the landlord than risking losing other tenants. Some families have divorced especially if a partner has failed to understand the situation of the pandemic.

Because of the stigmatization from colleagues, health workers feel they have developed a sense of abandonment by workmates. They feel they are not free with their workmates anymore, cannot share meals together as it used to be, and colleagues are shunning entering their rooms.

The health workers have also voiced a concern of missing their families. This is mostly professed by mainly those with young children. Others mention that they have missed their elderly parents whom they previously had a routine of visiting which is now impossible due to the stringent rules where traveling is impossible. The fact that they are high risk, it has even sometimes been impossible for health workers engaged in COVID-19 to visit sick relatives, especially due to the fear of infecting them with the disease as mentioned by a frontline health worker that:

> *You know, for example, one of my uncles was not well, was admitted and he somebody that I am very close to. I couldn't visit him as much but at least, I had to text him one day to let him know that the reason I am not visiting is because I am high risk.*

While health workers do miss their relatives, some of them are finding themselves in a confusion of whether to or not to visit relatives especially due to the fear of infecting family members. Correspondingly, some health workers are also pointing out that their relatives are scared and worried about their involvement in the COVID-19 response. The relatives keep calling the health workers beseeching them to keep safe. Those who were quarantined have received numerous calls from friends and relatives, some calls coming from people who have not called them for ages or those who had never called them in their life.

> *when we were quarantined, several calls where coming from people who never called you or probably had your number but imagine a number of years they have not called you but everybody want to call you, ask you of your wellbeing and some questions are very nauseating so you need to just ignore them.*

What is perplexing in the Ugandan case study is that when the health workers are taken home once after 3 days to talk to their children and to pick what they want, some family members are also rejecting them because they think it is risky to come near them since they have been exposed.

To some frontline health workers, COVID-19 has changed their social life and family routines. They cannot freely associate with people that they previously associated with and hugged in society, at church and in the hospital. Sometimes people cannot recognize you because you are putting on a mask. Some when you cannot recognize them they think you are bragging and using the mask as a scapegoat. They cannot freely check on friends. Those who used to freely interact and commiserate with patients by touching them and getting close to them have had to change all this. At home, some have had to change their routines with partners especially when children are at home rather than being at school. They have had to change the way they associate with their children as highlighted by one nurse:

> *My husband and I have to run shifts, so he goes to work early, his job is I mean he has full control of the flexibility. He will come and then watch over the kids and then I can come to work. And my social life is truncated. I cannot go to any place because anywhere I go, I have to go with my kids. There are things that I cannot do with my family again. I have stay away from holding my son and all that. Even normal day-to-day activities like my laundry has to be done differently.*

Behavioral mental health challenges faced by frontline health workers

Some frontline health workers have reported poor quality sleep. Among the sleep challenges mentioned include lack of enough of sleep, intermittent sleep, failure to sleep again after, change of sleeping pattern, that included inadequate sleep, and sleep disturbances. The predictors of poor quality sleep include change of environment especially for health workers who have been retained at their places of work and not sleeping in their homes and their beds. Others mentioned that the new beds are not comfortable, while to their minds are preoccupied with the following day's work given that they have two shifts hence necessitating waking up early to meet the new schedule. While others have thus equated the new sleep pattern to rest rather than sleep because it has been shortened. The anxiety associated with the COVID-19 disease has also been cited as another contributor to poor sleep.

> *You get a bit of some sleep though there's a kind of anxiety still in you that this person probably were in contact with coughed at a time I was giving out medication or may be when you are removing your gown because it's a procedure and you did not do it well. That kind of a thinking will come to you and sleep disappears.*

Feelings of nervousness and restlessness have been a common phenomenon for COVID-19 frontline health workers. Specifically, this transpired a week or two during the initial stages of reporting the COVID-19 pandemic cases especially when some frontline health workers such as the hygienists, laboratory personnel, physicians, and ambulance drivers had come into contact with people who at the time were not presumed to be infected but whose results later came out positive. In addition, at any moment a person suspected of having COVID-19 coughed as a reflex action during sample collection, this sparked off nervousness in those collecting the samples. The nervousness and restlessness deepened during the time the health workers who also had to undergo testing waited for the results until when their results were released and came out negative. The death of a person who may have had COVID-19 person in another hospital triggered restlessness among all health workers who had come into contact with the patient. In this case, nervousness and restlessness persevered until when the results of the samples taken from the dead body were released and were negative.

Whereas loss of appetite also known as anorexia has been emphasized as one of the symptoms of COVID-19, it has also manifested as one of the behavioral mental health challenges for frontline health workers. It featured prominently in the first phase of the pandemic at the time most of the mental health challenges were most felt. Like in other mental health problems discussed earlier, loss of appetite was also been triggered by having coming into contact with people who may have COVID-19. Besides loss of appetite, eating hurriedly because one is trying to avoid being in a large group of people or wants to move on to take over duty from a colleague or after having been called back on duty in the ward.

The coping mechanisms to overcome mental health and psychosocial challenges among frontline health workers during COVID-19

It is vital to ensure that the health workers cope with the mental health and psychosocial challenges they are facing, as these healthcare workers are risking themselves and their families to respond to the pandemic. These mechanisms are valuable in helping the health workers to adjust to challenges the health workers are facing mentally and to alleviate any mental or psychosocial events they may find themselves into. In this section we discuss mechanisms or the factors that have inherently helped health workers to manage the mental health and psychosocial challenges they are facing.

Generally, health workers utilized adaptive coping mechanisms. These are positive or healthy ways employed to handle the psychosocial and mental health challenges faced (Albott et al., 2020; Marroquín, Howard, & Stanton, 2017). These coping mechanisms have been characterized into either intrapersonal or interpersonal factors. The intrapersonal coping factors are strategies, actions, or deeds that are self-identified or individual based to handle demanding situations (Upton, 2013). They originate from within the individual. Interpersonal coping factors are the deeds or actions aimed at handling mental and psychosocial challenges faced encompassing the interaction of the individual with other individuals or groups of people and the environment (Upton, 2013).

In both intrapersonal and interpersonal coping, we establish that health workers used both problem solving and emotion-focused strategies to overcome the mental and psychosocial challenges that they faced. Regarding the problem-solving coping strategies, this is when solutions to the stressing factors are thought through, identify solutions, appraise the advantages and the disadvantages of the solutions, and thereafter implement what is best thought to remove the stressing factor (Marroquín et al., 2017; Sharma, 2003). On the other hand, emotion-focused coping strategies are an internal way of dealing with ill feelings about a debilitating condition (Sharma, 2003).

Interpersonal problem solving mechanisms

Most of these were effected at the organizational level and included the hospitals and governments of the respective countries through their ministries of health thinking through and determining what factors could cause mental health and psychosocial challenges to frontline health workers and their after applying policies and plans to alter the environment or the stressing situations.

Selection of the health workers to be part of the response team

First and foremost, health workers were selected ensuring that those who are resilient, fearless, and were willing to go an extra mile in handling the challenges that may be posed by a pandemic of COVID-19 magnitude and ready to serve to form part of the response teams. In Uganda's case, at the onset, a clear communication was made that no one was being forced to be part of the team. Much emphasis was to the younger health workers some of whom did not have children to carefully think about the challenges ahead as they considered joining the response team. It was emphasized that much as all had taken the Hippocratic Oath to treat the ill to the best of their ability, in this case no one was being forced to join the response team. The hospital leadership communicated that even the Ministry of Health was made aware that those who formed part of the response team were the ones willing to serve and fight the COVID-19 battle at the frontline. Consequently, to some health workers, this keeps them going in this time of fear, turbulence, and anxiety as pointed out by one frontline health worker that "*But as a person, what actually gives you courage, is that no one forced you to join.*"

Appropriate scheduling of duties

Duties have been scheduled and programed in a different way compared to the usual practice. In the Ugandan context, work has been scheduled in a way that each staff enters the treatment room at least only once a day so that one is not exposed constantly for the whole day. Duties are programmed so that time for each activity is adhered to, including time for watching news and time for exercise. This is meant to keep health workers busy and have their minds forget thinking about stressful consequences of the COVID-19.

In the Ghanaian case, at the time of response team formation, knowing that there were people enthusiastic to offer services to people who are being treated for COVID-19 like they had also done was motivating and comforting even when they felt like giving up. By acknowledging that there were health workers that were ready to support each other carry the burden of caring for people who are being treated for COVID-19 from one point to another was extremely cherished and encouraging. Besides, meeting people from other hospital departments with a like mind positively energized some to push on and serve as seen in this testimony

> *The opportunity to work with others I think it has affected my interests positively. I have got that impression that there are some other people I can work with to make a positive impact or a change in the narrative. I think the appreciation of the fact that there is somebody next to you who is willing for me. That is all I can explain. You are not in the fight alone. There is somebody who is standing next by you who is ready to carry on when you fall (Health worker, Tamale Teaching Hospital).*

Developing mutual support among the response team members

Creating mutual support and team work among health workers has been a helpful approach for building resilience toward stressing issues related to COVID-19 to health workers. It was suggested that sharing roles and allocating duties was very important. Anytime it was required to attend to people who are being treated for COVID-19, a team of around five health workers had to enter as a team, with each of them knowing the specific role to play or task they were to do. The one to take the vital signs, the one to take the history, the one to do whatever, and each one had a role to play. Mutual respect for one another is also emphasized because everyone is important in what the health workers termed as *"buddy style."* In this approach, donning and doffing of personal protective equipment is done in the presence of a colleague who has a checklist that he or she uses to monitor and ensure that the processes are executed properly (Cheng et al., 2020; Cook, 2020). Your associates or buddies are supposed to monitor you and you do the same to monitor and support your partners. With this system, health workers are encouraged to have mutual trust for each other in that whoever gives you information, you are obliged to believe it because each one went in for a particular role. The most dangerous part of care is when one is getting out of the PPE, since one has gotten into contact with people who are being treated for COVID-19. So, right there is somebody standing by you and serving as a guide and provide you with that supportive care, to ensure that you do the right things to stay safe. Therefore one could not tell that this one is a doctor, this is a hygienist, and this is a nurse, so everyone respects. For example, the hygienist was so important since he or she was the one to direct everyone on what to do, especially in donning and doffing. The buddies' approach has also been implemented in America by focused peer support to monitor stress, adhere to safety measures, as well as helping in creating resilient approaches to any mental health stressors (Albott et al., 2020; World Health Organization, 2020).

Good healthcare system leadership

Good leadership skills employed by the hospital leaders were vital in drumming up and offering mental and psychosocial support to the health workers. In Uganda's case, the hospital leaders underscored and shared a common goal that all health workers people had to know of treating people with COVID-19 and getting them better while maintaining the safety of the staff. In the Ugandan context, the hospital management team has every other day met health providers to establish and assess the challenges faced by the health workers and find ways on how to motivate the response team. One-on-one talks to health workers have been common to ensure that health workers are back to their normal senses. Some leaders have emphasized to health workers that their safety is paramount in this response to the pandemic. Leaders are trying their level best to provide what health workers need amid the scarcity of resources. In this period, hospital leaders have made their presence to respond to concerns of health workers a priority at any time as highlighted by one health worker

> *Since COVID-19 started, there are times we have to go and meet with my head of department to talk about any concerns arising. There are times we are talking at ten, eleven [in the night] and as a senior colleague. I will very much not want to be calling her that frequently especially that late but since this COVID-19 happened, we know that we have to give support, bring ideas, go to [the] administration, make sure that whatever we need have it.*

Interpersonal emotional building mechanisms

Engaging in hobbies that kill off stress

In their free time, health workers have engaged in hobbies that kill off stress including, reading books, surfing the internet, listening to music especially meditation music, listening to and watching television and movies. For example, in Entebbe Hospital, television screens were put in the isolation centers for the staff to watch and get the stress off their mind. The phone became an important personal tool as a source of entertainment, and make sure health workers were following what is going on around the world and the new information coming in. Talking to friends has also been helpful especially to avoid think about COVID-19 and loneliness either those they are working with or others through phone calls or using social media. When talking to friends, health workers get to hear narratives and feelings of others and how they overcome bad situations they have faced.

> *You know whenever you are alone, you may start thinking which again will bring you back to psychological torture. You come, we talk about it, and we laugh. Said one of the health workers.*

Prior experience in managing hemorrhagic fevers and outbreaks gave us pockets of experiences among some health workers and these very workers would rally their colleagues who appeared giving up.

Keeping staff together

The keeping of staff together in the Ugandan hospital was in its way done to make sure that unity and trust were created. In this way, health workers performed certain activities together. This also helped them to interact like having meals together, chatting, and laughing. This eventually helped the workers to overcome the despairs thoughts that they have when alone. This also helped to minimize the fear of going back and infecting family members. Besides the interaction, health workers were also engaged in exercises conducted by the physiotherapist which also emotionally helped in alleviating the worries that had come with the tasks they were involved. And once in a while, they are taken back home for a visit after ensuring that they are COVID-19 negative after getting negative test taken prior to the home visit. This is done to prevent thoughts of missing home and relatives.

Morale boosting from workmates

Several measures have been implemented to boost the morale of frontline health workers in the two hospitals. For example, health workers have had to morale boost their colleagues such as making light sentiments and jokes of the disease and call on others to adapt to the situation. Some other health workers with comical characters would humorously recount their tribulations and experiences to which others laughed about and move on. An experience is recounted for example of the team that participated in the Cesarean section where throughout the operation people kept making jokes and the mood of the operation was lightened up.

> *During the operation, I kept looking on for anything wrong that was going to happen. The good thing is that we had a very good team around. So, first, the mood was lightened because, they kept making jokes, and then because I was working with people who are really good, it lighted up the mood (Health worker, Uganda).*

In the Ugandan case study, since the health workers were staying together, morale boosting exercises were introduced every after 4 days conducted in the evening by the hospital physiotherapist which health workers were called on to attend. On other occasions, when colleagues spotted another colleague with low moods or restless, one would take the initiative to cheer-up such a colleague or immediately give him or her some counseling advice.

Family support

To most of the participants, family support was key in raising their moods at the time they felt dejected. The family members supported health workers, became their strength, became a source of inspiration and support. Family members periodically called to find out what was happening especially when they had heard of anything bad in the hospital had happened. To others, it was the community support and encouragement that they received that pushed them on during this hard time.

The intrapersonal coping strategies employed by frontline health workers in COVID-19

The intrapersonal coping mechanisms have also been classified as either being problem solving or emotional approach strategies (Marroquín et al., 2017). A problem solving is the dimension of coping aimed at resolving challenges brought about by a distressing problem while the emotional approach coping mechanism is dimension of regulating feelings that came with a traumatic event.

Adherence to infection prevention control and standard operating procedures

Health workers believe that they have had to be extra careful in whatever work they do and be more responsible than anybody else in order to be able to stay safe. This is premised on the conviction that this could have been the reason that has saved them from acquiring COVID-19 given that some of the health workers have unknowingly come into contact with people having COVID-19 especially during the early stages of the pandemic. Based on this, some have suggested that with adherence to the standard operating procedures and preventive guidelines, then one may easily avoid getting COVID-19. Certainly, some have reported adhering to dressing a face mask all the time removing it just before bed time. Some health workers have also stated that they have been very alert and watchful of any signs that are analogous to those of COVID-19 and have done everything possible to prevent them. For example, some have not allowed COVID-19 to take a toll on them for symptoms such as loss of appetite, anosmia, and loss of taste of food as this may heighten the fear for COVID-19. Consequently, even when they would not be eating, they try as much as possible to do so to avoid being characterized as having COVID-19 something that will also go on to disturb them mentally. This is exemplified in the quote by one health worker in Ghana who said that:

> *One of the issues about appetite and all that we are very cautious about include anosmia, that is inability to smell, and then inability to taste food is one of the main symptoms of COVID-19. So we are very alert with that. If you start losing appetite based on your inability to smell and taste, and your ability to taste and smell are the main boosters of appetite. If you start losing that we might have to check you so that if it means we test you properly then we do*

Staying away from family when one has been exposed

This is another of the intrapersonal behavioral response mechanisms geared to removing the fear of infecting family members. In Ghana where health workers kept coming from home daily to attend to COVID-19 work, each time health workers felt that they had been exposed and harbored the fear of infecting their family members, they decided to stay away from home. They would do this until when they got negative results of both themselves and those of the person they thought they had been exposed to.

> *Each time I have felt exposed, very much exposed. I stay away from home until when I get to know the results of the person I got exposed to would be, before I can get back home. I think that has been helpful.*

Others who thought that they were a danger to children of neighbors back at home would make a call for such children to be taken indoors before they came back home as highlighted by one of the health workers:

> *I have tried as much as possible to distance myself from them. Now if I close from work and am going to the house and I get to the gate and I realize that the children are there. I rather stay outside the gate and I call someone inside the gate to pick the children. So when I enter and go and bath everything and then I make sure that am ok. Then maybe I can come out and interact with the kids.*

The sense of calling to serve patients

Health workers have also drawn their coping to COVID-19 through altruistic devotion to their role as health workers who are called to serve and treat patients no matter the circumstances they find themselves in. Because of this, some health workers report that they have to get aware of their own emotions and control them, draw their own strength and courage to continue serving because, this is what they have been called to do and no one else will have to do it apart from them. Even where scarcity of resources as well as weaknesses in the response preparedness, plans, and policies may have dampened their psychological resilience, some health workers have devised means of neglecting these negative factors that would have dampened their spirits to serve as mentioned by one of the health workers in Ghana:

Ok, I have this mentality that no matter the situation, no matter how things are when I come to work my service is to the patient. Anything above me, is for those above me. So whether items are available or not I have to work and I have to ensure that a patient is comfortable in a situation she finds herself in or he finds himself in. So, actually I pay more attention to my people who are being treated for COVID-19 rather than what goes on around me in the hospital.

While the requirements of the Hippocratic oath were relaxed a bit to allow in only health workers willing to die a little for the cause, to some health workers, it is the same call to serve testified in the oath that pushed them on to hang in and cope with the challenges they faced. To some, by virtue of being in the health profession which is primary for saving life, this was a strong psychological stimulus for confronting the pandemic. It is a job they have chosen and could not run away from and this was the best time to showcase their calling as revealed by two health workers.

I will say my interest has increased because at the end of the day you have taken an oath to save lives. So if you have taken an oath to save lives what do you have to run away from it? I wouldn't say it has rather made me to feel a bit down but as I said earlier on that is the profession I have chosen to go into and the situation has come and I have to tackle it head on. Like I earlier on mentioned, you have taken an oath that this is your job. If you run away from it who else will come to do it? (Medical Officer, Tamale Teaching Hospital)

But I think I did not feel nervous reason being that there was this patient who needed for what I had to do. Even though I was not adequately protected, I felt that the need to save that life superseded everything else. And so, I took that step because nobody else was there to take the step (Nurse, Tamale Teaching Hospital).

Developed positive thinking

Developing a positive thinking is another of the coping strategies employed by the health workers. Some health workers reveal they have learned to calm down, relax, and give themselves positive hope as well as blocking their minds from thinking about COVID-19. In addition, it has been helpful to learn that the best way to save oneself as someone at the forefront from breaking down is by avoiding thinking negatively. On the other hand, others state that continuing to harbor fear in them could even affect their performance. For example, when a nurse who found herself in a stressful moment after getting into contact with a person who may have had COVID-19 consoled herself saying that:

I have a way of handling situations when it hits me so hard. I try to. So, I gave myself hope that ok, you know, though I had contact with her, she was asymptomatic. I mean I am very cautious with my hand hygiene.

Feeling of making a special contribution to the pandemic

Relatedly, some staff have been encouraged and energized to hang in with the conviction that they are making an important contribution to the pandemic response. For example, being part of the team that conducted a cesarean section on a mother who also had COVID-19 made some health workers euphoric, especially with the impression that possibly not very many people in Africa had made such a contribution. This is highlighted by one of the frontline health worker who says that

> *The whole time I was working in the first two weeks, it did not dawn on me that there is something I had really done. But now, but now I feel not everyone has done this. I am among the real people who have done this. I think I have been exposed for once for a better word before.*

Spirituality

In both countries, spirituality has been a major alleviator of mental health and psychosocial challenges. On Sunday Christians pray from TV with the live broadcasted services. In Uganda for example, at the time of writing this, no death had been reported. Consequently, some health workers believe that it is just by the grace of God that this has been so since Uganda's health system cannot be compared to that of developed nations with advanced health systems where deaths have been overwhelming. Consequently, in the Ugandan case study, after donning the personal protective equipment just before health workers go in to see people who are being treated for COVID-19 they first gather together as a team and pray together first before entering and after coming. Prayer has now become part of the hospital culture which gives the health workers courage and confidence to keep going in the mix of the stress. Health workers also mention that prayer gives them faith that all will be better. Prayer makes them stronger and gives them the audacity to keep moving on. It is that faith in God that health workers believe has partly contributed to having people who are being treated for COVID-19 get better and keep the case fatality low.

Believing that COVID-19 in the hospitals is less severe than earlier thought about

Some of the intrapersonal mechanisms were focused to emotion coping. For example, health workers also found solace in the fact that majority of the people who are being treated for COVID-19 who had been admitted were discharged and they were all right. Moreover, the health workers who had treated the people with COVID-19 were also testing negative. This even encouraged health workers who had originally hesitated to partake in the response team to change their mind and apply to work to give a hand. Some gained the courage to dispel fear and anxiety they had generated because they got somewhat convinced that even if they eventually got infected, they would be treated and get better. In addition, because most of the people who were treated for COVID-19 were not severely sick, and had majority of them came in with very mild symptoms or were asymptomatic, this also helped to somehow dispel the previous fear held that this was a fatal disease. A health worker expressed his feelings thus:

> *The people who are being treated for COVID-19 actually when you see them you wouldn't believe they are the ones apart from those who are on ventilators. They look normal like the way we look. They look normal and some of the people who are being treated for COVID-19 are asymptomatic they don't carry the symptoms so you wouldn't realize it. They can do their own activity it's not that they are bed ridden no they are not bed ridden and so far we have not had any patient who is on ventilator. It is just that this is a special condition which we have not encountered before but mentally it hasn't had any effect on my mental wellbeing.*

When comparisons are made between the fatalities of COVID-19 to that of Ebola by health workers who previously were part of the teams that treated people with Ebola and have also had the opportunity to treat people with COVID-19, this relaxed them a bit. A health worker spoke about the people who are being treated for COVID-19 as such that:

> *But for myself, probably the fact that the cases we have seen, have been mild to moderate, largely most of them have been doing well. It passes as a fruit. It is not like Ebola. I have it in mind that it's just like any other condition that we meet at the ward so it's just that this is special.*

Bearing in mind that one has no underlying medical condition that would put them at risk

Most people who were being treated for COVID-19 and died were reported to be those who had underlying medical conditions. Consequently, to most health workers at the frontline with no underlying medical condition, this was a factor that reduced their fear to the disease. Having no underlying medical condition was thus perceived that one was not in danger of death if they ever caught the disease. Closely related to this was the belief that when one is young, this was a factor that would save him from the extreme features of the disease. One nurse thus testified that: *and I know that I am young and given what I know about COVID-19, even if I am exposed to a positive patient, I believed I would get out of it.*

Adequate training and preparedness

Health workers who had received adequate training believed that this had given the adequate strength preparedness and psychologically positioned them well to deal with COVID-19 stressors because they know what to do and when to do it. *The training I have received, I think I am well positioned psychologically to deal with COVID.*

Taking COVID-19 as an opportunity to learn

To some health workers, COVID-19 has provided a practical experience and used it as an opportunity to learn about pandemics and communicable diseases prevention. This is mainly said by the health workers who are also in school either upgrading or taking additional courses. The pandemic is providing a chance to acquire knowledge on how to identify and measure disease outbreaks and the epidemiology of COVID-19. Hence, rather than hiding away from people who are being treated for COVID-19, such health workers find more time to be in the triaging centers. They then ask questions to get to know how triaging is done, how people who may have COVID-19 walk and outside of the hospital, how visitors come in and are handled, how the security check is conducted, and many other opportunities of learning that may be available.

> *The positive side in fact I have gotten the opportunity to learn more about COVID and I have gotten the opportunity to know that there are some actually conditions that are more dangerous than what we used to handle here in the ward Personally I am interested because as a public health student, this is a public health issue. I need to be interested. Usually, I visit the triage point, I. So I have been curious and once in a while I go to the holding bay to find out how people come in, how they are treated, how they are handling it.*

Discussion

This chapter has presented an in-depth understanding of how frontline health workers have been affected mentally and psychosocially and how they are coping with attending to people who are being treated for COVID-19. It has been shown that COVID-19 came with a range of negative emotional, psychosocial, and behavioral effects on the health workers. These have included fear, panic, worry, depression, stress, denial, and many others. Whereas these are not desirable, they were predictable as they have been reported in countries where COVID-19 first manifested (Chew et al., 2020; Cots, Alós, Bárcena, & Boleda, 2020; Khanal et al., 2020; Lam et al., 2020; Ornell, Halpern, Paim Kessler, & de Magalhães Narvaez, 2020; Ornell, Schuch, Sordi, & Kessler, 2020). The importance of revealing health workers emotions has previously been highlighted (Barello & Graffigna, 2020; Montemurro, 2020). It has been mentioned in that when health workers express their emotions especially in a pandemic like this one, those close to or responsible about them will get know how they are being affected so that appropriate help can be accorded to them (Barello & Graffigna, 2020). It has also been revealed that health workers remain focused, effective and likely to provide patient-centered care if they share their emotions with others which may eventually help them to get necessary help (Barello & Graffigna, 2020; Liu et al., 2020).

While the disease arrived late on the African continent, its psychosocial and mental health effects arrived much earlier. Before the first cases had been reported, fear, panic, stress, and worry have been the most predominant mental health issues, especially the fear of being infected and infecting others as well as the fear of failing to manage the pandemic because of inadequate capacity. As it has been observed in other countries (El-Hage et al., 2020; Spoorthy, 2020), fear in the two countries in this case study has partly been triggered by health workers zealously monitoring the physiological and biological health effects of the pandemic, including effects such as death, a behavior which detrimentally affected their mental health. Whereas in the world today people can still be connected via phones, social media, television, internet, and the various new technologies, physical separation from families for health workers especially those with children and aged relatives has proved to be a thorn in the psychosocial health of health workers. Fear especially that originating from observing the effects of the pandemic elsewhere was beneficial in a way that it helped health workers to appreciate that they were now faced with a serious problem that required adhering to standard operating procedures in order to prevent catching the disease. Similar thoughts have been echoed in previous studies where fear has been found to induce survival instincts when reacting to frightening events (Ornell, Schuch, et al., 2020).

The decision to quarantine or not to quarantine health workers who are attending to people who are being treated for COVID-19 has produced divergent effects. In Uganda health workers who have been quarantined for the time they are part of the response team are facing challenges of separation from the families which is leading to social exclusion especially for those who have young children. This decision also made most health workers decline the opportunity to be part of the response team. A similar situation has been reported in Ghana for health workers who were quarantined during the time they had been exposed. Health workers facing this family separation may lose concentration in their work as they keep thinking about what is happening at home. On the other hand, the resolution made in Ghana to let health workers attending to people who are being treated for COVID-19 to commute from home may have come with mixed reactions. In one way, frontline health workers commuting from home to work somehow removed the challenges associated with family separation. However, leaving frontline health workers to commute from home to work has presented other challenges such as social stigma and isolation by the community. It has also heightened the fears of infecting family members. The psychological resilience gained from previous outbreaks of hemorrhagic fevers such as Ebola has been helpful among health workers, especially in the early stages of COVID-19 response team formation. Studies conducted elsewhere have revealed that health workers who have formerly been part of outbreak response teams were helpful to build mental strength of other team members without prior outbreak experience (Liu et al., 2020; Mbonye et al., 2012). This is because such workers were assumed to have mental preparedness to handle the psychosocial challenges that come with COVID-19. Health workers who responded early to the call to be part of the COVID-19 response teams have been useful because their resilience was banked on by other health workers who initially had been scared to accept being part of the response teams but later gained confidence and accepted to join the response teams.

The lack of protective equipment has been a trigger for psychosocial and mental health challenges. While this not new in African settings and neither is it a solely African problem during this pandemic, it becomes a stressor especially in the event that this being a unique pandemic where given that most who are being treated for COVID-19 are asymptomatic, the risk of fear is heightened since anyone in one's environs can be a potential source of infection (Ornell, Schuch, et al., 2020). Therefore personal protective equipment do not only give physical protection but also provide a concealed but crucial layer of mental protection from COVID-19 (Lam et al., 2020). This is evident in the Ghanaian case study where health workers in the isolation treatment units feel much more mentally strong compared to their colleagues at the general wards who were reported to be deficient in personal protective protection. Besides, while being extra careful to prevent being infected was found to be a problem-solving coping strategy, its effectiveness as a coping mechanism is weakened when what are required to protect workers are insufficient.

Several factors have helped health workers to cope with the psychosocial effects—key among them the manifestation of the disease among the people who are being treated for COVID-19. In the face of the mental and psychosocial challenges health workers have faced, they have generally been adaptive at both intrapersonal and interpersonal level. A study in China has also established intrapersonal and interpersonal coping mechanisms by health workers and identified that (Ye et al., 2020). Resilience, good leadership, proper organization of work, proper and empathetic communication, and creating resilient teams are crucial in helping health workers to cope and to stay focused as observed in this COVID-19 pandemic and in the Ebola outbreak in West Africa and Uganda (Adams & Walls, 2020; Barba, Rosado, Pardo-Moreno, & Rey-Biel, 2020; Mühlenbernd, 2014; Okware et al., 2015). Most of these have been exhibited by leaders in the two hospitals. Getting cognizant of and anticipating the psychosocial effects is of great importance especially by putting into consideration the response plans that have been put forward to address the pandemic and how they may impact on the mindset of the health workers (Okware et al., 2015).

Conclusion

Fear, worry, anxiety, panic, and depression were mentioned as leading mental health and psychosocial issues mainly exacerbated by what health workers observed happening elsewhere before the pandemic hit the African continent. Health workers should be assured that feeling upset and having stress in circumstances like these is an expected anomaly. However, failure to address such anomalies is what shouldn't be allowed to suffice as this may jeopardize the response plan of not only institutions but countries at large. The COVID-19 pandemic has presented opportunities for building a better psychosocial strategy for frontline health workers during pandemics and outbreaks despite the negative effects it has brought. In future, it is incumbent to ministries of health to consider developing detailed mental health and psychosocial response plans that can be used in addressing challenges that may be faced by health workers. Besides, psychosocial resilience during pandemics and outbreaks should be incorporated into the education system to instill coping mechanisms into future health workers. This should assist in identifying culturally and socially relevant solutions. With the advancement in technology, governments would think of using communication media and technologies such as zoom, webinar, and Google meet to mention but a few to set up user friendly family connection communication centers where families can meet up their relatives and friends for chatting and reassure loved ones of their wellbeing. When the COVID-19 storm passes and the world is back to the new normal, better pandemics and outbreaks management will hinge on the lessons learned from the ability of the health systems to respond to the psychosocial and mental health effects faced by the health workers. Whether the two countries Ghana and Uganda emerge stronger from a mental health point of view for frontline health workers will depend on how best they capitalized on the opportunities that transpired more specifically the coping mechanisms at both individual and interpersonal level.

References

Adams, J. G., & Walls, R. M. (2020). Supporting the health care workforce during the COVID-19 global epidemic. *JAMA: Journal of the American Medical Association*, *323*(15), 1439–1440. https://doi.org/10.1001/jama.2020.3972.

Adhikari, S. P., Meng, S., Wu, Y., Mao, Y., Ye, R., Wang, Q., … Zhou, H. (2020). Epidemiology, causes, clinical manifestation and diagnosis, prevention and control of coronavirus disease (COVID-19) during the early outbreak period: A scoping review. *Infectious Diseases of Poverty*, *9*(29). https://doi.org/10.1186/s40249-020-00646-x.

Agyeman-Manu, K. (2020). *COVID-19 response: Ghana's experience*. Accra. Retrieved from https://apps.who.int/gb/COVID-19/pdf_files/07_05/Ghana.pdf.

Albott, C. S., Wozniak, J. R., McGlinch, B. P., Wall, M. H., Gold, B. S., & Vinogradov, S. (2020). Battle buddies: Rapid deployment of a psychological resilience intervention for healthcare workers during the COVID-19 pandemic. *Anesthesia and Analgesia*, *30*(12), 1–12. https://doi.org/10.1213/ANE.0000000000004912.

Aronson, J. (1999). A pragmatic view of thematic analysis. *The Qualitative Report*, *2*(1). Retrieved from: https://nsuworks.nova.edu/tqr/vol2/iss1/3.

Barba, R., Rosado, C., Pardo-Moreno, J., & Rey-Biel, J. (2020). Managing people, roles, and resources during Covid-19 Surge. *NEJM Catalyst*, 1–6. https://doi.org/10.1056/CAT.20.0152.

Barello, S., & Graffigna, G. (2020). Caring for health professionals in the COVID-19 pandemic emergency: Toward an "epidemic of empathy" in healthcare. *Frontiers in Psychology*, *11*, 1431. https://doi.org/10.3389/fpsyg.2020.01431.

Black Dog Institute. (2020). *Mental health ramifications of COVID-19: The Australian context*. Black Dog Institute. Retrieved from https://blackdoginstitute.org.au/docs/default-source/default-document-library/20200319_covid19-evidence-and-reccomendations.pdf.

Braun, V., & Clarke, V. (2006). Using thematic analysis in psychology. *Qualitative Research in Psychology*, *3*(2), 77–101. https://doi.org/10.1191/1478088706qp063oa.

Cheng, L., Chen, L., Xiao, L., Zhang, J., Cheng, Y., Zhou, L., … Liu, L. (2020). Problems and solutions of personal protective equipment doffing in COVID-19. *Open Medicine*, *15*(1), 605–612. https://doi.org/10.1515/med-2020-0172.

Chew, N. W. S., Lee, G. K. H., Tan, B. Y. Q., Jing, M., Goh, Y., Ngiam, N. J. H., … Sharma, V. K. (2020). A multinational, multicentre study on the psychological outcomes and associated physical symptoms amongst healthcare workers during COVID-19 outbreak. *Brain, Behavior, and Immunity*, *88*, 559–565. https://doi.org/10.1016/j.bbi.2020.04.049.

Cook, T. M. (2020). Personal protective equipment during the coronavirus disease (COVID) 2019 pandemic—A narrative review. *Anaesthesia*, *75*(7), 920–927. https://doi.org/10.1111/anae.15071.

Cots, J. M., Alós, J., Bárcena, M., & Boleda, X. (2020). Mental health of medical workers in Pakistan during the pandemic COVID-19 outbreak. *Asian Journal of Psychiatry*, *51*, 102080.

Dong, L., & Bouey, J. (2020). Public mental health crisis during COVID-19 pandemic, China. *Emerging Infectious Diseases*, *26*(7). https://doi.org/10.3201/eid2607.200407.

El-Hage, W., Hingray, C., Lemogne, C., Yrondi, A., Brunault, P., Bienvenu, T., … Aouizerate, B. (2020). Health professionals facing the coronavirus disease 2019 (COVID-19) pandemic: What are the mental health risks? *Encephale*, (January). https://doi.org/10.1016/j.encep.2020.04.008.

Ghana Health Services. (2020). *Updates on coronavirus disease (COVID-19) in Ghana as they happen*. Retrieved 24 August 2020, from https://www.ghanahealthservice.org/covid19/.

Groenewald, T. (2004). A phenomenological research design illustrated. *International Journal of Qualitative Methods*, *3*(1), 42–55. https://doi.org/10.1177/160940690400300104.

Hewlett, B. S., & Amolat, R. P. (2003). Cultural contexts of Ebola in Northern Uganda. *Emerging Infectious Diseases*, *9*(10), 1242–1248. https://doi.org/10.3201/eid0910.020493.

Jodi, A. (1994). A pragmatic view of thematic analysis. *The Qualitative Report*, *2*(1), 1–5. Retrieved from https://nsuworks.nova.edu/tqr/vol2/iss1/3.

Kaseje, N. (2020). *The World Economic Forum COVID Action Platform*. Retrieved 4 August 2020, from https://www.weforum.org/agenda/2020/03/why-sub-saharan-africa-needs-a-unique-response-to-covid-19.

Khanal, P., Devkota, N., Dahal, M., Paudel, K., & Joshi, D. (2020). *Mental health impacts among health workers during COVID-19 in a low resource setting: A cross-sectional survey from Nepal* (pp. 1–27).

Lam, S. C., Arora, T., Grey, I., Suen, L. K. P., Huang, E. Y., Li, D., & Lam, K. B. H. (2020). Perceived risk and protection from infection and depressive symptoms among healthcare workers in mainland China and Hong Kong during COVID-19. *Frontiers in Psychiatry*, *11*, 686. https://doi.org/10.3389/fpsyt.2020.00686.

Liu, Q., Luo, D., Haase, J. E., Guo, Q., Wang, X. Q., Liu, S., … Yang, B. X. (2020). The experiences of health-care providers during the COVID-19 crisis in China: A qualitative study. *The Lancet Global Health*, *8*(6), e790–e798. https://doi.org/10.1016/S2214-109X(20)30204-7.

Lone, S. A., & Ahmad, A. (2020). COVID-19 pandemic—An African perspective. *Emerging Microbes and Infections*, *9*(1), 1300–1308. https://doi.org/10.1080/22221751.2020.1775132.

Marroquín, B., Howard, T., & Stanton, A. L. (2017). Coping, emotion regulation, and well-being: Intrapersonal and interpersonal processes. In M. Robinson, & M. Eid (Eds.), *The happy mind: Cognitive contributions to well-being* (pp. 1–480). Los Angeles: Springer International Publishing AG. https://doi.org/10.1007/978-3-319-58763-9.

Mbonye, A., Wamala, J., Kaboyo, W., Tugumizemo, V., Aceng, J., & Makumbi, I. (2012). Repeated outbreaks of viral hemorrhagic fevers in Uganda. *African Health Sciences*, *12*(4), 579–583. https://doi.org/10.4314/ahs.v12i4.31.

McMahon, S. A., Ho, L. S., Brown, H., Miller, L., Ansumana, R., & Kennedy, C. E. (2016). Healthcare providers on the frontlines: A qualitative investigation of the social and emotional impact of delivering health services during Sierra Leone's Ebola epidemic. *Health Policy and Planning*, *31*(9), 1232–1239. https://doi.org/10.1093/heapol/czw055.

Ministry of Health. (2020a). *COVID-19 pandemic in Uganda*. Retrieved 24 August 2020, from https://www.health.go.ug/.

Ministry of Health. (2020b). *COVID-2019 pandemic in Uganda*. Retrieved 4 August 2020, from https://www.health.go.ug/covid/.

Ministry of Health. (2020c). *Update on the outbreak of COVID-I9 in Uganda*. Press Statement. Retrieved 23 August 2020, from https://www.health.go.ug/cause/update-on-the-outbreak-of-covid-19-in-uganda/.

Montemurro, N. (2020). The emotional impact of COVID-19: From medical staff to common people. *Brain, Behavior, and Immunity*, *87*, 23–24.

Mühlenbernd, R. (2014). Convention and innovation in social networks. *BMC Health Services Research*, *1283*, 317–328.

Munawar, K., & Choudhry, F. R. (2020). Exploring stress coping strategies of frontline emergency health workers dealing Covid-19 in Pakistan: A qualitative inquiry. *American Journal of Infection Control*. https://doi.org/10.1016/j.ajic.2020.06.214.

Okware, S. I., Omaswa, F., Talisuna, A., Amandua, J., Amone, J., Onek, P., … Thorkild, T. (2015). Managing Ebola from rural to urban slum settings: Experiences from Uganda. *African Health Sciences*, *15*(1), 312–321.

Olum, R., & Bongomin, F. (2020). Uganda's first 100 COVID-19 cases: Trends and lessons. *International Journal of Infectious Diseases*, *96*, 517–518.

Ornell, F., Halpern, S. C., Paim Kessler, F. H., & de Magalhães Narvaez, J. C. (2020). The impact of the COVID-19 pandemic on the mental health of healthcare professionals. *Cadernos De Saude Publica*, *36*(4), e00063520. https://doi.org/10.1590/0102-311X00063520.

Ornell, F., Schuch, J. B., Sordi, A. O., & Kessler, F. H. P. (2020). 'Pandemic fear' and COVID-19: Mental health burden and strategies. *Brazilian Journal of Psychiatry*, *42*(3), 232–235. https://doi.org/10.1590/1516-4446-2020-0008.

Sharma, M. (2003). Coping: Strategies. In N. A. Piotrowski (Ed.), *Vol. 2. Magill's encyclopedia of social science: Psychology: Data description-meditation and relaxation, volume 2* (pp. 1689–1699). University of California: Salem Press Editors. https://doi.org/10.1017/CBO9781107415324.004.

Spoorthy, M. S. (2020). Mental health problems faced by healthcare workers due to the COVID-19 pandemic—A review. *Asian Journal of Psychiatry*, *51*(January). https://doi.org/10.1016/j.ajp.2020.102119.

The Presidency of the Republic of Ghana. (2020). *Address to the nation by President Akufo-Addo on updates to Ghana's enhanced response to the Coronavirus pandemic, 5th April, 2020*. Retrieved 11 August 2020, from https://www.moh.gov.gh/address-to-the-nation-by-pres-akufo-addo/.

UNICEF GHANA. (2020). *COVID-19 situation report – number 2*. Accra. Retrieved from https://reliefweb.int/report/ghana/unicef-ghana-covid-19-situation-report-2-16th-april-30th-april-2020.

Upton, J. (2013). Psychosocial factors. In M. D. Gellman, & J. R. Turner (Eds.), *Encyclopedia of behavioral medicine* (13th ed., pp. 1580–1581). New York: Springer. https://doi.org/10.1007/978-1-4419-1005-9.

Vaismoradi, M., Jones, J., Turunen, H., & Snelgrove, S. (2016). Theme development in qualitative content analysis and thematic analysis. *Journal of Nursing Education and Practice*, *6*(5), 100–110. https://doi.org/10.5430/jnep.v6n5p100.

Vaismoradi, M., & Snelgrove, S. (2019). Theme in qualitative content analysis and thematic analysis. *Qualitative Social Research*, *20*(3). https://doi.org/10.17169/fqs-20.3.3376.

Wafula, P. (2020). COVID-19 frontline workers at Jinja Hospital strike over allowance. In *Daily monitor*. May 22, Retrieved from https://www.monitor.co.ug/News/National/COVID19-frontline-workers-Jinja-Hospital-strike-Tugumisirize/688334-5560412-xcq6b4/index.html.

WHO African Region. (2020). *COVID-19: Situation update for the WHO African Region*. Brazzaville: Republic of Congo. Retrieved from https://apps.who.int/iris/bitstream/handle/10665/333559/SITREP_COVID-19_WHOAFRO_20200729-eng.pdf.

World Health Organization. (2020). *Mental health and psychosocial considerations during COVID-19 outbreak*. Geneva: World Health Organization. Retrieved from https://www.who.int/docs/default-source/coronaviruse/mental-health-considerations.pdf?sfvrsn=6d3578af_2.

World Health Organization Regional Offices for Africa. (2020). *COVID-19 situation update for the WHO African region 19 August 2020: External situation report 25. Congo Brazzaville*. Retrieved from https://apps.who.int/iris/bitstream/handle/10665/333902/SITREP_COVID-19_WHOAFRO_20200819-eng.pdf.

Ye, Z., Yang, X., Zeng, C., Wang, Y., Shen, Z., Li, X., & Lin, D. (2020). Resilience, social support, and coping as mediators between COVID-19-related stressful experiences and acute stress disorder among college students in China. *Applied Psychology: Health and Well-Being*. https://doi.org/10.1111/aphw.12211.

Chapter 4

The psychosocial effect of COVID-19 on urban refugees: Narratives from Congolese refugees living in Kampala

Paul Bukuluki, Hadijah Mwenyango, Francis Kato, Agnes Kyamulabi, and Alex Bagabo
Department of Social Work and Social Administration, Makerere University, Kampala, Uganda

Introduction

Uganda's first Corona Virus Disease (COVID-19) case was confirmed on 21 March 2020, with cumulative confirmed cases indicating 1332 cases, 9 deaths, and 134 active cases as of August 13, 2020 (Ministry of Health Uganda, 2020). Like other countries, the Ugandan government instituted several containment measures such as the closure of public places and the country's borders, social distancing, stay home except for emergencies, and the banning of public transport. More public health measures as guided by WHO were also introduced, for instance, frequent handwashing with soap and water; use of alcohol-based sanitizers; avoiding touching of soft parts such as eyes, nose, and mouth; and mandatory quarantine of suspected cases and recent travelers and their contacts (Ministry of Health Uganda, 2020). Further, the Ugandan government also postponed the acceptance of new asylum seekers and closed all its refugee reception centers at the border points and the Department of Refugees (DOR) offices in Kampala and Old Kampala Police Desk Refugee Office (Sebagoro, Nyakabande, Matanda, Elegu, and Ntoroko) for 30 days from 25 March (Bukuluki, Mwenyango, Katongole, & Palattiyil, 2020; GoU, 2020). The effectiveness of these measures is perhaps seen in the fact that Uganda had so far registered 840 COVID-19 recoveries and had not recorded any COVID-19 related death as of July 2020 (Ministry of Health Uganda, 2020).

However, the risks carried by these measures especially against the vulnerable groups (such as the urban refugees) of the population are not well recorded

Mental Health Effects of COVID-19. https://doi.org/10.1016/B978-0-12-824289-6.00006-4

in Uganda. A usual mistake in the management of pandemics relates to the accentuation of the infection control measures at the expense of parallel disaster management interventions such as psychosocial support, collaboration, and networking (Hyun et al., 2020). Particularly for vulnerable groups (such as women, children, minorities, and refugees), the COVID-19 pandemic resulted in an upsurge of health care and socioeconomic disparities as well as a surge in the prepandemic issues such as discrimination, stigma, poverty, unemployment, and gender-based violence (Bukuluki et al., 2020).

The psychosocial impact of the COVID-19 pandemic has been recently studied by several scholars (Cerami et al., 2020; Dubey et al., 2020; Hyun et al., 2020; Kulyar, Bhutta, Shabbir, & Akhtar, 2020; Mackolil & Mackolil, 2020; Otu, Charles, & Yaya, 2020; Sun, Lin, & Operario, 2020). Psychosocial problems that could arise during pandemics include anxiety, uneasiness, mourning, helplessness, fatigue, impairment of concentration, sleep disorders, sexual dysfunction, infertility, psychological distress, and psychiatric disorders (Hyun et al., 2020). Studies in places like China and India reveal that migrants experience distress, death during migration, mass chemical spraying, and quarantine in inappropriate places which affects their physical and mental health (BBC, 2020; Qiu et al., 2020). These measures affect their human rights for health, dignity, and self-esteem. They also increase anger, disobedience, and long-lasting psychological stigma (Dubey et al., 2020). Quite several studies have focused on the psychosocial impact of pandemics (such as depression and PSTD) among frontline workers like health care staff and armed forces (Dubey et al., 2020). For instance, Dubey et al. (2020) state that Taiwanese nurses who worked in the SARS unit during the 2003 SARS outbreak suffered from more depressive symptoms and insomnia compared to those from non-SARS units (p. 781). Some of these studies have also concentrated on the psychosocial effects of COVID-19 on the general population. For example, Dubey et al. (2020) argue that COVID-19 has universally created mass hysteria, economic burden, and financial losses. However, these studies have not systematically studied the psychosocial effect of pandemics, particularly COVID-19 on vulnerable populations especially the urban refugees in low- and middle-income countries (LMICs) like Uganda.

Considering the lethal communicability of this pandemic, forcefully displaced people such as refugees are at heightened risk of contracting, spreading, and suffering the psychosocial issues stemming from the COVID-19 outbreak. Although refugees are generally found to have a high prevalence of common psychiatric disorders, like depression and a poor quality of life, these disorders are further exacerbated by governmentally imposed quarantine and lost income during the pandemic (Dubey et al., 2020). Urban refugees, in particular, live in places where public health infrastructure is already overstretched thus making these individuals vulnerable to exclusion, stigma, and discrimination (Bukuluki et al., 2020; Dubey et al., 2020). Furthermore, refugees tend to bear the stigma of being the source of the outbreak of the virus (Dubey et al., 2020).

Uganda is considered as a relatively favorable environment for refugees compared to other places in the world because refugees have free movement in the country and have better access to most rights (Bohnet & Schmitz-Pranghe, 2019; Crawford, O'Callaghan, Holloway, & Lowe, 2019). With 1.35 million refugees and asylum seekers, the country is ranked as the third largest refugee-hosting nation in the world. Refugees come from neighboring countries such as the Democratic Republic of Congo (DRC), South Sudan, Rwanda, Burundi, Ethiopia, Sudan, Eritrea, and Somalia (Mwenyango & Palattiyil, 2019). Although Uganda's Government's refugee policy requires refugees to settle in delineated settlements for them to access both Government and UNHCR assistance, over 100,000 refugees currently live on the outskirts of Kampala city and other towns in Uganda (Bukuluki et al., 2020). Urban centers attract refugees due to perceived opportunities for decent employment, education, and good infrastructure. Nevertheless, refugees who choose to live in urban centers are supposed to be self-sufficient in achieving all their needs. In this chapter, we examine the psychosocial consequences of COVID-19 on urban refugees in Uganda. We also explore indications of resilience among urban refugees.

Methodology

Design

The research employed a case study design and used the qualitative approaches of inquiry. We took a case study of Congolese refugees living in Kampala city to understand the effect of the lockdown and other related public and social measures instituted by the Government of Uganda in response to the COVID-19 global pandemic on the psychosocial wellbeing of urban refugees. The qualitative approach helped explore the lived experiences of urban refugees and how the lockdown and public health measures affected them. Our approach also facilitated exploration of how urban refugees made efforts to deal with the effects on the lockdown and public health measures.

Sample

The sample was generated through a blend of purposive and snowball sampling methods where the identification and recruitment of initial study participants were done with the help of community gatekeepers[a] who were also refugees. As we interviewed the initial urban refugees, they contacted their peers and we followed up by contacting those who were willing to be interviewed. In total, we identified and interviewed five males and five females. The ages of the study participants ranged from 21 to 40 years. The interviewees also varied in terms of the period of stay in Uganda ranging from 2 to 7 years. All the interviewees

a Community influencers who understand the community social, cultural, and political environment.

came from the Democratic Republic of Congo (DRC). They also followed different journeys, while some (7) had come directly from the border crossing points to Kampala, others (3) had first lived in a refugee settlement in Uganda before they relocated to Kampala.

The interviews were conducted at a time when the government had imposed strict public health and social measures such as stay at home orders and restrictions on movement (public transportation including the use of personal vehicles and motorcycles). As such, phone interviews were considered the most appropriate given the prevailing times—the context of a lockdown during a pandemic. Phone interviews are advanced as a viable option for qualitative research due to their logistical conveniences and the ability to facilitate reaching geographies (and population) with access limitations (Drabble, Trocki, Salcedo, Walker, & Korcha, 2016). Moreover, Trier-Bieniek (2012) has shown phone interviews to enable the interviewees to remain in (relatively) safe and comfortable settings during the interview conversation. However, the research team acknowledges the limitation of using phone interviews. For example, it was not possible to observe the nonverbal communication cues that are possible with face-to-face interviews.

Procedures

The research team first identified a community mobilizer who is member and leader within the refugee community in Kampala—this was a refugee from the Democratic Republic of Congo who later supported the identification and mobilization of the initial potential study participants. To facilitate the community mobilizer's role, the study team explained the purpose, the methods (phone interviews), and the ethics and emphasized that only those willing to volunteer to participate should be recruited. Subsequently, the community mobilizer returned a list of potential study participants who indicated a willingness to participate with their telephone contacts. For those who were recommended to us by their peers whom we had already interviewed, we asked them to provide their telephone contacts to call them and request their voluntary participation in the study.

Before initiating telephone calls, several efforts were made to facilitate the ease of communication with prospective interviewees. The research team worked with the mobilizer and in some cases the study participants to indicate the language of preference with each of the identified potential participants. Our study participants were able to speak English, Swahili, and a little Luganda. They sometimes used Luganda or English and in others, it was a combination of the two languages to facilitate understanding for both the interviewer and interviewee during the conversation.

The research team made the initial phone calls to establish rapport and further explain the study and take the study participants through an informed consent process. This process aimed at seeking interviewees' voluntary participation, explains possible risks and benefits, and provided clarity on any issues related to privacy and confidentiality, and confirm their willingness to be interviewed and set up an agreeable time for the interview in advance. Verbal consent was obtained from all the interviewees. Although some of the potential interviewees had to change schedules for the interviews to take place, none of the (10) identified members turned down the request for an interview. While the research team had prepared and familiarized with the data collection instrument—the interview guide, at least two members of the research team participated in the first two interviews to support each other, further familiarize and appreciate dynamics of the interview, reflect on personal reactions, examine what went well, what needs improvement, and identify opportunities for improving the subsequent interviews.

Interviews were conducted in May 2020. A semistructured interview guide was used, which included 11 primary questions and follow-up probes related to the interviewees (urban refugees) "life experiences of the COVID-19 global pandemic and the impact of corresponding government-led public health and social (prevention and mitigation) measures in several areas of their mental and psychosocial wellbeing. "These included social networks/relationships, social support, resilience and personal coping mechanisms, socioeconomic and psychological status, family dynamics and sociodemographic data. Interviews generally ranged from approximately 30 to 56 min. At the end of each interview, the respondents were provided a token of 10,000 Uganda shillings (close to 3 US$) as a way of appreciating their valued time. The interviews were audio-recorded, transcribed, and processed into Microsoft word document to facilitate analysis and presentation of findings. Data analysis used open coding (Flick, 2009) following thematic analysis.

Thematic analysis (Braun & Clarke, 2012) was used to draw emerging themes and subthemes linked to the research issues. Interviews were audio-recorded, transcribed, and those conducted in Luganda were translated into English and entered into MS Word software for editing as the first step to "formal" analysis. Data were then categorized according to key themes, subthemes, and codes that were emerging. Some direct quotes from study participants were abstracted from the data and used as evidence to substantiate the study findings. Pseudo names have been used to refer to study participants to maintain confidentiality.

Results

Key findings: Psychosocial impact of COVID-19 on urban refugees

In Table 1, we present the sociodemographic characteristics of the interviewees who participated in this research. The information was gathered as part of the interview. This is important because it provides a context with which to appreciate the emerging issues from the phone interviews.

TABLE 1 Sociodemographic characteristics of the interviewees.

#	Pseudo name of participant	Gender	Marital status	Age in years	Work status before COVID-19	# of people in household		When came to UG	Education
						< 18	18+		
01	Phoebe	Female	Single	26	Saloon	6	5	2012	University
02	Philip	Male	Married	35	Broker	3	3	2016	University
03	Elizabeth	Female	Married	28	Tailor	6	5	2015	University
04	Christine	Female	Married	29	Vending	2	5	2016	University
05	Paul	Male	Single	23	Paparazzi	1	0	2015	University
06	Aline	Female	Single	18	No. work	3	4	2015	P7
07	Eddie	Male	Single	32	Music distributor	2	2	2012	University
08	Beatrice	Female	Single	21	Unemployed	4	7	2016	Secondary
09	Mathew	Male	Single	30	Graphic designer	1	0	2016	University
10	Felix	Male	Cohabiting	40	Broker	6	2	2013	University

The narratives from refugees revealed specific psychosocial experiences including fear, anger/irritability, socioeconomic distress, anxiety, insomnia, isolation/detachment, loss of social support, and failure to meet social roles. These are explained in detail in the following section.

Fear of COVID-19

Generally, outbreaks are a source of fear and distress for everybody. Likewise, the narratives in the current study showed a high perception of the danger related to COVID-19 as a major concern for the urban refugees. The imagined danger was sought to be much higher than what the leaders expressed which in turn prompted a sense of fear and panic among some of the urban refugees. This is revealed in the following expression.

> *Even if here in Uganda they told us that those 400 [COVID-19] cases that up to now no one is dead with the COVID-19, but for sure we know that African leaders are lying… I can't allow even my children to go out, I can't allow even my wife to go out, am the one who goes out because we are fearing.*
>
> [Philip]

Although the statement explicitly reflects fear about contracting COVID-19, this could also be due to distrust likely resulting from unclear information (such as about the COVID-19 cases, recoveries, and deaths) and communication about the pandemic. Besides, fear in a way is associated with panic though it was not mentioned. However, the statement of not allowing children to go out brings out the panic element that is likely to raise tensions in the family.

Anger/irritability

Difficult periods trigger emotions of which some could be harmful. This research found experiences of anger and irritation among Congolese urban refugees because of the COVID-19 pandemic. The anger is related to the competing demands and related difficulties to meet outstanding needs. For example, some Congolese parents who participated in the study labeled their children as disturbing due to the children's endless demands amid lack of means. This clarity cannot overly be put better than it is in both Christine's and Elizabeth's account of the reported behavioral changes, which seemed to cause a level of irritation on the part of some (Congolese refugee) parents as can be seen in the following excerpts:

> *These days they (children) can over disturb, you don't have anything, 'uh mummy they told us that our hands-we wash them with soap' yet you don't have even soap, they say, 'you want us to wash our hands without soap' and when you tell them to go and wash the hands, they say 'but there is no soap' and you find yourself slapping the child.*
>
> [Christine]

When you don't have something you change naturally, you can change haha because they [children] can ask for something that I don't have for the first time, the second time, third time, I feel angry.

[Elizabeth]

These excerpts mirror the feeling of loss of control in the face of adversity associated with insufficient supply of essentials, the uncertainty of disease progression, financial losses, and increased perception of risk and vulnerability to the pandemic. The scarcity of sufficient, safe, and affordable water supply plus soap makes refugees fail to comply with public health measures such as basic hand hygiene regulations emphasized by the government and the World Health Organisation. This increases feelings of deprivation, neglect, and exclusion (Dubey et al., 2020), and it also affects the relationship of parents and their children.

Financial distress

Like other countries, Uganda implemented lockdown measures to abate the spread of COVID-19. This increased despair in people who receive day-to-day income, specifically concerning the loss of jobs and heightened poverty. Our respondents narrated the loss of jobs and income. For example, one refugee grieved that:

My job which has been moving our life is no longer there, I stay at home, a person who has been struggling to get what the children eat...I have been going to town to get 'bitenge' [cloth material] and I go and sell them, I take back the money, there they give me a small percentage and I also get something little but these days they have closed and I don't know whether when they come back, they will take [employ] me back.

[Christine]

This statement shows that refugees have lost wages and incomes due to the closure of businesses which has affected their livelihood. Exposure to such losses is associated with immediate and long-term psychological effects including post-traumatic stress disorder (PTSD) and sometimes suicide (Dubey et al., 2020).

Anxiety

Anxiety is linked to other factors such as stress reactions and a lack of common information about a specific condition (Mackolil & Mackolil, 2020). This research found indications of anxiety among the Congolese urban refugees. Some resulted from fear of contracting the disease as explained by one of the participants:

The first day that we started hearing that here in Uganda, there are some [COVID-19] cases, it started traumatising me. I started having signs of it, the headache, flu, coughing, fever and I started fearing that maybe I have got, it but I didn't know.

[Phoebe]

This account demonstrates an association with the broadcasted symptoms of the disease without having any COVID-19 related diseases. It is argued that that the continual flow of information particularly through online and social networks causes adverse psychosomatic issues (WHO, 2020). On the other hand, some respondents expressed worry not particularly related to contracting the virus but with its impact. For example, some were uncertain of how to settle their recurrent debts and their sustenance, yet they lost their sources of income. One respondent expressed his concern about the burden related to COVID-19 and said,

My wife has a lot of stress since this COVID-19 started and our lives have changed…if we want to eat we must look for someone to lend us some money and now, we have borrowed from many people so we ask ourselves, how shall we pay all the debts.

[Philip]

In a similar tone, another participant expressed concern about the postpandemic period and said,

Things may not be as they used to be before [the pandemic], so that thing worries me most because I overthink about it and I end up asking myself that, but will things go back as they used to be, business moving as before, everything moving as they used to be done, the laws?

This statement indicates hopelessness in the face of the pandemic. The accumulation of such critical and sometimes negative thoughts could also lead to a reduction in the quality of life. This situation is further jeopardized by governmentally imposed quarantine and lost income during the pandemic (Dubey et al., 2020).

Sleep disorders

Good sleep depends on the ability to relax the mind. There were reports of sleep disorders relating to insomnia and hallucinations among urban refugees. For the parents, this was due to thoughts concerning their failure to meet parental roles and excessive bills during and after COVID-19 such as rent. One of the respondents explained how her children and herself were affected and said,

A child sleeps only for 5 minutes and he starts to knock [at the door] 'mummy I want food; I want to eat' and if you don't have, you remove him out of the way so that he can go back to sleep so, after that, you go back to sleep and then another one comes, 'mother' and there, you lose sleep.

[Christine]

This is an expression of the difficulty to have a good rest when occupied with indigent thoughts. This was the same revelation from other participant:

I can go to bed around 9 pm when I want to sleep but I end up sleeping at around 1 am when am just wondering a lot how I will live after this corona.

[Philip]

If I came a bit early (before COVID-19), it would be 10 pm, I would come very tired that is when I slept, then wake up very early… but this time [during COVID-19], I don't get that feeling of sleeping because I think a lot about life.

[Phoebe]

Those who did not mention changes in their sleeping routines instead experienced nightmares. This was disclosed by one of the participants in his description of a dream that troubled him:

I saw people were on a burial but the person who was dead was me… all these [messages] we see of COVID-19—the pictures that they are showing us of people who are dead, I don't know whether it is connected.

[Mathew]

This reveals the risk of being exposed to excessive information and sometimes misinformation about COVID-19 and its impact. Sleep disorders combined with worry about the outbreak of the virus are associated with an upsurge in mental health issues (WHO, 2020).

Social and physical isolation

COVID-19 has exacerbated the social and physical isolation of refugees by reducing their interaction with key resourceful social networks. Refugees in this study felt lonely. This was due to lockdown measures relating to confinement at homes, social distancing, curfew on movement from 7 p.m. to 6.30 a.m., and restriction of public transport at the time. This was revealed in one interview:

There is no way I can move to meet with my friends because there is no transport… and it's very difficult for me to communicate with them because I have no phone

[Agnes]

This physical isolation is combined with social isolation as explained by another participant that:

You can't see them [friends] anymore; you can't meet them so that you share ideas with them and to tell them the way you may want them to help you.

[Christine]

These two statements indicate the importance of social interactions with significant others. Although previous research indicates that the COVID-19 lockdown strengthens family bonds (Mackolil & Mackolil, 2020), strict control measures such as restriction of public transport and lockdown of public places (such as churches) deprive refugees of the opportunity to utilize their support networks which intensified their suffering. This finding emulates the claim that refugees devote considerable time to social circles of people with whom they have commonalities and similar experiences (Kluge, Jakab, Bartovic, D'Anna, & Severoni, 2020). Many of our respondents showed a greater connection to God/ Supernatural Being before places of worship were closed. For instance, one participant disclosed that:

> *When I had problems, I could go there and tell him [pastor] to pray for me so they [pastors] would do it as counselling but nowadays meeting is not easy.*
>
> [Mathew]

Beatrice's statement was not much different from **Mathew**'s tribulation:

> *Before COVID-19, I used to meet the pastor and the pastor prayed for me, advised me and maybe preached to me and now this time there is no way I can meet the pastor.*

The closure of religious places deprived refugees of community-based support which provided the needed coping skills. Although refugees still showed greater connection through the continuation of prayers in their families and reliance of God for providence, the extended prohibition of such gatherings could result in reemergence of painful memories and displacement trauma.

Loss of social support

Although refugees lose their original support due to relocation, many of them form new relationships in their destination places (Mwenyango & Palattiyil, 2019). Some who are fortunate to keep families and friends depend on them for maintenance. Bukuluki et al. (2020) state that most urban refugees depend on informal support systems such as remittances from relatives outside Uganda (such as Sweden and the United States of America). Likewise, our respondents were unanimous about receiving emotional and financial support from relatives and friends before COVID-19. However, they complained that the lockdown due to the pandemic has deprived them of such support. For example, two participants regretted that,

> *You can't get a person who can help you in this situation of COVID-19, everybody first cares for his/her life, ...everybody is at their home for us these days we are very poor... there is no relative you can depend on and say that this usually gives me because everyone now wants to start with his family.*
>
> Ariani

> *It is difficult for us to get what to feed the children, something to pay [bills], aah even this is my 2 [second] or 3 [third] month I can't even pay the rent but before COVID-19, I couldn't even spend a week without someone in Congo sending some money.*
>
> [Philip]

The statements indicate that social networks are a great source of financial and emotional support. However, difficult times constrain and weaken existing social bonds (Hyun et al., 2020) because people tend to preserve their belongings instead of devoting to helping others. This creates additional challenges for people depending on networks for their livelihood.

Social malfunction

Many of the refugees complained of their inability to fulfill their parental roles. This is due to the sudden loss of jobs implying that they could not secure necessities for their upkeep and their families. One of the participants said:

> *I can say that the way we live now, it is so hard for us to get food, we live by the grace of God, there is no food, staying at home no working, the prices for things have increased.*
>
> [Phoebe]

This reflects an increase in social pressure due to a lack of income and is escalated due to rising costs. This was reflected in another interview:

> *For us refugees, we just want to have something to eat, rent and security but now to get what to eat is not easy, to pay rent is also not easy.*
>
> [Elizabeth]

Another respondent specifically pointed out his frustration with changes in family nutrition as they are no more able to provide a proper diet in their families. He said,

> *I was 75kgs before COVID 19 but today am 60kgs or 69kgs…my appetite isn't good, am eating somethings I couldn't eat…in my house we wouldn't eat mukene [silver fish] but now, we are eating mukene because of corona. Things have changed, you can eat because you are hungry but without appetite, you just eat to survive.*
>
> [Philip]

These statements indicate exposure to aggravated health problems resulting from family pressure and dietary complications. Further consequences from such could be psychological stress and gender-based violence in homes due to the inability to meet personal and family demands (Bukuluki et al., 2020).

Resilience and personal coping mechanisms

People need resources to cope with adversity (Ungar & Herrenkohl, 2013). Although most of the data indicate exposure of urban refugees to hurdles (due to lack of physical and emotional resources) during the COVID-19 period, some were able to maintain balance—a sign of resilience. This was through several coping measures including reducing expenditure on nonessential items (such as alcohol), continued observance of prayers during the lockdown, and participation in small group interactions such as sharing tales, indoor games, and watching television. Such measures helped them to overcome negative thoughts and stress. These were reflected in the following expressions:

> *If I'm not okay, I tell the younger-ones stories, we talk together, all of us laugh and then we relax a little bit.*
>
> [Arian]

> *I make myself busy, sometimes, I can forget [problems] a bit with playing Ludo [board game], sometimes watching TV.*
>
> [Beatrice]

> *I can pray at home if I want to, we can sing a small song at home, we can do everything at home...we try to pray together like, we do it for 3 hours or we pray for 2 hours.*
>
> [Elizabeth]

While the earlier excerpts show interpersonal resilience, there were other narratives from participants that revealed intrapersonal resilience among some of the refugees.

> *This COVID is teaching me how to use the money whichever little I may get like for me I could not spend [a day] without taking my beer, I would spend more on drinking...I told my wife that after this [pandemic] the program [of drinking] will be only on Saturday... I can see how she [wife] is also very economical on how to treat even our visitors.*
>
> [Philip]

These statements reflect the development of adaptive strategies (such as reduced expenditure) to the circumstances. Awareness and acceptance of the existing conditions are key facets of resilience. It is stated that in situations of adversity, resilience is observed when individuals engage in behaviors that help them to navigate their way to the resources they need (Ungar & Herrenkohl, 2013).

Discussion

Global pandemics are known sources of aggravated mental health issues (Dubey et al., 2020; Kulyar et al., 2020). This research reveals the existence of psychosocial problems among urban refugees including anxiety, sleep disorders, psychological distress, and psychiatric disorders. For example, excessive information concerning susceptibility to certain risks (in this case COVID-19) affects mental health. WHO (2020) cautions that the sudden and continuous stream of news reports about an outbreak causes extreme worry. In recent times, this information is inaccurate, yet it is associated with the escalation of social stigma, discrimination, and stress (Hyun et al., 2020). For instance, research indicates that the COVID-19 pandemic has aggravated the use of derogatory statements against Chinese nationals worldwide, specifically, linked to their values and food (Dubey et al., 2020). In the next section, we contextualize their narratives into three main themes: social role limitations and lost identity; ruptured lives and loss of control, to provide a clearer description of their psychosocial state.

Social role limitations and lost identity

People need to feel functional within their families and the community. Our findings show that urban refugees are no longer able to fulfill their social and health responsibilities such as childcare, medical care, feeding their families, and paying their bills which have contributed to collective fear and anxiety. They have lost their sources of survival, accumulated debts, and experience isolation and hopelessness. Despite social networks being a great source of support and livelihood, our findings, like Hyun et al. (2020), confirm that control measures such as social distancing or quarantine deprive families and communities of emotional bonds and weaken their support network. Such distress could be expected as Bukuluki et al. (2020) describe that urban refugees depend on the informal market economy and small enterprises such as artisans, tailoring, hairdressing, and vending of food and second-hand clothes which were not exonerated by the lockdown directives. Although this could be perceived as a widespread problem in the urban centers because of general dependence on small and medium enterprises, refugees suffer most due to a lack of alternative means of survival and limited access to social support networks. And unlike refugees in organized settlements who receive assistance (food and material items) from the government and UNHCR, our participants are not benefiting from the current food distribution (ongoing efforts by the government to lessen starvation in Kampala and Wakiso townships resulting from the closure of businesses) which jeopardies their wellbeing and coping capacities. Sudden misfortunes (such as the loss of emotional bonds) are associated with increased guilt, frustration, depression, and mental suffering, ultimately leading to functional impairment and increased rates of suicide (Subbaraman et al., 2014). Further, the failure to meet parental and social roles contributes to loss of respect, confidence, and identity as responsible adults. Although the participants indicated signs of resilience by cutting their expenditure on nonessential items like alcohol (which is perhaps a better transformation in terms of improving health) and reducing the number of meals, it is difficult for their children to adjust. This resulted in feelings of numbness and insignificance because of the inability to meet their children's demands. Though it is important to meet essential items such as food for personal and family members, negative emotions (resulting from the incapacity to meet these demands) bring about mental health disorders such as depression, anxiety, dementia, and disorientation (Dubey et al., 2020).

Ruptured lives

The lockdown has not only broken refugee social networks but has also shattered their survival/lives. Being in a new environment, it is not uncommon for refugees to experience loss of relationships, personal control, and identity. However, without meeting their networks which they have rebuilt in host environments implies a great loss not only of friendship but also of subsistence. The attitude of prioritizing personal care and immediate family members is also exacerbated by physical and social isolation since people are unaware of events in the families of their significant others. Moreover, the impact of collapsing businesses on which refugees depended is not only affecting individuals but also communities. Lost employment and income during the pandemic entail immediate and long-term consequences on the recovery and resilience of refugees. For instance, the failure to acquire food reverses progress in achieving Sustainable Development Goal (SDG2) underlining the significance of food security. Besides the WHO stresses the importance of keeping regular sleep routines and eating healthy food to increase immunity against the virus (WHO, 2020). However, the findings indicate an increase in risk exposure and psychological stress due to the inability to meet personal and family demands. Unresolved family problems could result in depression, substance abuse, sexual abuse, and violence. Research shows that failure to meet ascribed roles in traditional societies intensifies gender inequalities, causing anger and frustration which aggravate emotional and physical violence (Bukuluki et al., 2020).

Loss of personal control

The psychosocial experiences of participants relating to fear and anxiety indicate a state of emotions taking over the lives of refugees. Some statements from the participants reflect fear about contracting COVID-19 due to distrust likely resulting from unclear information and communication from the authorities. COVID-19 related fear has been described as "coronaphobia" in some studies (Dubey et al., 2020, p. 1). Known causes of fear include exposure to COVID-19 cases, being quarantined, the death or illness of a relative, or friend from COVID-19 (Dubey et al., 2020). Similarly, refugees in the current study seemed helpless and perhaps are experiencing a situation where they have lost hope for the future. However, the feelings of fear reported by the participants could be beyond COVID-19 illness to perceived consequences for contracting the diseases such as isolation, discrimination, stigma, and marginalization with all its social and economic ramifications such as the account of the participant who stated that his wife would not tolerate him moving out to meet friends who would render him support. Now such descriptions indicate helplessness. Dubey et al. (2020) state that such extreme emotions such as those relating to stigma diminishes people's will to seek important services such as medical support. This, in turn, intensifies the transmission of COVID-19 within communities.

Resilience and coping mechanisms

Boyden and Mann (2005, p. 4) describe resilience as the capacity to recover from, adapt, and remain strong in the face of adversity. In their conceptualization of resilience, Ungar and colleagues describe four factors including navigation, negotiation, resources (opportunity), and meaning (Ungar & Herrenkohl, 2013, p. 256). It involves both coping ability and adaptive capacity. Coping ability indicates short-term ability to survive while adaptive capacity denotes more sustainable responses to adversity (Gallopín, 2006). The pandemic and government directives to combat the spread of COVID-19 have exposed refugees to difficult experiences that threaten personal, family, and community coping mechanisms and led to the destruction of social and cultural norms as well as protective factors. Despite that, some participants have adapted and responded positively to such setbacks and deprivation. While most of their external resources (such as the extended family, friends and neighbors) are constrained by the pandemic, refugees exhibit resilience based on personal and collective strengths. Important attributes that contributed to resilience were personality, optimism about the future, and spirituality. As explained by Boyden and Mann (2005), refugee resilience must be one of the touchstones for supporting them.

Do refugees need psychosocial support?

The psychosocial impacts of COVID-19 to the Congolese urban refugees in Uganda highlighted have led to posing the question of what should be done to protect urban refugees from suffering harm during the pandemic? Refugees need psychosocial support for their psychological and emotional wellbeing, as well as their social and physical wellbeing. This should involve an evaluation of their mental health, social status, and functional capacity within their families and the community. The refugees revealed a lack of access to necessities resulting in socioeconomic distress and perceived social malfunction. Local and refugee leaders can identify the most vulnerable households, and these should benefit from government assistance (food, water, and face masks) distributed by the National Task Force on COVID-19.

Some refugees as highlighted in the prior sections need additional, specific psychosocial support including structured counseling and motivational enhancement. In some places like Korea, mental health professionals have provided the needed mental health support including, stress management, tips on how to calm down, overcoming adversities guidelines on adults caring for children, improving resilience during quarantine, meditation, dealing with stigma, and getting back to normalcy (Hyun et al., 2020). These are helpful measures that could be adapted to the psychosocial needs of urban refugees in Uganda. We are also aware that such could necessitate intensified capacity building for frontline workers such as health care staff and other social care workers (such as social workers and mental health experts) to appreciate the specific immediate and long-term needs of urban refugees resulting from the pandemic. As explained previously, participants experienced serious anxiety problems due to recurrent debts and their survival during the postpandemic period. For instance, it is important to create a sense of security (in terms of legal aspects and assistance) to eliminate the helplessness. Such integrative assessment can be achieved via modern communication platforms such as social media/telephone services and voice recordings on psychosocial support (Kulyar et al., 2020). The WHO has also issued specific advice for the reduction in COVID-19 related psychosocial issues. For example, people need to limit their exposure to news about COVID-19. This could be through minimization of watching, reading, or listening to news about COVID-19; securing information updates only from trusted sources (such as WHO website) at specific times twice or once a day; and taking practical preparedness and protective steps for self and loved ones. Likewise our participants highlighted the importance of social interactions, which necessitates professionals and authorities to encourage vulnerable groups (such as refugees) to stay connected to maintain social networks and being empathetic to all those who are affected by COVID-19.

Mass sensitization along with mass media should take responsibility for providing the correct information. Bukuluki et al. (2020) advise that community engagement could be an important route for channeling timely and accurate information concerning the causes, symptoms, and control measures of COVID-19. This is vital in curbing fear experienced by the participants concerning contracting the disease. Refugees must have access to relevant information in appropriate languages to ensure full inclusion in the national COVID-19 prevention and response measures (Walker, 2020). Moreover, creating effective communication systems mitigates the risk of inappropriate behavior (such as disobeying public health directives) resulting from the COVID-19 "infordemic" as described by the WHO.

Conclusion

Findings in the current study have shown the existence of psychosocial problems (including anxiety, sleep disorders, psychological distress, and psychiatric disorders) among urban refugees due to the COVID-19 pandemic and the public health measures instituted by the government to curb its spread. These reveal an urgent need for the assessment of the psychosocial needs of urban refugees. Authorities need to accentuate psychosocial support as much as COVID-19 containment measures, for instance without adequate food supplies, refugees are susceptible to contracting other illnesses as much as COVID-19. Working together with mental health and other professionals (such as social workers) trained in refugee management and protection, the government should strengthen its protective services for refugees in urban cities.

About resilience and coping mechanisms, more effort is needed to further strengthen the resource systems for refugees and interpersonal connections. Intrapersonal coping mechanisms need to be strengthened through increasing access to mental health and psychosocial support services. Given the effect of COVID-19 on livelihoods, special social protection programs like cash for work or public works would be critical in helping revive the livelihoods of urban refugees. Programs to mitigate the effects of COVID-19 should consider the needs and vulnerability of refugees living outside formal refugee settlements who do not access the full package of services provided by UNHCR and other CSOs. There is a need to prioritize urban refugee's access to psychosocial support services to further build their resilience to cope with the impact of the COVID-19 pandemic.

References

BBC. (2020). Coronavirus: anger as migrants sprayed with disinfectant in India. *BBC (March 31, 2020)*. Available at: https://www.bbc.com/news/world-asia-india-52093220.

Bohnet, H., & Schmitz-Pranghe, C. (2019). *Uganda: A role model for refugee integration?*. Vol. 2/2019, 2/2019. Available from: https://www.ssoar.info/ssoar/handle/document/62871.

Boyden, J., & Mann, G. (2005). Children's risk, resilience, and coping in extreme situations. In *Handbook for working with children and youth: Pathways to resilience across cultures and contexts* (pp. 3–26). SAGE Publications Inc.

Braun, V., & Clarke, V. (2012). Thematic analysis. In H. Cooper, P. M. Camic, D. L. Long, A. T. Panter, D. Rindskopf, & K. J. Sher (Eds.), *Research designs: Quantitative, qualitative, neuropsychological, and biological: Vol. 2. APA handbooks in psychology®. APA handbook of research methods in psychology* (pp. 57–71). American Psychological Association. https://doi.org/10.1037/13620-004.

Bukuluki, P., Mwenyango, H., Katongole, S. P., & Palattiyil, G. (2020). The socio-economic and psychosocial impact of COVID-19 pandemic on urban refugees in Uganda. *Humanities and Social Sciences*. https://doi.org/10.1016/j.ssaho.2020.100045.

Cerami, C., Santi, G. C., Galandra, C., Dodich, A., Cappa, S. F., Vecchi, T., et al. (2020). COVID-19 outbreak in Italy: Are we ready for the psychosocial and the economic crisis? Baseline findings from the PsyCovid study. *Frontiers in Psychiatry*, *11*, 556. https://doi.org/10.3389/fpsyt.2020.00556.

Crawford, N., O'Callaghan, S., Holloway, K., & Lowe, C. (2019). *The comprehensive refugee response framework: Progress in Uganda*. Report No.: CC BY-NC-ND 4.0.

Drabble, L., Trocki, K. F., Salcedo, B., Walker, P. C., & Korcha, R. A. (2016). Conducting qualitative interviews by telephone: Lessons learned from a study of alcohol use among sexual minority and heterosexual women. *Qualitative Social Work*, *15*(1), 118–133.

Dubey, S., Biswas, P., Ghosh, R., Chatterjee, S., Dubey, M. J., Chatterjee, S., et al. (2020). Psychosocial impact of COVID-19. *Diabetes and Metabolic Syndrome: Clinical Research and Reviews*, *14*(5), 779–788.

Flick, O. (2009). *An introduction to qualitative research*. Sage Publications.

Gallopín, G. C. (2006). Linkages between vulnerability, resilience, and adaptive capacity. *Global Environmental Change*, *16*(3), 293–303.

Hyun, J., You, S., Sohn, S., Kim, S. J., Bae, J., Baik, M., et al. (2020). Psychosocial support during the COVID-19 outbreak in Korea: Activities of multidisciplinary mental health professionals. *Journal of Korean Medical Science*, *35*(22), 1–13.

Kluge, H. H. P., Jakab, Z., Bartovic, J., D'Anna, V., & Severoni, S. (2020). Refugee and migrant health in the COVID-19 response. *Lancet*, *6736*(20), 1237–1239.

Kulyar, M. F. E. A., Bhutta, Z. A., Shabbir, S., & Akhtar, M. (2020). Psychosocial impact of COVID-19 outbreak on international students living in Hubei province, China. *Travel Medicine and Infectious Disease*, 101712. Available at: https://scholar.google.com/scholar?hl=en&as_sdt=0%2C5&q=Kulyar%2C+M.+F.+E.+A.%2C+Bhutta%2C+Z.+A.%2C+Shabbir%2C+S.%2C+%26+Akhtar%2C+M.+%282020%29.+Psychosocial+impact+of+COVID19+outbreak+on+international+students+living+in+Hubei+province%2C+China.+Travel+Medicine+and+Infectious+Disease.&btnG=#d=gs_cit&u=%2Fscholar%3Fq%3Dinfo%3A0yOXdBkLDZ8J%3Ascholar.google.com%2F%26output%3Dcite%26scirp%3D0%26hl%3Den (Accessed 3 June 2020).

Mackolil, J., & Mackolil, J. (2020). Addressing psychosocial problems associated with the COVID-19 lockdown. *Asian Journal of Psychiatry*, *51*, 102156.

Ministry of Health Uganda. (2020). *MoH Uganda: COVID-19 information portal.* [cited 2020 Apr 10]. Available from: https://covid19.gou.go.ug/.

Mwenyango, H., & Palattiyil, G. (2019). Health needs and challenges of women and children in Uganda's refugee settlements: Conceptualising a role for social work. *International Social Work*, *62*(6), 1535–1547.

Otu, A., Charles, C. H., & Yaya, S. (2020). Mental health and psychosocial well-being during the COVID-19 pandemic: The invisible elephant in the room. *International Journal of Mental Health Systems*, *14*(1), 1–5.

Qiu, J., Shen, B., Zhao, M., Wang, Z., Xie, B., & Xu, Y. (2020). A nationwide survey of psychological distress among Chinese people in the COVID-19 epidemic: Implications and policy recommendations. *General Psychiatry*, *33*, e100213.

Subbaraman, R., Nolan, L., Shitole, T., Sawant, K., Shitole, S., Sood, K., et al. (2014). The psychological toll of slum living in Mumbai, India: A mixed methods study. *Social Science & Medicine*, *119*, 155–169.

Trier-Bieniek, A. (2012). Framing the telephone interview as a participant-centred tool for qualitative research: A methodological discussion. *Qualitative Research*, *12*(6), 630–644.

Sun, S., Lin, D., & Operario, D. (2020). Need for a population health approach to understand and address psychosocial consequences of COVID-19. *Psychological Trauma: Theory, Research, Practice, and Policy*, *12*(S1), S25.

Ungar, M., & Herrenkohl, T. I. (2013). Resilience, trauma, context, and culture. *Trauma, Violence, & Abuse*, *14*(3), 255–266.

Walker, K. (2020). *Refugees and displaced highly vulnerable to COVID-19.* Available at: https://www.natureasia.com/en/nmiddleeast/article/10.1038/nmiddleeast.2020.39?utm_campaign=NatureMidE_&utm_source=twitter&utm_medium=social&utm_account=NatureMidE&sf231791576=1 (Accessed 24 April 2020).

World Health Organization. (2020). *Mental health and psychosocial considerations during the COVID-19 outbreak.* 18 March 2020. Available at: https://apps.who.int/iris/bitstream/handle/10665/331490/WHO-2019-nCoV-MentalHealth-2020.1-eng.pdf?sequence=1&isAllowed=y (Accessed 10 July 2020).

Chapter 5

Psychological distress, social support, and psychological flexibility during COVID-19

Richard Tindle[a,b] and Ahmed A. Moustafa[c,d]

[a]*Faculty of Business, Justice and Behavioural Sciences, School of Psychology, Charles Sturt University, Port Macquarie, NSW, Australia,* [b]*School of Health and Behavioural Sciences, Discipline of Psychology, University of the Sunshine Coast, Sippy Downs, QLD, Australia,* [c]*Department of Psychiatry, Wroclaw Medical University, Wroclaw, Poland,* [d]*School of Psychology & Marcs Institute for Brain and Behaviour, Western Sydney University, Sydney, NSW, Australia*

Due to the novel Coronavirus Disease 2019 (COVID-19), society has needed to adjust to government social distancing and quarantine measures to help restrict the spread of the virus. Due to these restrictions, social isolation has increased and limited individuals' access to social support from friends, family, and their extended social networks. As a consequence, individuals must adjust to increased feelings of loneliness, anxiousness, frustration, and depression. Those who are unable to effectively cope with negative emotions (i.e., have low psychological flexibility), lack social support, and have lower levels of resilience are more likely to report higher levels of psychological distress and poor psychological well-being (Dawson & Golijani-Moghaddam, 2020).

The 2003 Severe Acute Respiratory Syndrome (SARS) was labeled as a mental health catastrophe (Mak et al., 2009; Maunder, 2009). Indeed, the World Health Organization warned that the mental health problems associated with the 2003 SARS outbreak should be taken as a "*...dress rehearsal for the catastrophe that could emerge with the long-overdue influenza pandemic [10]... if we are not better prepared next time*" (Maunder, 2009, pp. 316). The psychological outcomes of the 2003 SARS epidemic showed that the stress associated with quarantine measures, being infected with a disease, social isolation, can have severe psychological impacts within society (Lancee, Maunder, & Goldbloom, 2008; Mak et al., 2009; Marjanovic, Greenglass, & Coffey, 2007; Maunder, 2009; Nandi et al., 2008; Zhang, Wang, Rauch, & Wei, 2020). Indeed, healthcare workers in Hong Kong and Canada were still reporting high levels of psychological distress and mental illness two years after the outbreak (Lancee et al., 2008; Maunder, 2009). Given the scale of the COVID-19 pandemic and the strict isolation measures placed on society, we can expect to observe high levels

Mental Health Effects of COVID-19. https://doi.org/10.1016/B978-0-12-824289-6.00012-X

of psychological distress and mental illness for many years after the pandemic has ended. Therefore it is important to understand the extent of psychological distress and ways we can help reduce the psychological impacts on society and individuals. In this chapter, we will focus on the mitigating role of social support and psychological flexibility on psychological distress and psychological health during the COVID-19 pandemic.

Psychological distress during COVID-19

Before COVID-19, there were already some concerning levels of psychological distress in the general population. For example, from 2017 to 2018 approximately 13% of the Australian population were experiencing high or very high levels of psychological distress (Australian Bureau of Statistics, 2019), which is an increase from 2011 to 2012 (10.8%) and 2014 to 2015 (11.7%). This suggests an increasing trend of psychological distress in the general population. These figures are similar in other countries, for example, 12% in Canada (Enticott et al., 2018), 18.3% in the UK (Davillas & Jones, 2020), and 14.7% in China reported high to very high levels of psychological distress (Feng et al., 2020). In 2011–2012, 8.7% of the United States population reported poor mental health (Mojtabai & Jorm, 2015), figures on psychological distress indicated that 3.7% of the population were at risk of severe mental illness (Tomitaka et al., 2019). However, since the COVID-19 outbreak, we have observed increases in the levels of psychological distress among the general population (McGinty, Presskreischer, Han, & Barry, 2020). High levels of psychological distress can lead to a reduction in work and academic performance (Sharp & Theiler, 2018), the development of unhealthy behaviors (e.g., smoking, alcohol, poor diet, and hygiene; Lund, Reider, Whiting, & Prichard, 2010; Robotham and Julian, 2006; St-Pierre, Sinclair, Elgbeili, Bernard, & Dancause, 2019), and an increased risk of developing mental health problems (Caron & Liu, 2010; Payton, 2009; Stallman & Shochet, 2009).

Initial research conducted in China investigated the levels of psychological distress among the general population (e.g., Chao, Chen, Liu, Yang, & Hall, 2020; Feng et al., 2020; Qiu et al., 2020; Zhang, Lu, et al., 2020; Zhang, Wang, et al., 2020). Qiu et al. (2020) conducted the first nationwide psychological distress survey from a sample of 52,730 Chinese participants across 36 provinces. Their results indicated that 35% of respondents were experiencing psychological distress, with approximately 5% showing responses indicative of severe distress. More concerning was the higher levels of distress reported in regional Chinese provinces. Their study suggested that the knowledge that COVID-19 could be transmitted between humans, WHO labeling the outbreak an international public health emergency, and strict quarantine may have contributed to the elevated levels of psychological distress.

Levels of psychological distress are expected to increase during the COVID-19 pandemic. In the USA, there has been a significant increase in the prevalence of psychological distress within the general population (McGinty et al., 2020). In 2018 only 3.8% of the population reported serious psychological distress, compared to 13.6% in April 2020 (McGinty et al., 2020). Due to quarantine measures, 13.8% also reported feelings of loneliness, an increase of 2.8% from 2018 (i.e., 11%). In an Argentinian sample, a latent profile analysis showed that during quarantine, a majority of individuals were classified as having mild (40.9%) or severe (41.0%) distress. These two groups also reported higher levels of depression and anxiety (Fernández, Crivelli, Guimet, Allegri, & Pedreira, 2020). Studies in Europe have also shown higher than normal levels of psychological distress during the COVID-19 pandemic (Casagrande, Favieri, Tambelli, & Forte, 2020). A German study showed 50% of the sample reported concerns about anxiety, depression, and psychological distress related to COVID-19 (Petzold et al., 2020). In Italy, 41.8% of individuals reported high levels of psychological distress (Casagrande et al., 2020). Across the world, individuals are showing concerning increases in their reported levels of psychological distress during the COVID-19 pandemic. A majority of these studies also reported that females, young adults, those with existing medical conditions, minority groups, and the unemployed are at a higher risk of experiencing psychological distress during the pandemic (Brooks et al., 2020; Casagrande et al., 2020; Fernández et al., 2020; Petzold et al., 2020; Qiu et al., 2020; Zhang, Lu, et al., 2020). However, the strongest predictor of psychological distress during the COVID-19 pandemic appears to be the impact of quarantining and social isolation (Brooks et al., 2020; Casagrande et al., 2020; Feng et al., 2020; Qiu et al., 2020; Rogers et al., 2020; Zhang, Wang, et al., 2020).

The effect of quarantine, self-isolation, and social distancing should be considered when assessing the increase in psychological distress associated with the COVID-19 pandemic. The evidence before COVID-19 showed that isolation and quarantine increase psychological distress (Bergomi et al., 2017; Mak et al., 2009; Nandi et al., 2008). For example, studies conducted during the 2002–2004 SARS outbreak found that being quarantined predicted the development of symptoms related to acute stress disorder (Bai et al., 2004; Brooks et al., 2020). Brooks's et al. (2020) conducted a systematic review of 24 articles assessing the psychological impact of quarantine during virus outbreaks (e.g., SARS, COVID-19, MERS, and Ebola). Their results confirmed that the longer the quarantine duration, the higher the risk of developing negative psychological health. One study showed that quarantines lasting longer than 10 days significantly increase the risk of developing high levels of psychological distress and posttraumatic stress symptoms (Hawryluck et al., 2004). Given the isolation period for COVID-19 is 14 days and the continual social isolation from others, psychological distress may continue to increase.

Due to the COVID-19 pandemic, we have observed a significant increase in psychological distress within the global population. While quarantine measures, self-isolation, and social distancing restrictions remain, we can expect the prevalence of psychological distress to increase. Given the known association between psychological distress and poor mental health, it is important to identify how individuals might reduce psychological distress and what psychological mechanisms can be learned to combat high levels of psychological distress.

Social support

Social support from family, friends, and colleagues can act as a buffer between a stressful event and negative feelings (i.e., depression, anxiety, and distress; Cohen & Willis, 1985; Field & Schuldberg, 2011; Raffaelli et al., 2012). The buffering hypothesis is a robust phenomenon where the perceived availability of social support is related to stress and quality of life (Cohen & Willis, 1985). That is, when an individual perceives they have access to social support, they are more likely to experience a higher quality of life and lower stress (Chao, 2012; Cohen & Willis, 1985; Field & Schuldberg, 2011; Raffaelli et al., 2012; Saltzman, Hansel, & Bordnick, 2020). Conversely, when perceived social support is low, stress is higher and quality of life is lower. However, better quality and higher frequencies of social interactions with others are also associated with lower psychological distress (Galatzer-Levy, Burton, & Bonanno, 2012). Forming and accessing social support with others is a strong predictor of positive psychological well-being and reduced levels of distress (Çivitci, 2015; Robbins et al., 2004). Due to current COVID-19 social restrictions, the perceived access to social support might be limited. The reduction in social support is likely to have a detrimental impact on psychological well-being, distress, and quality of life.

Government policies on COVID-19 have largely focused on measures to prevent spread, such as social distancing, quarantining, or self-isolation and the enforcement of penalties (i.e., legal). As such, it is unsurprising that there is an increased sense of loneliness and a reduction in social support (McGinty et al., 2020; Saltzman et al., 2020). A similar pattern was observed during the 2003 SARS epidemic, where a reduction in social support from friends and family was negatively associated with mental health (Leigh-Hunt et al., 2017; Mak et al., 2009). For example, individuals who experienced social isolation also showed an increase in feelings of loneliness, poor mental health, and increasing levels of psychological distress (Mak et al., 2009). More concerning is that a lack of social support has been associated with an increase in the development of symptoms related to depression and anxiety, but also increases the severity of existing mental illnesses such as bipolar and schizophrenia (Wang, Mann, Lloyd-Evans, Ma, & Johnson, 2018). Social support during the COVID-19 pandemic should be considered necessary to help reduce the psychological impacts of isolation and enhance an individual's resources to cope with the situation.

Mak et al. (2009) conducted a study to investigate how self-care self-efficacy mediates the relationship between social support and mental health among SARS survivors. 'Self-care self-efficacy' refers to an individual's confidence that they can effectively carry out relevant self-care activities

(Lev & Owen, 1996; Tsay & Healstead, 2002). Their results showed that the effect of social support from family and friends on mental health was mediated by self-care self-efficacy. This suggests that having strong social support networks from family and friends can increase our perception of how well we can cope with the current pandemic and improve our mental health. Conversely, without social support, individuals may feel as though they do not have the resources to effectively cope with the situation and experience poorer mental health. During COVID-19, support from family and friends has been reduced due to strict social restrictions limiting the number of people who can visit households. This could indicate that mental health may deteriorate if individuals do not have access to social support to improve self-care self-efficacy to help protect against the negative psychological impacts arising during COVID-19.

A recent longitudinal study investigated the prevalence and predictors of loneliness during the COVID-19 pandemic (Bu, Steptoe, & Fancourt, 2020). Using a sample of 35,000, 14% of participants were in the highest category of loneliness compared to only 6.1% of adults before COVID-19. Their study showed that levels of loneliness did not improve during the first few weeks of COVID-19 lockdowns. Most concerning was that individuals who showed high levels of loneliness at baseline reported significant increases in pandemic-related loneliness as the study progressed. Those most at risk of developing high levels of loneliness were young people, females, unemployed or low-income earners, students, and those with a preexisting mental health condition. However, protective factors against loneliness were rurality and social support (i.e., perceived social support, living with others, and having more close friends). An interesting outcome of their study was that participants who had high face-to-face contact before COVID-19 did not report higher levels of loneliness once they were required to cease contact. The authors suggest that the forced changes to social behaviors are not risk factors for high levels of loneliness during COVID-19. These results emphasize the importance of social support during COVID-19 to cope with loneliness. However, social support does not necessarily need to be through face-to-face contact. This finding is echoed by previous research which has used online interventions and social media as an avenue for social support (Blake, Bermingham, Johnson, & Tabner, 2020; Cole, Nick, Zelkowitz, Roeder, & Spinelli, 2017; Lechner et al., 2020).

The recent literature during the COVID-19 pandemic and previous epidemics has highlighted the importance of social support during periods of isolation, quarantine, social distancing, and reduced contact with friends, family, and colleagues. Consequences of poor social support include increased feelings of distress, loneliness, and mental health that can last for years after the end of the pandemic (Lancee et al., 2008; Maunder, 2009). More research is needed to develop opportunities for social contact and developing and maintaining social support beyond traditional face-to-face contact. If social restrictions remain in place for extended periods it will be necessary to provide the appropriate social support for those at risk of developing poor mental health. Doing so will help individuals develop appropriate social networks needed to improve self-care self-efficacy and reduce the negative psychological impacts of social isolation.

Psychological flexibility

Psychological flexibility refers to an individual's ability to cope with, accept, and adjust to difficult situations (Burton & Bonanno, 2016; Kashdan, Barrios, Forsyth, & Steger, 2006; Kashdan & Rottenberg, 2010; Kashdan et al., 2006). When experiencing stressful life events psychological flexibility is protective against negative feelings and can promote positive mental health (Masuda et al., 2011). That is, psychological flexibility can act as a buffer between stress and negative psychological outcomes (Gloster, Meyer, & Lieb, 2017). For example, those who are more psychologically flexible typically report lower levels of depression, anxiety, and distress during stressful life events (Masuda et al., 2011). Understanding the role of psychological flexibility during the COVID-19 pandemic will help identify how well an individual can successfully navigate the negative effects of quarantine, self-isolation, and social distancing. Further, identifying how psychological flexibility can be used to build resilience and reduce negative psychological outcomes (i.e., distress) during COVID-19 could have important clinical and therapeutic implications (Kroska, Roche, Adamowicz, & Stegall, 2020).

Kroska et al. (2020) investigated the association between psychological flexibility, pandemic-related adversity, and psychological distress. A hierarchical regression confirmed previous research that COVID-19 circumstances significantly increase levels of psychological distress (Casagrande et al., 2020; Fernández et al., 2020; Kroska et al., 2020; Petzold et al., 2020; Satici, Gocet-Tekin, Deniz, & Satici, 2020; Zhang, Wang, et al., 2020)—this remained significant after adding psychological flexibility to the model. However, higher levels of psychological flexibility were significantly associated with lower levels of psychological distress. These results show the importance of psychological flexibility within the context of COVID-19. For example, where an individual is lacking social support and experiencing high levels of psychological distress, targeted interventions could be developed to promote psychological flexibility. While there may be some distress still present due to the current situation, building psychological flexibility could significantly reduce overall levels of psychological distress.

Several studies have investigated the mitigating role of psychological flexibility during the COVID-19 pandemic (e.g., Arslan et al., 2020; Dawson & Golijani-Moghaddam, 2020; Kroska et al., 2020). These studies have focused on identifying how psychological flexibility can enhance well-being, psychological health, and reduce psychological distress. During the pandemic, psychological flexibility seems to moderate the negative effects of COVID-19 on mental health (Pakenham & Bursnall, 2006). Whereby, the effects of COVID-19 (i.e., lockdowns, quarantine, and self-isolation) on mental health outcomes are dependent on psychological flexibility. The protective nature of psychological flexibility can be observed when an individual is more self-aware and flexible on different perspectives (i.e., self-as-context), have a strong connection to personal values, and can recognize their feelings but not ruminate on those feelings (i.e., diffusion; Pakenham et al., 2020). Conversely, psychological inflexibility can exacerbate the effects of COVID-19 on mental health outcomes (Pakenham et al., 2020). Specifically, rigid beliefs, an unwillingness to adapt to the changing social restrictions, and ruminating on negative thoughts will increase psychological distress and lead to poor mental health.

Psychological inflexibility might mediate the relationship between COVID-19 related stress and psychological problems (Arslan et al., 2020). For example, COVID-19 related stress directly impacts on psychological problems (i.e., depression, anxiety, and distress) but also indirectly through psychological inflexibility. This suggests that the negative impact of COVID-19 stress on depression, anxiety, and distress is exacerbated when an individual is psychologically inflexible. Further, psychological inflexibility is also moderated by pessimism which can contribute to more psychological problems associated with COVID-19 stress. Conversely, therapeutic techniques aimed at modifying psychological flexibility and promoting optimism could help individuals reduce feelings of depression, anxiety, and distress. Taken together, when an individual is psychologically flexible and optimistic the negative impacts of COVID-19 on psychological problems can be mitigated or reduced. Psychological flexibility is an important factor to consider within the context of COVID-19 and reducing the negative psychological impacts of the pandemic.

The aforementioned studies have found that psychological flexibility mediates the effects of distress, psychological health. However, a person's level of psychological flexibility can also contribute to the type of coping strategies they will employ when they face with a stressful event. For instance, psychological inflexibility is associated with more avoidant coping styles (i.e., self-distraction, denial, substance use, behavioral disengagement, venting, and self-blaming; Eisenberg, Shen, Schwarz, & Mallon, 2012) and an increase in psychological distress. Conversely, psychological flexibility is associated with approach coping styles (i.e., emotional support, instrumental support, positive reframing, planning, and acceptance; Eisenberg, Shen, Schwarz, & Mallon, 2012).

Dawson and Golijani-Moghaddam (2020) investigated how coping mechanisms mediate the relationship between psychological flexibility and COVID-19 outcomes (i.e., well-being, anxiety, depression, distress, and worry). Using mediation analysis, they showed that psychological inflexibility indirectly and directly increased psychological distress through avoidant coping styles. Further mediation analyses found similar results where well-being was significantly reduced by psychological inflexibility through avoidant coping. This study has important implications for how we conceptualize psychological flexibility, especially within the context of COVID-19. The authors argue that while psychological flexibility directly impacts on psychological distress and is related to coping strategies, psychological flexibility is not necessarily a coping strategy but might determine the type of coping strategy an individual employs. As such, the way an individual navigates the negative impacts of COVID-19 will be determined by their level of psychological flexibility and their selection of appropriate coping strategies. In terms of therapeutic intervention, consideration should be given to identifying a person's psychological flexibility as well as their current coping strategies.

Psychological flexibility is an important factor to consider when identifying the effects of COVID-19 on the psychological well-being of individuals. Psychological inflexibility should be considered a risk factor given its association with higher levels of distress and a tendency to choose maladaptive coping strategies. Therapeutic interventions such as acceptance and commitment therapy which typically target psychological flexibility may be useful during the COVID-19 pandemic (Frinking et al., 2019; Kashdan & Rottenberg, 2010, Kashdan et al., 2006; Kroska et al., 2020)—especially given that individuals are unable to change the current circumstance.

Conclusions

In this chapter, we have identified that psychological distress has increased significantly across multiple countries as a result of the COVID-19 pandemic. The increase in psychological distress is likely to have lasting impacts on the psychological health of those most at risk for many years after the pandemic has ended. One of the strongest predictors of psychological distress is the effect of quarantining and social isolation (Brooks et al., 2020). When individuals were forced to socially distance, self-isolate, and withdraw from frequent social contact with friends and family, there was an observed reduction in the perceived availability of social support.

As social support is an important buffer between stressful events and psychological distress, the immediate reduction in perceived social support during COVID-19 restrictions could be contributing to increased levels of psychological distress. However, those most at risk are individuals who do not have preexisting social support networks and were experiencing high levels of loneliness before the COVID-19 outbreak. While social support is an important buffer, face-to-face contact does not seem to be completely necessary to maintain social support from friends, family, and colleagues. Encouraging individuals to participate in alternative methods to maintain frequent and quality social support might contribute to reducing current levels of psychological distress. Social support can increase our perception of how well we can cope with the current pandemic, increase psychological flexibility, and improve mental health.

Psychological flexibility seems to moderate and mediate the relationship between COVID-19 stressors and our overall levels of psychological distress and well-being. There are important clinical and therapeutic implications for acknowledging the impact of psychological flexibility during a global pandemic. Given that individuals are unable to change the COVID-19 situation, being psychologically flexible will help cope with, accept, and adjust to the current COVID-19 pandemic. Consideration should be given to how psychological inflexibility is related to maladaptive coping styles to limit the effects of the pandemic. Building cognitive abilities to promote psychologically flexible individuals who can choose adaptive coping mechanisms could be a useful avenue to help reduce the negative psychological impacts resulting from the COVID-19 pandemic. Social support and psychological flexibility can both buffer the effects of COVID-19 on psychological distress and mental health. Further consideration should be given to identify if increased social support will contribute to psychological flexibility and reduce the levels of distress during the global COVID-19 pandemic.

References

Arslan, G., Yıldırım, M., Tanhan, A., Buluş, M., & Allen, K. A. (2020). Coronavirus stress, optimism-pessimism, psychological inflexibility, and psychological health: Psychometric properties of the coronavirus stress measure. *International Journal of Mental Health and Addiction*, *2*. https://doi.org/10.1007/s11469-020-00337-6 (Who).

Australian Bureau of Statistics. (2019). National Health Survey: First results. *cat. no. 4102.0*. https://www.abs.gov.au/statistics/health/health-conditions-and-risks/national-health-survey-first-results/latest-release.

Bai, Y. M., Lin, C. C., Lin, C. Y., Chen, J. Y., Chue, C. M., & Chou, P. (2004). Survey of stress reactions among health care workers involved with the SARS outbreak. *Psychiatric Services*, *55*(9), 1055–1057. https://doi.org/10.1176/appi.ps.55.9.1055.

Bergomi, M., Modenese, A., Ferretti, E., Ferrari, A., Licitra, G., Vivoli, R., ... Aggazzotti, G. (2017). Work-related stress and role of personality in a sample of Italian bus drivers. *Work*, *57*(3), 433–440. https://doi.org/10.3233/WOR-172581.

Blake, H., Bermingham, F., Johnson, G., & Tabner, A. (2020). Mitigating the psychological impact of covid-19 on healthcare workers: A digital learning package. *International Journal of Environmental Research and Public Health*, *17*(9). https://doi.org/10.3390/ijerph17092997.

Brooks, S. K., Webster, R. K., Smith, L. E., Woodland, L., Wessely, S., Greenberg, N., & Rubin, G. J. (2020). The psychological impact of quarantine and how to reduce it: Rapid review of the evidence. *The Lancet*, *395*(10227), 912–920. https://doi.org/10.1016/S0140-6736(20)30460-8.

Bu, F., Steptoe, A., & Fancourt, D. (2020). Loneliness during lockdown: Trajectories and predictors during the COVID-19 pandemic in 35,712 adults in the UK. *MedRxiv*. https://doi.org/10.1101/2020.05.29.20116657. 2020.05.29.20116657.

Burton, C. L., & Bonanno, G. A. (2016). Supplemental material for measuring ability to enhance and suppress emotional expression: The flexible regulation of emotional expression (FREE) scale. *Psychological Assessment*, *28*(8), 929–941. https://doi.org/10.1037/pas0000231.supp.

Caron, J., & Liu, A. (2010). A descriptive study of the prevalence of psychological distress and mental disorders in the Canadian population: Comparison between low-income and non-low-income populations. *Chronic Diseases in Canada*, *30*(3), 84–94.

Casagrande, M., Favieri, F., Tambelli, R., & Forte, G. (2020). The enemy who sealed the world: Effects quarantine due to the COVID-19 on sleep quality, anxiety, and psychological distress in the Italian population. *Sleep Medicine*. https://doi.org/10.1016/j.sleep.2020.05.011.

Chao, R. C. L. (2012). Managing perceived stress among college students: The roles of social support and dysfunctional coping. *Journal of College Counseling*, *15*(1), 5–21. https://doi.org/10.1002/j.2161-1882.2012.00002.x.

Chao, M., Chen, X., Liu, T., Yang, H., & Hall, B. J. (2020). Psychological distress and state boredom during the COVID-19 outbreak in China: The role of meaning in life and media use. *European Journal of Psychotraumatology*, *11*(1). https://doi.org/10.1080/20008198.2020.1769379.

Çivitci, A. (2015). The moderating role of positive and negative affect on the relationship between perceived social support and stress in college students. *Kuram ve Uygulamada Egitim Bilimleri*, *15*(3), 565–573. https://doi.org/10.12738/estp.2015.3.2553.

Cohen, S., & Willis, T. A. (1985). Stress, social support, and the buffering hypothesis. *Psychological Bulletin*, *98*(2). https://doi.org/10.1037/0033-2909.98.2.310.

Cole, D. A., Nick, E. A., Zelkowitz, R. L., Roeder, K. M., & Spinelli, T. (2017). Online social support for young people: Does it recapitulate in-person social support; can it help? *Computers in Human Behavior*, *68*, 456–464. https://doi.org/10.1016/j.chb.2016.11.058.

Davillas, A., & Jones, A. M. (2020). The COVID-19 pandemic and its impact on inequality of opportunity in psychological distress in the UK. *SSRN Electronic Journal*, *567*, 1–14. https://doi.org/10.2139/ssrn.3614940.

Dawson, D. L., & Golijani-Moghaddam, N. (2020). COVID-19: Psychological flexibility, coping, mental health, and wellbeing in the UK during the pandemic. *Journal of Contextual Behavioral Science*, *17*(July), 126–134. https://doi.org/10.1016/j.jcbs.2020.07.010.

Eisenberg, S. A., Shen, B. J., Schwarz, E. R., & Mallon, S. (2012). Avoidant coping moderates the association between anxiety and patient-rated physical functioning in heart failure patients. *Journal of Behavioral Medicine*, *35*(3), 253–261. https://doi.org/10.1007/s10865-011-9358-0.

Enticott, J. C., Lin, E., Shawyer, F., Russell, G., Inder, B., Patten, S., & Meadows, G. (2018). Prevalence of psychological distress: How do Australia and Canada compare? *Australian and New Zealand Journal of Psychiatry*, *52*(3), 227–238. https://doi.org/10.1177/0004867417708612.

Feng, L.s., Dong, Z.j., Yan, R.y., Wu, X.q., Zhang, L., Ma, J., & Zeng, Y. (2020). Psychological distress in the shadow of the COVID-19 pandemic: Preliminary development of an assessment scale. *Psychiatry Research*, *291*(June). https://doi.org/10.1016/j.psychres.2020.113202, 113202.

Fernández, R. S., Crivelli, L., Guimet, N. M., Allegri, R. F., & Pedreira, M. E. (2020). Psychological distress associated with COVID-19 quarantine: Latent profile analysis, Outcome Prediction and Mediation Analysis. *Journal of Affective Disorders*, *277*(August), 75–84. https://doi.org/10.1016/j.jad.2020.07.133.

Field, R. J., & Schuldberg, D. (2011). Social-support moderated stress: A nonlinear dynamical model and the stress-buffering hypothesis. *Nonlinear Dynamics, Psychology, and Life Sciences*, *15*(1), 53–85.

Frinking, E., Jans-Beken, L., Janssens, M., Peeters, S., Lataster, J., Jacobs, N., & Reijnders, J. (2019). Gratitude and loneliness in adults over 40 years: Examining the role of psychological flexibility and engaged living. *Aging and Mental Health*, *0*(0), 1–8. https://doi.org/10.1080/13607863.2019.1673309.

Galatzer-Levy, I. R., Burton, C. L., & Bonanno, G. A. (2012). Coping flexibility, potentially traumatic life events, and resilience: A prospective study of college student adjustment. *Journal of Social and Clinical Psychology*, *31*(6), 542–567. https://doi.org/10.1521/jscp.2012.31.6.542.

Gloster, A. T., Meyer, A. H., & Lieb, R. (2017). Psychological flexibility as a malleable public health target: Evidence from a representative sample. *Journal of Contextual Behavioral Science*, *6*(2), 166–171. https://doi.org/10.1016/j.jcbs.2017.02.003.

Hawryluck, L., Gold, W. L., Robinson, S., Pogorski, S., Galea, S., & Styra, R. (2004). SARS control and psychological effects of quarantine, Toronto, Canada. *Emerging Infectious Diseases*, *10*(7), 1206–1212. https://doi.org/10.3201/eid1007.030703.

Kashdan, T. B., Barrios, V., Forsyth, J. P., & Steger, M. F. (2006). Experiential avoidance as a generalized psychological vulnerability: Comparisons with coping and emotion regulation strategies. *Behaviour Research and Therapy*, *44*(9), 1301–1320. https://doi.org/10.1016/j.brat.2005.10.003.

Kashdan, T. B., & Rottenberg, J. (2010). Psychological flexibility as a fundamental aspect of health. *Clinical Psychology Review*, *30*(4), 865–878. https://doi.org/10.1016/j.cpr.2010.03.001.

Kroska, E. B., Roche, A. I., Adamowicz, J. L., & Stegall, M. S. (2020). Psychological flexibility in the context of COVID-19 adversity: Associations with distress. *Journal of Contextual Behavioral Science*. https://doi.org/10.1016/j.jcbs.2020.07.011.

Lancee, W. J., Maunder, R. G., & Goldbloom, D. S. (2008). Prevalence of psychiatric disorders among Toronto hospital workers one to two years after the SARS outbreak. *Psychiatric Services (Washington, D.C.)*, *59*(1), 91–95. https://doi.org/10.1176/ps.2008.59.1.91.

Lechner, W. V., Laurene, K. R., Patel, S., Anderson, M., Grega, C., & Kenne, D. R. (2020). Addictive behaviors changes in alcohol use as a function of psychological distress and social support following COVID-19 related university closings. *Addictive Behaviors*, *110*(May). https://doi.org/10.1016/j.addbeh.2020.106527, 106527.

Leigh-Hunt, N., Bagguley, D., Bash, K., Turner, V., Turnbull, S., Valtorta, N., & Caan, W. (2017). An overview of systematic reviews on the public health consequences of social isolation and loneliness. *Public Health*, *152*, 157–171. https://doi.org/10.1016/j.puhe.2017.07.035.

Lev, E. L., & Owen, S. V. (1996). A measure of self-care self-efficacy. *Research in Nursing and Health*, *19*(5), 421–429. https://doi.org/10.1002/(sici)1098-240x(199610)19:5<421::aid-nur6>3.0.co;2-s.

Lund, H. G., Reider, B. D., Whiting, A. B., & Prichard, J. R. (2010). Sleep patterns and predictors of disturbed sleep in a large population of college students. *Journal of Adolescent Health*, *46*(2), 124–132. https://doi.org/10.1016/j.jadohealth.2009.06.016.

Mak, W. W. S., Law, R. W., Woo, J., Cheung, F. M., Lee, D., ... Lee, D. (2009). *Social support and psychological adjustment to SARS : The mediating role of self-care self-efficacy*. https://doi.org/10.1080/08870440701447649. 0446.

Marjanovic, Z., Greenglass, E. R., & Coffey, S. (2007). The relevance of psychosocial variables and working conditions in predicting nurses' coping strategies during the SARS crisis: An online questionnaire survey. *International Journal of Nursing Studies*, *44*(6), 991–998. https://doi.org/10.1016/j.ijnurstu.2006.02.012.

Masuda, A., Anderson, P. L., Wendell, J. W., Chou, Y. Y., Price, M., & Feinstein, A. B. (2011). Psychological flexibility mediates the relations between self-concealment and negative psychological outcomes. *Personality and Individual Differences*, *50*(2), 243–247. https://doi.org/10.1016/j.paid.2010.09.037.

Maunder, R. G. (2009). Was SARS a mental health catastrophe? *General Hospital Psychiatry*, *31*(January), 316–317. https://doi.org/10.1016/j.genhosppsych.2009.04.004.

McGinty, E. E., Presskreischer, R., Han, H., & Barry, C. L. (2020). Psychological distress and loneliness reported by US adults in 2018 and April 2020. *JAMA: The Journal of the American Medical Association*, *324*(1), 93–94. https://doi.org/10.1001/jama.2020.9740.

Mojtabai, R., & Jorm, A. F. (2015). Trends in psychological distress, depressive episodes and mental health treatment-seeking in the United States: 2001-2012. *Journal of Affective Disorders*, *174*, 556–561. https://doi.org/10.1016/j.jad.2014.12.039.

Nandi, A., Tracy, M., Aiello, A., Jarlais, D., Des, C., & Galea, S. (2008). Social support and response to AIDS and severe acute respiratory syndrome. *Emerging Infectious Diseases*, *14*(5), 825–827. https://doi.org/10.1080/08870440701447649.

Pakenham, K. I., & Bursnall, S. (2006). Relations between social support, appraisal and coping and both positive and negative outcomes for children of a parent with multiple sclerosis and comparisons with children of healthy parents. *Clinical Rehabilitation*, *20*(8), 709–723. https://doi.org/10.1191/0269215506cre976oa.

Pakenham, K. I., Landi, G, Boccolini, G, Furlani, A, Grandi, S, & Tossani, E. (2020). The moderating roles of psychological flexibility and inflexibility on the mental health impacts of COVID-19 pandemic and lockdown in Italy. *Journal of Contextual Behavioral Science*, *17*, 109–118. https://doi.org/10.1016/j.jcbs.2020.07.003.

Payton, A. R. (2009). Mental health, mental illness, and psychological distress: Same continuum or distinct phenomena? *Journal of Health and Social Behavior*, *50*(2), 213–227. https://doi.org/10.1177/002214650905000207.

Petzold, M. B., Bendau, A., Plag, J., Pyrkosch, L., Mascarell Maricic, L., Betzler, F., … Ströhle, A. (2020). Risk, resilience, psychological distress, and anxiety at the beginning of the COVID-19 pandemic in Germany. *Brain and behavior*, *10*(9), e01745. https://doi.org/10.1002/brb3.1745.

Qiu, J., Shen, B., Zhao, M., Wang, Z., Xie, B., & Xu, Y. (2020). A nationwide survey of psychological distress among Chinese people in the COVID-19 epidemic: Implications and policy recommendations. *General Psychiatry*, *33*(2), 19–21. https://doi.org/10.1136/gpsych-2020-100213.

Raffaelli, M., Andrade, F. C. D., Wiley, A. R., Sanchez-armass, O., Edwards, L. L., & Aradillas-garcia, C. (2012). Stress, social support, and depression: A test of the stress-buffering hypothesis in a Mexican sample. *Journal of Research on Adolescence*, *23*(2), 283–289. https://doi.org/10.1111/jora.12006.

Robbins, S. B., Le, H., Davis, D., Lauver, K., Langley, R., & Carlstrom, A. (2004). Do psychosocial and study skill factors predict college outcomes? A meta-analysis. *Psychological Bulletin*, *130*(2), 261–288. https://doi.org/10.1037/0033-2909.130.2.261.

Robotham, D., & Julian, C. (2006). Stress and the higher education student: A critical review of the literature. *Journal of Further and Higher Education*, *30*(2), 107–117. https://doi.org/10.1080/03098770600617513.

Rogers, J. P., Chesney, E., Oliver, D., Pollak, T. A., Mcguire, P., Fusar-poli, P., & Lewis, G. (2020). Psychiatric and neuropsychiatric presentations associated with severe coronavirus infections : A systematic review and meta-analysis with comparison to the COVID-19 pandemic. *The Lancet Psychiatry*, *7*(7), 611–627. https://doi.org/10.1016/S2215-0366(20)30203-0.

Saltzman, L. Y., Hansel, T. C., & Bordnick, P. S. (2020). Loneliness, isolation, and social support factors in post-COVID-19 mental health. *Psychological Trauma Theory Research Practice and Policy*, *12*(S1), 55–57. https://doi.org/10.1037/tra0000703.

Satici, B., Gocet-Tekin, E., Deniz, M. E., & Satici, S. A. (2020). Adaptation of the fear of COVID-19 scale: Its association with psychological distress and life satisfaction in Turkey. *International Journal of Mental Health and Addiction*. https://doi.org/10.1007/s11469-020-00294-0.

Sharp, J., & Theiler, S. (2018). A review of psychological distress among university students: Pervasiveness, implications and potential points of intervention. *International Journal for the Advancement of Counselling*, *40*(3), 193–212. https://doi.org/10.1007/s10447-018-9321-7.

Stallman, H. M., & Shochet, I. (2009). Prevalence of mental health problems in Australian university health services. *Australian Psychologist*, *44*(2), 122–127. https://doi.org/10.1080/00050060902733727.

St-Pierre, M., Sinclair, I., Elgbeili, G., Bernard, P., & Dancause, K. N. (2019). Relationships between psychological distress and health behaviors among Canadian adults: Differences based on gender, income, education, immigrant status, and ethnicity. *SSM—Population Health*, *7*(June 2018), 100385. https://doi.org/10.1016/j.ssmph.2019.100385.

Tomitaka, S., Kawasaki, Y., Ide, K., Akutagawa, M., Ono, Y., & Furukawa, T. A. (2019). Distribution of psychological distress is stable in recent decades and follows an exponential pattern in the US population. *Scientific Reports*, *9*(1), 1–10. https://doi.org/10.1038/s41598-019-47322-1.

Tsay, S. L., & Healstead, M. (2002). Self-care self-efficacy, depression, and quality of life among patients receiving hemodialysis in Taiwan. *International Journal of Nursing Studies*, *39*(3), 245–251. https://doi.org/10.1016/S0020-7489(01)00030-X.

Wang, J, Mann, F, Lloyd-Evans, B, Ma, R, & Johnson, S. (2018). Associations between loneliness and perceived social support and outcomes of mental health problems: A systematic review. *BMC Psychiatry*, *18*(156). https://doi.org/10.1186/s12888-018-1736-5.

Zhang, J., Lu, H., Zeng, H., Zhang, S., Du, Q., Jiang, T., & Du, B. (2020, July). The differential psychological distress of populations affected by the COVID-19 pandemic. *Brain, Behavior, and Immunity*. https://doi.org/10.1016/j.bbi.2020.04.031.

Zhang, S. X., Wang, Y., Rauch, A., & Wei, F. (2020). Unprecedented disruption of lives and work: Health, distress and life satisfaction of working adults in China one month into the COVID-19 outbreak. *Psychiatry Research*, *288*(March). https://doi.org/10.1016/j.psychres.2020.112958, 112958.

Chapter 6

The impact of COVID-19 social restrictions on culture and psychosocial well-being: The Ghanaian experience

Alfred Dickson Dai-Kosi[a], Victoria Akuorkor Acquaye[b], Kingsley Kwadwo Asare Pereko[c], Paa-Kwesi Blankson[d], and Christian Ackom[b]

[a]*Department of Community and Preventive Dentistry, School of Medicine and Dentistry, University of Ghana, Legon, Ghana,* [b]*Department of Psychological Medicine and Mental Health, School of Medical Sciences, College of Health and Allied Sciences, University of Cape Coast, Cape Coast, Ghana,* [c]*Department of Community Medicine, School of Medical Sciences, College of Health and Allied Sciences, University of Cape Coast, Cape Coast, Ghana,* [d]*Department of Oral and Maxillofacial Surgery, Korle-Bu Teaching Hospital, Accra, Ghana*

Introduction

In December 2019 what began as local transmission of a novel coronavirus disease in the Wuhan Province of China has escalated into a global pandemic as declared by the World Health Organization (WHO). The first reported case of Coronavirus (COVID-19) in Ghana was recorded on 12th March 2020 when two persons tested positive to the virus (MoH, 2020). As of 16th July 2020 the disease had spread exponentially to a new global record of 13,378, 853 cases with 580,045 deaths. In Ghana, as of the same 16th July 2020, 26,125 persons were infected while 139 had lost their lives (WHO, 2020). This chapter looks at the concept of COVID-19 lockdown and restrictions especially their influence on the sociocultural life of Ghanaians. It also evaluates the impacts of coronavirus on the individuals in relation to social support in a highly communal society. In addition, the chapter reviews the health belief and health-seeking attitudes of the people of Ghana considering the threat of coronavirus. Finally, it proffers strategies to help bring coronavirus under control while the people go about their daily activities.

The coronavirus continues to ravage humanity across all the continents of the world in terms of social, economic, political, education, and health. The rate of devastation of the disease was so pronounced that the World Health

Mental Health Effects of COVID-19. https://doi.org/10.1016/B978-0-12-824289-6.00003-9

Organization (WHO) in the last week of March 2020 was compelled to classify it as Public Health Emergency of International Concern (PHEIC). This classification then places coronavirus, in relation to other disease conditions, as the sixth PHEIC in accordance with the International Health Regulations. Others that preceded coronavirus in that classification include H1N1 Influenza (2009), Polio (2014), Ebola in West Africa (2014), Zika (2016), and Ebola which ravaged many lives in the Democratic Republic of Congo (2019) (WHO, 2020). Thereafter, on February 11, 2020, WHO after careful analysis of the rate of spread of the coronavirus, officially declared it as "pandemic" and subsequently prescribed a number of protocols including regular hand-washing under running water with soap, regular temperature checks, and maintaining physical distance popularly referred to as "social distancing" of at least 2 m from others. These were some of the important protocols (Khan et al., 2020). The spread of the coronavirus started emerging by 16th April 2020. The rate of new infection and the concomitant spread have declined in Europe, notably Spain and Germany, and some Asian countries including China. However, the USA, Brazil, and India continue to struggle with the virus (International, 2020). The threat of coronavirus in Africa is also a reality as many states are recording increasing cases of new infection. In a desperate attempt to bring the disease under control, many countries instituted draconian measures to curb the disease from spiraling out of control including lockdown and restrictions of the movement of their citizens. These restrictions, to a large extent, have helped stem the tide of the spread of the pandemic but the level of psychological impact on the life of the people has not been explored. This, basically, is the focal point of this chapter.

COVID-19 lockdowns and restrictions

In the absence of a vaccine to treat the virus, one of the alternative methods considered effective in containing the pandemic and prescribed by WHO and other health professionals is lockdown and also the enforcement of social/physical distancing. In the case of COVID-19, the use of lockdown and physical distancing was adopted globally and different countries implemented either partial or total lockdown at the start of the pandemic. China was one of the first countries to introduce the lockdown in order to control the spread of the coronavirus in the province of Wuhan. Most likely, these measures were inspired by the belief that the lockdown and the social distancing protocols could be the most effective strategies to bring the virus under control in the short term. As it would turn out, many countries adopted the lockdown and physical distancing measures as containment of the pandemic despite their dire socioeconomic impacts on the countries (Armitage & Nellums, 2020; Brooks et al., 2020). It should be pointed out that the economic impacts have affected both the developed and developing countries. According to Lewnard and Lo (2020), the pandemic brought in its trail dire economic devastation among both developed and developing countries. These economic challenges were in the form of mass unemployment and collapse of manufacturing companies. Others comprised weakening of the fundamentals of the global economy as witnessed in the United States (US) and China, as well as threat of possible collapse of new and developing economies, especially in the short term. There were other major challenges such as deterioration of the public health that could lead to socioeconomic difficulties and the anxiety associated with social isolation and quarantine (Armitage & Nellums, 2020). Social restrictions including isolation and lockdown to a communally oriented society such as Ghana and for that matter Africans could pose a number of cultural and psychological problems.

COVID-19 and sociocultural challenges of Ghanaians

Culturally, Ghanaians have been oriented to live communally (Falade, 2018). According to Idang (2015), culture entails the sum total of behavior in terms of traits and characters that are akin to a group of people setting them apart from other people or societies. Some of these specific traits include language, dress code, food, music, dance, work attitude, religious and spiritual activities. The belief system of the people and how they observe social norms, values, and daily living are highly influenced by their cultural orientation. Values, for instance, can be explained as people's beliefs about what is right and wrong as well as what they perceive to be important in life. Gyekye (2003) aptly explains that culture plays an important role in the life of people and covers other important areas such as marriage, customs, and traditions. He emphasizes that there are many standards set by cultural boundaries to guide the way of life of different cultural groups. Indeed since these cultural norms have become the embodiment of the Ghanaians who live in close relationship with one another, how would the social restrictions affect them? Some of the communal activities which most Ghanaians engage in but have been affected by the restrictions include daily connectivity with family and friends, observation of rites of marriage, puberty, funerals, child naming, and many more.

Culture from the clinical perspective can be defined as the discipline under psychiatry/clinical psychology that covers the various interrelationships between culture and psychiatry (American Psychiatric Association, 2013). It seeks to understand variations relating to incidence, prevalence, clinical expression, course of the disease, and/or outcome of certain psychiatric disorders as they affect different cultural groups and societies. The objective of the emphasis on understanding clinical/psychiatric cases in line with culture is to make accurate diagnosis with more efficacious treatment being situated within the cultural circumstances of the patients. The American Psychiatric Association (2013) has recognized the pivotal role of culture in the treatment of psychiatric disorders by addressing cultural differences that exist in the description of most of the major psychiatric disorders listed in the Diagnostic *and Statistical Manual of Mental Disorders*, Fifth Edition (DSM-V). It also provides comprehensive guidance regarding the development of cultural formulations.

The restriction of the mobility and the inability of the people to freely go about their activities might be a major source of psychological distress. One common mental health problem identified in relation with the COVID-19 pandemic is psychological distress (Asiamah et al., 2020). Psychological distress is a state of emotional suffering that is characterized by symptoms of depression and anxiety (Mirowsky & Ross, 2002). The symptoms of psychological distress are varied and may depend on the perceptions of persons involved. Some of the common symptoms include a loss of interest in activities previously enjoyed, sadness; hopelessness, restlessness; and feeling tense (Lebel et al., 2011).

The onset of such mental health problems could be triggered by the sudden halt in daily activities of individuals. Cumming and Henry who propounded the disengagement theory of aging indicates that retirement or disengagement from work should be gradual. Disengagement theory explains the process of withdrawal from established social life that individuals experience as a result of aging. It indicates that such withdrawal process should be gradual so as to prepare the person involved to accept the change in order to psychologically integrate into the new life (Cumming & Henry, 1961). In the event where the disengagement from work or daily activities emanates from sudden stoppage such as lockdown, anxiety and other mental health problems could be triggered (Cumming & Henry, 1961). The implementations of lockdowns and restrictions necessitated by the outbreak of COVID-19 did not make room for any form of gradual preparation for stoppage of work or daily activities that people previously engaged in. Therefore, with associated social isolation and quarantine as well as the novel nature of the disease, it could lead to anxiety and other mental health challenges among the citizenry. In fact, short-term social isolation and other forms of restrictions can cause major changes in health behaviors leading to deterioration of health and general well-being. Malcolm, Frost, and Cowie (2019) agree with Armitage and Nellums (2020) that a decline in mental health is one likely consequence of social isolation caused by an unexpected event such as the outbreak of a disease. The occurrence of such mental health challenges becomes more evident because of the fear and apprehension associated with novel diseases such as COVID-19. People may become anxious and worried about the causes and possible impact of diseases which can significantly affect their level of anxiety (Armitage & Nellums, 2020).

Also worthy of mention is anxiety which has been detected among patients with COVID-19. McManus, Bebbington, Jenkins, and Brugha (2016) confirm that a disease such as COVID-19 has both direct and indirect psychological and social impacts on individuals. The authors further stress that the effect of the disease could be very pervasive and might have both short- and long-term effects on the mental health of individuals. Anxiety and depression among patients is heightened as a result of waiting time during which the diagnosis and treatment of a particular disease commence. In the management of COVID-19 in Ghana, it takes a reasonable time for the collection of sample and test results to be relayed to suspected members of community and that could substantially increase their anxiety (Fogarty & Cronin, 2008; Paul et al., 2011). Undoubtedly, patients awaiting the result of their laboratory tests might experience significant levels of anxiety. It is very important to handle this delicate process carefully in order not to expose members to such anxiety. The fact that the lockdown could lead to anxiety and other forms of mental health problems can also be explained in line with the Fogg behavior model (FBM) propounded by Fogg (2009) which stipulated that a pandemic of the magnitude of COVID-19 that leads to sudden lockdowns may evoke intense fear and panic among people as they struggle to cope with the disease. In addition, the rate of infection among health personnel is also a major worry to the populace. The most painful aspect was the loss of three of Ghana's most experienced doctors to the coronavirus pandemic and over 779 other health workers infected with the virus in Ghana (MoH, 2020). The fear this situation evokes among other health workers could undermine their efficiency. As a result, anxiety among healthcare workers globally is high. For instance, in a Chinese study to assess the effect of the disease on healthcare workers, out of the 1257 health workers comprising nurses and physicians directly treating patients with the disease, 41.5% had developed depression, anxiety, insomnia, and distress as compared to their colleagues who were not directly in charge of such patients (Lai, Ma, Wang, et al., 2020). Similarly, a study conducted in Singapore in April 2020 reveals that out of the 500 healthcare workers attending to COVID-19 patients, 14.5%, 8.9%, and 6.6% of them experienced anxiety, depression, and stress, respectively, while 7.7% also had posttraumatic stress disorder (Tan et al., 2020). Aside the psychological distress caused as a result of the restrictions and the lockdown, the virus also poses other possible threats. One of such threats is that the severe acute respiratory syndrome coronavirus 2 (SARS-CoV-2), the causative virus of COVID-19, might also attack the brain or affect the immune system. That in turn might have negative effect on brain functions leading to psychiatric disorders (McManus et al., 2016).

COVID-19 lockdown and restrictions as well as other related challenges could affect an individual in a number of ways. Firstly, fear of the disease and associated restrictions may trigger anxiety and other psychological indicators. Secondly, in terms of sociocultural impacts, the restrictions limit individual's ability to interact with his or her social circles. In effect, social support may be greatly limited in a communal society such as Ghana, and this could have dire consequences.

Influence of restrictions and lockdowns on individuals

Social support is one of the most effective methods to cope with stressful events. When people come together to comfort distressed individuals in the form of hope and encouragement, the level of the distress is significantly reduced (Howren, Christensen, Karnell, & Funk, 2010). Social support, in the form of help from spouses, parents, and siblings, plays important roles in coping with psychological distress. In addition, another important form of social support emanates from external sources including friends, work colleagues, and members of the larger society. These forms of help also confirm the communal nature of Ghanaians in offering help to their compatriots as part of their cultural upbringing (Assimeng, 2007). The sad aspect of COVID-19 pandemic is that these forms of social support could not benefit patients in isolation as they are quarantined due to the contagious nature of the disease.

There has been a widely held view in literature on the effectiveness of social support in moderating distressed situations. Social support, in the form of help from spouses, parents, and siblings, plays important roles in moderating psychological distress experienced by patients. In addition, supports from friends, work colleagues, and members of society also provide good measure of help to patients. These forms of help also confirm the communal nature of Ghanaians and for that matter other African people as well.

Other forms of coping mechanisms usually adopted during difficult situations include hope in the healing power of God and prayer (Twumasi, 1975). Majority of Ghanaians believe that their psychological distress could be resolved through divine intervention and therefore rely heavily on prayer as a tool for God's intervention. In many cultural settings in Ghana, after the diagnosis of a disease without a known cause, a significant majority of clients turn to possible spiritual cause of their diseases. In their attempts to identify causes of such diseases, some people reflect over their lives, looking for something they might have done which could incur a curse on them (Katz & Hawley, 2005). This reaction and health-seeking behavior are largely determined by the cultural background of the patients involved. Katz and Hawley (2005) identify cultural values as significant variables in the treatment preferences of individuals with a strong spiritual belief that the outcome of their disease is under God's control. Hope and belief in the efficacy of God's healing power have been established as one of the most reliable means of dealing with diseases among Ghanaians in particular, and Africans in general. This belief in God's healing powers by many Africans was identified by Mbiti (1990) that Africans are highly religious. They, therefore, have a hope that whatever challenge that may confront them could be resolved by turning to God in prayer (Mbiti, 1990). The fact that many people believe in the efficacy of prayer but could not congregate to pray as a result of COVID-19 restrictions may be a source of worry. In that regard, anxiety among believers could significantly increase concerning the uncertainty about when they can freely congregate and worship to nourish their spirituality (Anarfi et al., 2016). In addition, cultural practices such as the traditional methods of greeting and converging to fraternize have all been negatively affected by the coronavirus restrictions. Traditional greetings and meetings among community members offer some of the most effective social support and avenue for sharing one's burden with others (Banda, 2017). The traditional handshake involves two people engaged in a long handshake in which each of the fingers temporarily becomes interlocked for a few seconds before disentangling one's palm. In the end, the thumbs are clasped together to produce an echolike sound signaling the end of the handshake. Members thereafter continue with enquiries about the health of each family and even clan which provide the opportunity to learn about the welfare of each community member (Banda, 2017). This practice is a major stress reliever for members and contributes to enhancing their mental well-being.

Conceptualization of health problems and COVID-19 compliance

It is very important to understand the perception of people when it comes to interpretation, appraisal, and health-seeking behavior in relation to diseases such as COVID-19. The health belief model is a psychological health behavior change model that was developed by Hochbaum (1958) to explain and predict how individuals behave in health-related matters pertaining to a particular disease (Sohler, Jerant, & Franks, 2015). It was first used to evaluate American citizens' interest in a free tuberculosis screening program. The model comprises four constructs that influence patients' disease perception and behavior as illustrated in Fig. 1.

The first construct assessed by the health belief model is the perceived susceptibility to a disease. The theory explains an individual's evaluation of whether he or she is susceptible to contract a particular disease and then a

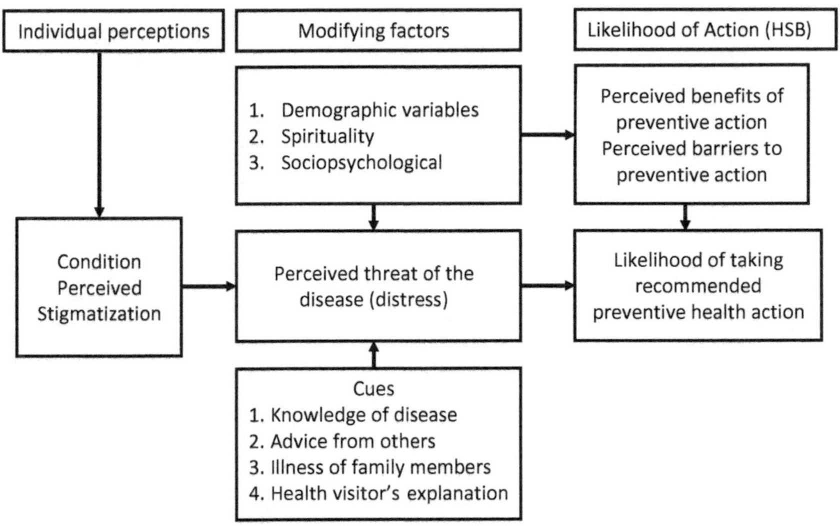

FIG. 1 Health belief model of health-seeking behavior among patients. *Adapted from Hochbaum, G. M. (1958). Public participation in medical screening programs: A socio-psychological study. US Department of Health, Education, and Welfare, Public Health Service, Bureau of State Services, Division of Special Health Services, Tuberculosis Program.*

subsequent action to seek treatment may be initiated by the person (Lewis & Merched, 2014). According to Glanz, Rimer, and Viswanath (2008), people's motivation to act in a particular manner in relation to treat diseases that infect them depends largely on their health belief and perceptions of the threat posed by the disease. Glanz et al. (2008) are of the view that proper and prudent health behaviors are determined by the individual's health belief. Therefore if there is any form of public health policy and education, they have to be targeted at the health belief of patients. Perception of the severity of the disease is the second construct in which the person appraises the level of danger posed by the condition. If the risk level of getting a particular disease is appraised to be very high by a patient, the likelihood of taking steps for immediate medical attention is higher than if the risk is considered low. The thought of the benefits to be derived from embarking on such action forms the basis for the third construct. The perception of negative obstacles as barriers to a specific health action to be undertaken by the individual is also considered. Further, the steps necessary to actualize the decision by the individual are also critically reviewed before an action is taken (Rawlett, 2011). The influence of demographic factors and determinants of health action are considered as needs factors. This model is very appropriate in explaining behavior of people toward COVID-19 because it is applicable to health behaviors that are under the control of an individual patient. For instance, an individual who identifies certain symptoms relating to the virus has the ability to assess the severity of the disease and take appropriate course of actions (Lewis & Merched, 2014). The patient's health-seeking behavior therefore largely depends on the interplay among the factors he or she considers important and relevant to the treatment of the disease. The health belief model is very appropriate for explaining health-related behavior among patients with coronavirus in Ghana because people's health-seeking behavior is influenced by their health belief and advice from friends and family (Amegbor, 2014; Gyasi et al., 2016). If an individual considers that the symptoms resemble that of COVID-19 but appraises that they are not severe or feels stigmatized, he or she may avoid seeking help from health professionals (Andisheh-Tadbir, Mehrabani, & Heydari, 2008).

One single important determinant is the perception of the level of threat the disease poses to the patient. This appraisal largely depends on the danger that confronts the patient and likely outcome if he or she does not act appropriately. In Ghana a section of the public believes that the coronavirus does not pose any major threat to them because they do not have other health challenges. One report presented by the authorities managing the disease indicates that it appears that most of the deaths occurred due to underlying comorbidities such as diabetes, hypertension, and cancer (MoH, 2020). Some people unfortunately misinterpret this assertion to mean that once they do not have any known comorbidities they cannot get infected by the disease and become careless. The public needs to know that early reporting for testing and care for those who test positive is a sure way to win the battle against the virus. It will also prevent asymptomatic patients from spreading the disease to others. Early and rapid testing is the way to control the disease as has been recommended globally. In view of that, testing using saliva samples is currently going on trial in the United Kingdom (Robert, 2020). Experts revealed that the virus shows in the saliva before other respiratory channels such as the nose and throat and the results could be ready within 2 h. Further, perceived susceptibility to a disease comprises another important component of the health belief model. If a person appraises that the risk of contracting a disease is highly probable then such a person may take practical measures to prevent the infection. There are some people who believe that protection comes from God and therefore they are protected against the virus.

Relating health belief model to COVID-19, even though the disease has biogenic basis the limited knowledge and novel nature may lead some patients to appraise it from different perspectives. Some people may even doubt literature on the causes and impact of the disease and that can influence their attitude toward health-seeking behavior. All forms of obstacles that impede smooth operations of health delivery are classified as barriers to healthcare. These barriers include access to healthcare especially in situations where patients are willing to seek healthcare but unavailability of facilities prevents patients to benefit from such services. In Ghana, there are several people who wish to be tested but may not have the opportunity due to unavailability of testing kits. Others who need hospital in-service care are allowed to receive care from home which may compromise the laid down protocols especially on infecting others. In addition, long waiting period at health facilities serves as another barrier to healthcare and health-seeking behavior (Afolabi, Daropale, Irinoye, & Adegoke, 2013).

The perceptions of individuals about etiology of a particular disease determine their attitude and health-seeking behavior. The main classification of illness from the perspective of Kleinman and Seeman's (2000) specifies that experience of illness is geared toward consciousness of the individual who has the health problem but not only biogenic indicators in the body. This assertion is contrary to the position of the biomedical model which explains disease conditions as a structural abnormality of any organ in the individual patient. The illness model illustrates that illness experience is based on the patient's experience in relation to his or her sociocultural background (Kleinman & Seeman, 2000). It is clear from the ongoing analysis that the perspective of significant number of Ghanaians about coronavirus might not exactly follow the advice of the health authorities. As per this view, such people could perceive themselves as not ill but the disease may be present and they would therefore carry the virus as asymptomatic patients. People who have such perceptions about the COVID-19 pandemic may not be willing to abide by the protocols. Health professionals and managers of the pandemic need to approach the fight against the disease in line with the cultural background of the people.

Another category of perceiving health is sickness which refers to how other people label a patient due to ill health condition. This label is usually done with reference to the sociocultural abilities of such a patient (Twaddle, 1994). Normally, certain social roles are assigned to a person who is regarded to be sick and such a person may assume the "sick role" according to the particular society he or she belongs to. These roles may exclude the individual from socioeconomic activities until the person is deemed healthy to return to normal societal activities. Many societies consider a sick person as a form of deviation from the "healthy population" (Parsons, 1951). In view of such interpretation of a sick role, when a member of a society is unwell with any socially recognizable illness or disease, society members carry out certain duties to aid the recovery process. Parsons (1951) explains that a sick person faces some obligatory conducts and is made to accept the moral responsibility regarding him or her as undesirable and as a situation which should be overcome as soon as possible. It is based on the acceptance of the sick role that the person then is encouraged to seek competent help from a physician and obliged to cooperate with the physician in order to recover completely. The healing process of a sick member of a particular society is very much influenced by culture. Members assess the effectiveness of measures applied to restore the sick back to healthy state of health and the level of recovery to judge whether the individual has improved or deteriorated. The restoration of health of the sick can be influenced by spiritual, psychosocial, and biological disposition of the patient. Patient's acceptance of treatment depends largely on the effectiveness of medical care in addressing both the disease and illness components of their health problem.

One other factor that may influence people's attitude toward health is stigmatization which continues to be a major problem impeding quality healthcare in Ghana. Experts bemoan late health-seeking among patients with diseases such as breast cancer and believed that stigmatization was the main reason for the delay (Clegg-Lamptey & Hodasi, 2007). When etiology and impacts of diseases are not readily known it can lead to myths surrounding such diseases in a highly spiritual society as Ghana. With such high levels of stigmatization, it is clear that many people will prefer to remain silent about their COVID-19 status. This situation makes it much more difficult for people to voluntarily avail themselves for testing and subsequent treatment. It is not surprising that some people were not willing to meet with the COVID-19 taskforce to be tested during the contact tracing and community surveillance in Ghana (MoH, 2020). Vivien and Noor (2013) revealed that if patients of a disease consider it as a type of illness, rather than disease, the disease and the subjective illness feeling as well as the disease need to be tackled. It is not surprising that some Ghanaians claimed they did not believe coronavirus actually exists and that the officials are only hyping it for their personal interests (Oppong-Nkrumah, 2020). The managers of the health services need to understand that perceptions of health problems by the lay person might be different from the medical models and be guided by that in their approach to education and treatment of the coronavirus pandemic. One of the most effective approaches to influence patients' perception toward positive health-seeking behavior is education. Education should be targeted at understanding the link between susceptibility and risk of the disease and acceptance of the protocols in order to reduce the infection rate. Redefining the manifestation of coronavirus based on the cultural background, especially in the label of illness and presence of actual disease, is very crucial in accepting the existence of a disease such as coronavirus (Amegbor, 2014). Finally, conscious and consistent effort to reduce stigmatization of patients with coronavirus can greatly help people to visit the health facilities or report to the COVID-19 task force when they suspect they have coronavirus.

Conclusion

In conclusion, in order to control people's health behavior, their health belief and attitude need to be understood by the authorities. The cultural background of many Ghanaians indicates that perceptions of diseases are not only based on the biomedical model but it is much more complicated with religiosity being also involved. Thus the coronavirus comes with several psychological problems and the authorities need to embark on more education and attitudinal change among Ghanaians to win the fight against the coronavirus.

References

Afolabi, M. O., Daropale, V. O., Irinoye, A. I., & Adegoke, A. A. (2013). Health-seeking behaviour and students' perception of health care services in a university community in Nigeria. *Health and Science Research*, *5*(5), 817–824.

Amegbor, P. M. (2014). *Health seeking behaviour in Asikuma Odoben-Brakwa district: A pluralistic health perspective*. Norway: University of Oslo. (Master's thesis) Retrieved from: https://www.duo.uio.no/bitstream/handle/10852/40395/1. Retrieved on 15th August, 2020.

American Psychiatric Association. (2013). *Diagnostic and statistical manual of mental disorders* (5th ed.). Washington, DC: American Psychiatric Association.

Anarfi, K. J., Badasu, D. M., Yawson, A., Atobra, D., Abuosi, A. A., & Adzei, F. A. (2016). Religious affiliation and health-seeking behavior related to non-communicable diseases among children in Ghana. *International Journal of Healthcare*, *2*(2).

Andisheh-Tadbir, A., Mehrabani, D., & Heydari, S. T. (2008). Epidemiology of squamous cell carcinoma of the oral cavity in Iran. *The Journal of Craniofacial Surgery*, *19*(6), 1699–1702.

Armitage, R., & Nellums, L. B. (2020). COVID-19 and the consequences of isolating the elderly. *The Lancet Public Health*. https://doi.org/10.1016/s2468-2667(20)30061-x. Retrieved 16/07/2020.

Asiamah, N., Opuni, F. F., Mends-Brew, E., Mensah, S. W., Mensah, H. K., & Quansah, F. (2020). *Short-term changes in behaviors resulting from COVID-19-related social isolation and their influences on mental health*. Posted, Research square.

Assimeng, M. (2007). *Social structure of Ghana* (2nd ed.). Accra: Ghana Publishing Corporation.

Banda, R. (2017). *Twelve traditions and customs only Ghanaians can understand*. Culture trip. https://theculturetrip.com/africa/ghana/articles/12-traditions-and-customs. Retrieved on 16th August, 2020.

Brooks, S. K., Webster, R. K., Smith, L. E., Woodland, L., Wessely, S., Greenberg, N., et al. (2020). The psychological impact of quarantine and how to reduce it: Rapid review of the evidence. *The Lancet*, *395*, 913–920.

Clegg-Lamptey, J. N. A., & Hodasi, W. M. (2007). A study of breast cancer in Korle-bu Teaching Hospital: Assessing the impact of health education. *Ghana Medical Journal, 41*(2), 72–77.

Cumming, E., & Henry, W. E. (1961). *Growing old* (p. 227). New York: Basic.

Falade, B. (2018). Cultural differences and confidence in institutions: Comparing Africa and the USA. *South African Journal of Science, 114*(5/6). https://doi.org/10.17159/sajs.2018/20170135. #2017–0135. ISSN 0038–2353.

Fogarty, C., & Cronin, P. (2008). Waiting for healthcare: A concept analysis. *Journal of Advanced Nursing, 61*(4), 463–471.

Fogg, B. J. (2009). Behavior model for persuasive design. In *A Proceedings of the 4th international conference on persuasive technology, Persuasive, New York* (pp. 401–407). NY, USA: ACM.

Glanz, K., Rimer, B. K., & Viswanath, K. (2008). *Health behavior and health education: Theory, research and practice* (4th ed., pp. 67–92). Jossey-Bass publisher: San Francisco.

Gyasi, R. M., Asante, F., Yeboah, J. Y., Abass, K., Mensah, C. M., & Siaw, L. P. (2016). Pulled in or pushed out? Understanding the complexities of motivation for alternative therapies use in Ghana. *International Journal of Qualitative Studies on Health and Well-Being, 11*, 1–12. https://doi.org/10.3402/qhw.v11.29667.

Gyekye, K. (2003). *African cultural values: An introduction* (5th ed.). Accra: Sankofa, Publishing Company.

Hochbaum, G. M. (1958). *Public participation in medical screening programs: A socio-psychological study*. US Department of Health, Education, and Welfare, Public Health Service, Bureau of State Services, Division of Special Health Services. Tuberculosis Program.

Howren, M. B., Christensen, A. J., Karnell, L. H., & Funk, G. F. (2010). Health-related quality of life in head and neck cancer survivors: Impact of pretreatment depressive symptoms. *Health Psychology, 29*, 65–71.

Idang, G. E. (2015). African culture and values. *Phronimon, 16*(2), 97–111. ISSN 2413–3086.

International. (2020). *Governments are starting to ease restrictions: The Economist*. https://www.economist.com/international/2020/04/16/governments. (Accessed 16 August 2020).

Katz, S. J., & Hawley, S. T. (2005). From policy to patients and back: Surgical treatment decision making for patients with breast cancer. *Health Affairs, 26*, 761–769.

Khan, S., Siddique, R., Ali, A., Bai, Q., Li, Z., Li, H., et al. (2020). The spread of novel coronavirus has created an alarming situation worldwide. *Journal of Infection and Public Health*. pii: S1876 0341(20)30405–6.

Kleinman, A., & Seeman, D. (2000). Personal experience of illness. In G. Albrecht, R. Fitzpatrick, & S. Scrimshaw (Eds.), *Handbook of social studies in health and medicine* (pp. 230–243). London: SAGE Publications Ltd.

Lai, J., Ma, S., Wang, Y., et al. (2020). Factors associated with mental health outcomes among health care workers exposed to coronavirus disease 2019. *JAMA Network Open, 3*, e203976.

Lebel, S., Castonguay, M., Mackness, G., Irish, J., Bezjak, A., & Devins, G. M. (2011). The psychosocial impact of stigma in people with head, neck or lung cancer. *Psycho-Oncology, 86*, 456–462.

Lewis, M., & Merched, A. J. (2014). Tumor-associated macrophages, inflammation and pathogenesis of hepatocellular carcinoma. *Journal of Molecular and Genetic Medicine, 8*(3), 1–5.

Lewnard, J. A., & Lo, N. C. (2020). Scientific and ethical basis for social-distancing interventions against COVID-19. *The Lancet Infectious Diseases, 20*, 631–633.

Malcolm, M., Frost, H., & Cowie, J. (2019). Loneliness and social isolation causal association with health-related lifestyle risk in older adults: A systematic review and meta-analysis protocol. *Systematic Reviews, 8*(1), 1–8.

Mbiti, J. S. (1990). *African religions and philosophy*. Oxford, United Kingdom: Heinemann Educational.

McManus, S., Bebbington, P., Jenkins, R., & Brugha, T. (2016). *Mental health and wellbeing in England: Adult Psychiatric Morbidity Survey 2014*. https://files.digital.nhs.uk/pdf/q/3/mental_health_and_wellbeing_in_england_full_report.pdf. (Accessed 11 April 2020).

Mirowsky, J., & Ross, C. E. (2002). Measurement for a human science. *Journal of Health and Social Behavior*, *43*, 152–170.

MoH. (2020). *Provisional standard treatment guidelines for novel coronavirus infection*. https://www.moh.gov.gh/wp-content/uploads/2016/02/COVID-19-STG-JUNE-2020-1.pdf. (Accessed 6 August 2020).

Oppong-Nkrumah, K. (2020). *About 20% of Ghanaians don't believe that coronavirus exists*. UTV. https://www.youtube.com/watch. Retrieved 12/08/20.

Parsons, T. (1951). *The social system*. Glencoe, IL: The Free Press.

Paul, C., Carey, M., Anderson, A., Mackenzie, L., Sanson-Fisher, R., Courtney, R., et al. (2011). Cancer Patients' concerns regarding access to cancer care: Perceived impact of waiting times along the diagnosis and treatment journey. *European Journal of Cancer Care*, *21*, 321–329.

Rawlett, K. E. (2011). Analytical evaluation of the health belief model and the vulnerable populations conceptual model applied to a medically underserved, rural population. *International Journal of Applied Science and Technology*, *1*(2), 34–46.

Robert, M. (2020). *'Do it at home' coronavirus saliva test trial*. BBC News. https://www.bbc.com/news/health-53131237. (Accessed 20 July 2020).

Sohler, N. L., Jerant, A., & Franks, P. (2015). Socio-psychological factors in the expanded health belief model and subsequent colorectal cancer screening. *Patient Education and Counselling*, *98*(7), 901–907.

Tan, B. Y., Chew, N. W., Lee, G. K., Jing, M., Goh, Y., Yeo, L. L., et al. (2020). Psychological impact of the COVID-19 pandemic on health care workers in Singapore. *Annals of Internal Medicine*, *56*(9), 23–45.

Twaddle, A. C. (1994). Disease, illness and sickness revisited. In A. Twaddle, & L. Nordenfelt (Eds.), *Vol. 18. Disease, illness and sickness: Three central concepts in the theory of health* (pp. 1–18). Linköping: Studies on Health and Society.

Twumasi, P. A. (1975). *Medical systems in Ghana: A study in medical sociology*. Tema: Ghana Publishing Corporation.

Vivien, Y. W. C., & Noor, N. A. M. (2013). An examination of sociocultural factors influencing lifestyle, health and health-seeking behaviour—A case study of Malaysia Chinese Cancer Survivors. In *Proceeding of the international conference on social science research, ICSSR 2013, 4–5 June 2013, Penang, Malaysia*.

World Health Organization. (2020). *Coronavirus disease 2019 (COVID-19) situation report-64*. World Health Organization. Available from: https://www.who.int/docs/default-source/coronaviruse/situationreports/20200324-sitrep-64-covid-19.pdf?sfvrsn=703b2c40_2. (Accessed 18 July 2020).

Chapter 7

"Alone, but not lonely": The impact of COVID-19 on older persons and the role of technology in staying connected

Ceylan Okan, Gabrielle Weidemann, and Phoebe E. Bailey
School of Psychology, Western Sydney University, Sydney, NSW, Australia

Introduction

Chapter overview

An emerging social and health challenge is the aging of the global population, and the difficulty this poses for appropriate resource allocation specific to the needs of older adults. The World Health Organization predicts a twofold growth in the older adult population by 2050, such that adults over the age of 60 will make up 22% of the world's population; currently there are 125 million people aged 80+ (World Health Organization, 2018). The population aged 65 years and over in Australia has also increased, with baby boomers comprising 15.9% of the Australian population in 2019, up from 12.3% in 1999 (ABS, Australian Bureau of Statistics, 2017). As we age, a variety of things change, including our physical capabilities, energy levels, retiring from work, children leaving the family home, relocation to more suitable housing, and death of loved ones. This can leave older adults feeling lonely, and adjusting to these changes may be challenging, particularly given the altered social circumstances that many of these changes necessitate. For example, retiring from work does not only result in stress as a result of losing a sense of purpose (Bleidorn & Schwaba, 2018), but it can also dramatically change the size of people's social networks (Börsch-Supan & Schuth, 2014). Thus, feeling lonely due to being socially isolated from former social circles may have a significant negative impact on mental health, including an increased risk of depression (Pinquart, 2002a, 2002b). The costs of the negative impacts associated with aging include increased health care expenditure to manage geriatric diseases (Counsell, Callahan, Tu, Stump, & Arling, 2009), as well as the cost of facilitating community engagement among older adults, who may otherwise lead isolated lives (Collom, 2008).

Mental Health Effects of COVID-19. https://doi.org/10.1016/B978-0-12-824289-6.00017-9

The emergence of the novel coronavirus (SARS-CoV-2), the virus that causes COVID-19, in late 2019 and its rapid spread around the world in early 2020 has had extraordinary and unforeseen physical and mental health consequences for older adults. In March 2020, the Center for Disease Control and Prevention (CDC COVID-19 Response Team, 2020) reported approximately 80% of COVID-19 deaths in China and the USA were among older adults, aged over 65 years. At the same time, the estimated global death toll from COVID-19 was 7000 spread across approximately 150 countries. By 8 July 2020, the World Health Organization pandemic website (World Health Organization, 2020) reported 11,669,259 confirmed global cases and 539,906 confirmed deaths across 216 countries. Alarmingly, the cases and deaths continue to rise while scientists scramble to find beneficial treatments and develop an effective vaccine. However, a widely available vaccine is not likely to be accessible in the foreseeable future and many more deaths are expected. Globally, aged care facilities and hospices have reported devastatingly high contagion rates and deaths as a result of the spread of COVID-19, often brought into the facilities by staff members, and visiting friends and families who may have been completely unaware that they were doing so, as many infected individuals can remain completely asymptomatic (Hu et al., 2020). It has been suggested that in some European countries, as many as 50% of deaths in the elderly due to COVID-19 are residents of aged care homes (Comas-Herrera et al., 2020).

Global measures taken to prevent the spread of the novel virus include full or partial lockdowns, where residents are forbidden from leaving their home except under very restricted conditions (e.g., for health care or purchasing essential items). Other measures include *Social Distancing*, whereby social interaction involving close physical contact is prohibited. Older adults are particularly encouraged to self-isolate, given a heightened vulnerability to the virus, as a result of their declining immune systems and higher likelihood of having a chronic condition (Wu, 2020). Social and physical distancing may cause an exacerbation of existing feelings of loneliness for many older adults. This chapter explores the unique challenges that COVID-19 poses for the mental health of older adults, particularly the effects of enforced social distancing and physical isolation. The potential for online communication technologies to ameliorate some negative effects of physical isolation among older adults is also explored.

Loneliness in older age and mental health implications

Social isolation has traditionally been defined as an objective lack of integration into social networks (Rook, 1984) and an absence of specific role relationships, such as being an active partner, parent, or grandparent (Chappell & Badger, 1989). Social isolation may not necessarily be by choice and is a grim reality faced by many older adults, both in general and especially during the coronavirus pandemic. In general, the reality of retirement for many is an isolating experience, entailing a reduced sense of purpose (e.g., the loss of employment can reduce motivation to achieve goals), loss of relationships with work colleagues, and the loss of social support and health benefits of working (Topa & Valero, 2017). There may also be a need to relocate to more affordable housing to secure a financially sustainable retirement. For those needing a higher level of care or with a preference for community engagement, there is the growing demand for retirement villages, independent living units, and nursing home care facilities (Adams, Sanders, & Auth, 2004). However, this can result in a sense of isolation from family, and an increased risk of financial exploitation and abuse (Wilber & Reynolds, 1997). The COVID-19 pandemic has added additional layers of complexity to the social isolation experienced by older adults due to both geographical distancing (i.e., laws preventing traveling between towns, states, and/or countries) and social distancing (i.e., prevention of social visits with close physical contact) (Stanley et al., 2010). In contrast, having full- or part-time work and being a valuable contributor to society is commonly associated with having a sense of purpose and better health outcomes (Avendano & Cylus, 2019). Working also increases opportunities for partaking in regular fulfilling social contact with others (Pinquart, 2002a, 2002b). This is also true for older adults who engage in volunteering roles, who report experiencing a similar sense of purpose and motivation as those who are engaged in paid work (Greenfield & Marks, 2004).

Some general growing trends in the older population include increasing sense of loneliness (Pinquart & Sorensen, 2001), sense of social isolation (Cornwell & Waite, 2009), perceived social disconnection (i.e., thwarted belongingness), and feeling they are a burden to others (i.e., perceived burdensomeness) (Van Orden, Cukrowicz, Witte, & Joiner Jr, 2012). As a result, older adults are at an increased risk of developing clinical depression (Fiske, Wetherell, & Gatz, 2009) and of experiencing suicidality (Almeida et al., 2012). In Australia, men aged over 85 have the highest suicide rate of all demographic groups, with a rate of 39.3 deaths per 100,000 people, almost double the rate of teenagers, and eight times the rate of women in the same age group (ABS, Australian Bureau of Statistics, 2016). This trend is replicated in other countries, with Baby Boomers in the U.S.A (Phillips, 2014), Greece, the Republic of Korea, UK, and the Netherlands (Alicandro et al., 2019) also demonstrating an increase in older age suicides, particularly following the global recession from 2008 to 2015. However, other countries report a decline in older adult suicides, such as in Italy (De Leo, Vichi, Kolves, & Pompili, 2020) and Japan (Dhungel, Sugai, & Gilmour, 2019), possibly due to improved health care receiving nursing and care assistance, and increased quality of life. It will be important for countries to monitor suicide rates among older adults during and following the coronavirus pandemic social isolation periods.

Though it is difficult to gauge the exact relationship between loneliness, depression, and suicidality, feeling lonely and disconnected from support is a large risk factor for suicidal ideation in the older population (Liu, Gou, & Zuo, 2016). Prior studies recognize the significance of supportive social relationships as a strong predictor of healthy aging (Vanderhorst & McLaren, 2005). The positive impact of supportive social connections is evident among older adults who are in long-term marriages or relationships, where this connection has fostered a sense of belonging and purpose (McLaren, Gomez, Gill, & Chesler, 2015). Interestingly, having a poorer sense of belongingness within a marriage has a detrimental effect on mental health, and this may strengthen the relationship between increased age and greater suicidal ideation. Having a sense of belongingness is a key factor in reducing the risk of suicide in older adults residing in the community (Heisel, Neufeld, & Flett, 2016). Indeed, Vanderhorst and McLaren (2005) investigated whether marital status, social support, and sense of belonging are predictors of mental health (i.e., levels of depression and suicidal ideation) in a community sample of older adults. They found a strong negative relationship between social support resources and levels of suicidal ideation and depression symptoms. This highlights the importance of enhancing social support resources for older adults in general, and is even more important during the pandemic.

Nevertheless, the time pressure that younger generations face due to work commitments and other personal obligations contributes to reduced social contact with older adults (Dunbar, 2016). In the changing social landscape, and due to the physical and social distancing measures to prevent the spread of COVID-19, face-to-face interactions between older adults and their family and local community are even more infrequent than usual. This has led to the coronavirus pandemic being described as "a lonely pandemic" (Hartt, 2020), whereby older adults are more likely to feel lonely due to the strict restrictions placed on socializing. Therefore continued social contact through other means, such as video conference calling, will be crucial for maintaining the psychological wellbeing of older adults.

Loneliness and mental health impacts during the coronavirus pandemic

A growing number of investigations have been published during the COVID-19 pandemic, which explore the trends of older adults' mental health and their experiences during the coronavirus pandemic and lockdown periods. A large survey of Spanish people (aged 18–88 years; $N = 1310$) conducted during the COVID-19 lockdown period showed that, intriguingly, increasing age was associated with reduced distress and loneliness (Losada-Baltar et al., 2020). However, it was also shown that negative self-perceptions about aging were associated with greater distress and loneliness during this period. It appears that positive self-perceptions in older age may ameliorate the negative mental health effects of social isolation. Losada-Baltar et al. (2020) also noted that participants in their study were all users of online technologies which could have reduced the effect of age on loneliness and distress.

In line with Losada-Baltar et al. (2020), at the time of the coronavirus pandemic, Israeli older adults demonstrated a stronger positive association between loneliness and anxiety, depression, and distress, if they reported an older subjective age (Shrira, Hoffman, Bodner, & Palgi, 2020). Subjective age refers to the extent to which people feel younger or older than their chronological age and is typically measured by asking people how old they *feel* (Alonso Debreczeni & Bailey, 2020). In other words, older adults who reported feeling younger than their chronological age were less likely to experience negative psychological effects of loneliness. Labeling theory suggests that negative age stereotypes are integrated into self-evaluations which then contribute to poor self-perceptions among older adults (Pinquart, 2002a, 2002b). According to stereotype embodiment theory, age stereotypes become self-relevant through extensive exposure in the surrounding social and cultural environment (Levy, 2009). Therefore older adults with a more negative perception of their own age group may be more likely to incorporate negative age stereotypes into the way they evaluate themselves. Negative stereotypes of older adults as helpless, frail, and unable to contribute to society were perpetuated by the press, government public announcements, and social media during the coronavirus pandemic (Ayalon et al., 2020). In some cases, a trade-off between protecting the lives of the elderly versus keeping the economy open was portrayed as being the most acceptable and balanced option for the benefit of Australia and other countries. Given that older adults with negative self-perceptions are likely to be more vulnerable to the effects of negative age stereotypes, COVID-19 related ageism may have had a particularly detrimental effect on the psychiatric symptoms of these older adults.

Setting aside the moderating role of negative self-perceptions in influencing the association between age and mental health outcomes during the coronavirus pandemic, further studies have provided evidence for reduced psychological distress among older cohorts. Consistent with maintained (and in some cases improved) emotion regulation in older age, Barber and Kim (2020) showed that community-dwelling older adults in the US, and particularly older men, reported less worry than young adults about the potential consequences of COVID-19. Reduced worry is beneficial to mental health, but also predicted fewer behavior changes, suggesting a need for COVID-19 behavioral change interventions targeted at older men. A further survey of a large US national lifespan sample (aged 18–100 years; $N=6666$) showed that older age was associated with less depression and anxiety in response to the emerging COVID-19 crisis (Bruine de Bruin, 2020). Similarly, Swedish older adults rated their wellbeing during the early stages of the pandemic as high as, or even higher than, in the past 5 years (Kivi, Hansson, & Bjälkebring, 2020).

We surveyed a convenience sample of younger ($N=101$, M age $=20.6$ years; 51 female) and older ($N=99$, M age $=73.4$ years; 56 female) adult Australians in May to July 2020. The younger adults were undergraduate students at Western Sydney University, whereas the older adults were community dwelling. We asked, on a scale from 1 (not at all) to 3 (a moderate amount) to 5 (a great deal), "How distressing have you found the coronavirus situation?", and "How lonely have you been during the coronavirus social isolation period?". Loneliness scores were higher among younger ($M=2.9$, $SD=1.22$) than older ($M=2.1$, $SD=1.06$) adults, $F(1, 198)=25.25$, $P<0.001$. Levels of distress were moderate but not significantly different for younger ($M=2.9$, $SD=1.07$) and older ($M=2.8$, $SD=1.07$) adults, $F(1, 198)=0.46$, $P=0.497$. One of our older participants remarked, "at this point in time neither my wife nor I are suffering any mental health issues due to the shutdown. In fact, we are quite enjoying the break from what has been our busy retirement life and we are now looking at ways on how we can keep it that way for whenever life will return to normal."

Socioemotional selectivity theory predicts that, as time remaining in life is perceived as becoming limited, motivations shift from achieving future-oriented goals (e.g., accumulation of resources) to maximizing emotional wellbeing in the present (Carstensen, 2006). However, the strength and vulnerability model suggests that serious or prolonged stressors may make it more difficult for older adults to maintain their psychological wellbeing, as levels of increased vulnerability would outweigh diminishing strength in their coping mechanisms (Charles, 2010). It may be that, relative to younger adults, older adults cope well with social isolation and physical distancing in the initial stages of the pandemic. One possible explanation for this is that shorter intervals of being alone is something they may have previously experienced or experience on a regular basis. However, as the pandemic situation progresses and the length of physical and social isolation increases, their ability to regulate negative affect may decline. Thus a decline in the mental health of older adults may be expected in the coming months and years as the pandemic progresses beyond their coping resources.

It should be acknowledged that older adults from countries such as Brazil, Italy, Spain, the UK, and USA have experienced a much higher mortality rate as a proportion of the population than other countries such as Australia and New Zealand (World Health Organization, 2020). Periods of physical isolation and lockdown rules also vary depending on location (Mækelæ et al., 2020). Older adults are a heterogeneous group, and country of residence added another dimension to this heterogeneity during the coronavirus pandemic. In addition, the experience of older adults at different life stages, or with differing health profiles or living situations, is also likely to have varied. One study of the impact of social distancing on US older adults aged 60 to 85+ years ($N=833$) found that 42.9% reported feeling lonely on some or most days, and 30.9% reported feeling more lonely than prior to social distancing (Emerson, 2020). However, those living alone reported greater increases in loneliness. Nursing home residents have particularly suffered in Australia due to the significantly higher mortality rate and stricter lockdown measures during the pandemic (Pachana, Beattie, Byrne, & Brodaty, 2020). Furthermore, the participants in most COVID-19 studies to date completed surveys online, suggesting easy access to the internet. Responses may differ for older adults without internet access or the technical ability or willingness to connect online. Taken together, older adults living alone or in nursing homes, or with poor mental health prior to the pandemic, or in countries with high mortality rates may be especially vulnerable to the adverse effects of isolation and physical distancing.

According to the interpersonal theory of suicide, suicidal desire increases if both thwarted belongingness and perceived burdensomeness are experienced by the individual; this increases the risk of suicide due to the sense of hopelessness and this suicidal desire is separate from capability to commit suicide (Van Orden et al., 2012). During the pandemic, older people, particularly those in places with a high number of COVID-19 cases, were explicitly made aware that they may not receive treatment due to resource rationing, potentially contributing to perceived burdensomeness (Wand, Zhong, Chiu, Draper, & De Leo, 2020). Feelings of thwarted belongingness are also likely to have increased due to physical distancing and social isolation. As such, the Australian Psychological Society suggested using various methods of telecommunication for coping with social distancing. These online technologies can contribute to a sense of belonging and social support to offset the risk of suicide (Armitage & Nellumns, 2020). However, a large proportion of older adults either do not have access to technology or do not have the skills to adequately use social networking technology (such as video calling through smartphone apps). Carers in nursing homes also have limited time and resources available to assist older adults with these technologies. There are concerns that the so-called *Digital Divide* may exacerbate issues associated with isolation, loneliness, and bereavement in older age (Holmes et al., 2020), and worryingly, Australians aged 65+ years have been described as the most digitally excluded age group (Thomas et al., 2017).

Alternative ways to socialize? Online communication and social media use by older adults

Technological developments in communication together with the age of social media have brought about changes in how we communicate, both as individuals and as members of a social group. People separated by geographical distance are able to access low cost synchronous and asynchronous conversations via text, image, and voice, and the developing nature of technology means there are more communication options for internet users including voice and video calls. These are usually free, or at minimal cost, when compared with traditional landline telephone calls, which are particularly expensive for making international calls. For example, WhatsApp, FaceTime, Skype, and Zoom make video conferencing freely available to anyone with internet access and an account. A longitudinal study involving a nationally representative sample ($N = 1424$) of US adults with an average age of 64.8 years evaluated the influence of various communication technologies on depressive symptoms (Teo, Markwardt, & Hinton, 2019). Users of video chat (e.g., Skype) had half the level of depressive symptoms at two-year follow-up relative to nonusers of communication technologies, or those who used email only. Email, social media, and instant messaging were not associated with reduced symptoms of depression. This suggests that the "richer" a communication tool is (e.g., interactive live video where you can see the other person v. nonlive and inanimate, standard phone calls or emails), the better it is at promoting social and emotional connectedness.

With much research focused on the impact of social media usage among the young, there is a relative scarcity of research concerning older adult's use of social media. Limited use of social media may have protected older adults against ageism and general exposure to information about the harms of COVID-19. At least one study has shown that frequent exposure to social media during the coronavirus pandemic among Chinese citizens aged 18+ years was associated with increased depression and anxiety (Gao et al., 2020). At the same time, the potential benefits of social media for connection and social support may not have been realized among older adults who tend to engage less than younger adults with social media.

Research with adolescents has identified that social media use is associated with low self-esteem and self-confidence due to social comparisons and impression management (Vogel, Rose, Roberts, & Eckles, 2014). In contrast, recent studies with older adults, however, suggest that there are various benefits to using social media. One such study with a convenience sample of northern Israeli adults aged 50 and over found that internet use reduces loneliness and increases subjective quality of life (Khalaila & Vitman-Schorr, 2018). Similarly, a study conducted with Turkish older adults ($N=563$) found that using the internet to stay connected reduces self-reported loneliness relative to those who do not use the internet (Şar, Göktürk, Tura, & Kazaz, 2012). Despite these mental health benefits, older adults do not commonly use social media—previous studies have found 7% of people aged 65 years and above maintained social media profiles, compared to a large 75% of young adults aged 18–24 years (Lenhart, 2009). However, the number of older adults using social media is rapidly rising. More recent statistics from the U.S. show that 60% of older adults use the internet, and of these, 46% use social networking sites (Smith, 2014). A significant barrier to the use of social media is that older adults generally do not possess the digital literacy required to navigate the internet on their own (Momeni, Hariri, Nobahar, & Noshinfard, 2018). *Digital literacy* is defined as an individual's ability to search, find, evaluate, and compose clear information through typing, writing, tapping, and by using other mediums (e.g., multimedia videos, video calling, and messaging) on various digital platforms, which requires a basic level of computer competency (Bawden, 2008). However, given that many older adults reported feeling lonelier than usual during COVID-19 social distancing (Emerson, 2020), social media may be a viable option for increasing social engagement and decreasing loneliness. Indeed, more than two-thirds of adults aged 60–85 years ($N=833$) reported using more social media than usual, as well as spending more time on computers/tablets and emailing or texting friends and family (Emerson, 2020). This highlights the need for evidence to establish the efficacy of online communication tools and social media use as tool for decreasing loneliness that older adults may experience due to the pandemic.

Although not a lot of research within this area exists due to low uptake of social media (such as Instagram and Facebook) by older adults, some studies have shown benefits for older adults using social media platforms. One such study explored the social connectedness of Nigerian older adults aged over 50 who reported already being active users of social media networking sites, such as Facebook (Ciboh, 2017). These older adults benefited from being active users of Facebook, a free social media networking platform, through the continuation of their existing relationships. They also connected with global friends and family with whom they did not have regular face-to-face interaction. Ciboh (2017) concluded that using Facebook to keep in touch with their friend and family networks increases the older adults' social capital. In Nigeria, Ciboh (2017) outlines how *social capital* involves not only a network of social relationships, but also includes capital exchange (i.e., the close bonds that help friends solve financial problems, intimate personal problems, group problems, and assist with broadening worldviews). However, the study used a sample already rich in social capital, consisting of social media users who were mainly white-collar, professional government ministry employees, with participants reporting many significant personal relationships.

Further studies report that Facebook use increases older adult users' sense of social connectedness, similar to the levels more frequently reported in studies with younger samples (Sinclair & Grieve, 2017). It has been shown that older adults who use Facebook experience not only social benefits, but also improvements in cognition compared with their peers who do not use Facebook. A small amount of decline in memory processing is expected with age (Grady & Craik, 2000), and aspects of working memory are improved in older adults who use Facebook, relative to those who do not (Myhre, Mehl, & Glisky, 2017). Older adults who use the internet also harbor a stronger sense of community, compared to their peers who are not internet users (Sum, Mathews, Pourghasem, & Hughes, 2009). Thus, aside from being an alternative way for older adults to retain social engagement during the COVID-19 pandemic, maintaining digital literacy and socially interacting with others using social networking platforms may also be of general cognitive and mental health benefit to the aging population. The coronavirus pandemic highlights an urgent need for more research. At the same time, it offers a unique opportunity to establish the role of online connectedness in short- and long-term cognitive, emotional, social, and mental health benefits among older adults.

Virtual reality (VR) technology is also proving useful for ameliorating the negative effects of loneliness in older age. One study explored the use of VR to engage older adults in an aged care facility (Baker et al., 2020). A promising finding was that VR gave older adults a reason to reconnect with friends and family. It gave them something to talk about. An older resident who used Google Earth VR to "visit" the address of her granddaughter was "thrilled" and phoned her immediately to tell her all about it. VR may also provide an opportunity for older adults to simply escape the confines of a nursing home or the place where they are in lockdown during the pandemic. And although results for the utility of socially assistive robot (SAR) technology for social facilitation in aged care are inconclusive (Abdi, Al-Hindawi, Ng, & Vizcaychipi, 2018), research could assess whether robots may provide another solution to social isolation and may help keep older adults socially engaged during lockdown periods. With the ever-evolving nature of technology, it is important that adaptations are made for the technology to suit individual needs. For example, exergame (a term used for video games that are also a form of exercise) devices such as Nintendo Wii and Xbox Kinect have been used to prevent falls in the elderly by creating an interactive intervention opportunity aimed to improve balance and mobility, similar to physical therapy (Choi, Guo, Kang, & Xiong, 2017). These are tools that could help older adults to maintain physical fitness during social isolation.

Older adults and online communication during the coronavirus pandemic

Given the consequences associated with COVID-19 and its impact on traditional ways of socializing and staying connected, it is prudent that future studies and programs are aimed at minimizing the "social" distance between people, thus increasing social connectedness without bringing people physically together. While COVID-19 is currently having a physical, emotional, psychological, and financial toll, there may be ways in which to minimize this impact on older adults. The social distancing and digital technology struggles of older adults during COVID-19 have been dubbed a "double burden of exclusion" (Seifert, Cotten, & Xie, 2020), as many older adults either do not have access to technology required to maintain social connection, or do not have the knowledge to use such technology.

Recommendations for clinicians to address loneliness and depressive symptoms as a result of social isolation include promoting digital literacy in older adults by asking if they own technology and if they know how to use it, and to also be fluent with using the tools themselves to demonstrate to the older adults how to use them (Gould & Hantke, 2020). For example, a clinician working with older adults on reducing depression and anxiety during the pandemic should give recommendations for smartphone applications (e.g., Headspace, Calm, Smiling Minds, COVID coach) based on the need of the older adult and their level of digital literacy. After using clinical judgment regarding the usefulness of the app, clinicians must then be able to demonstrate how to use it. Some of these recommendations could include the 15 inexpensive and accessible apps summarized by Banskota, Healy, and Goldberg (2020) as the best apps for older adults based on reviews and features that address specific needs (such as hearing or visual impairment). These included Facetime and Skype for social networking; Teladoc and K Health for Telemedicine; Calm, Headspace, Yoga: Down Dog, and MyFitness Pal for health and fitness; and Be My Eyes, and Glide, for vision and hearing impairment.

Conclusion

The COVID-19 pandemic presents many challenges to older adults, and social distancing as a form of disease prevention may have mental health consequences. The current review shows that, in the early stages of the pandemic, older adults appear to be coping well relative to young adults. However, the negative mental health problems due to social distancing may increase in older adults living alone or in nursing homes, or who are already feeling lonely, with a low sense of purpose, or with a negative perception of aging.

Future studies are needed to examine the effects of social distancing for those with limited access to online communication, as well as the effect of ongoing social distancing over an extended timeframe, both of which may be associated with more negative outcomes for older adults. Future research must take into account the heterogeneous experiences of older adults with different living situations and social support structures, or who are located in countries that vary in terms of COVID-19 mortality rates or lockdown rules. In particular, this review highlights the need for studies examining the validity of online communication and social engagement tools for ameliorating the ill effects of physical distancing, and enhancing overall quality of life, among older adults.

References

Abdi, J., Al-Hindawi, A., Ng, T., & Vizcaychipi, M. P. (2018). Scoping review on the use of socially assistive robot technology in elderly care. *BMJ Open*, *8*. https://doi.org/10.1136/bmjopen-2017-018815, e018815.

ABS, Australian Bureau of Statistics. (2016). *3303.0—Causes of death, Australia, 2015*. Retrieved on 18th June 2019 from: https://www.abs.gov.au/ausstats/abs@.nsf/Lookup/by%20Subject/3303.0~2015~Main%20Features~Intentional%20self-harm:%20key%20characteristics~8.

ABS, Australian Bureau of Statistics. (2017). *3101.0 Australian Demographic Statistics, June 2019. ABS cat. no. 3101.0*. Canberra: ABS. Retrieved on 12th August 2020 from: https://www.abs.gov.au/ausstats/abs@.nsf/0/1CD2B1952AFC5E7ACA257298000F2E76?OpenDocument.

Adams, K. B., Sanders, S., & Auth, E. A. (2004). Loneliness and depression in independent living retirement communities: Risk and resilience factors. *Aging & Mental Health*, *8*, 475–485.

Alicandro, G., Malvezzi, M., Gallus, S., La Vecchia, C., Negri, E., & Bertuccio, P. (2019). Worldwide trends in suicide mortality from 1990 to 2015 with a focus on the global recession time frame. *International Journal of Public Health*, *64*, 785–795. https://doi.org/10.1007/s00038-019-01219-y.

Almeida, O. P., Draper, B., Snowdon, J., Lautenschlager, N. T., Pirkis, J., Byrne, G., et al. (2012). Factors associated with suicidal thoughts in a large community study of older adults. *The British Journal of Psychiatry*, *201*, 466–472.

Alonso Debreczeni, F., & Bailey, P. E. (2020). A systematic review and meta-analysis of subjective age and the association with cognition, subjective wellbeing, and depression. *The Journals of Gerontology, Series B: Psychological Sciences and Social Sciences*. https://doi.org/10.1093/geronb/gbaa069. Advance online publication.

Armitage, R., & Nellumns, L. (2020). Considering inequalities in the school closure response to COVID-19. In *Lancet global health 2020: Correspondence*.

Avendano, M., & Cylus, J. (2019). *Working at older ages: Why it's important, how it affects health, and the policy op.tions to support health capacity for work*. Copenhagen (Denmark): European Observatory on Health Systems and Policies.

Ayalon, L., Chasteen, A., Diehl, M., Levy, B., Neupert, S. D., Rothermund, K., et al. (2020). Aging in times of the COVID-19 pandemic: Avoiding ageism and fostering intergenerational solidarity. *The Journals of Gerontology: Series B*. https://doi.org/10.1093/geronb/gbaa051.

Baker, S., Waycott, J., Robertson, E., Carrasco, R., Neves, B. B., Hampson, R., et al. (2020). Evaluating the use of interactive virtual reality technology with older adults living in residential aged care. *Information Processing & Management*, *57*, 102105. https://doi.org/10.1016/j.ipm.2019.102105.

Banskota, S., Healy, M., & Goldberg, E. M. (2020). 15 smartphone apps for older adults to use while in isolation during the COVID-19 pandemic. *The Western Journal of Emergency Medicine*, *21*, 514–525. https://doi.org/10.5811/westjem.2020.4.47372.

Barber, S. J., & Kim, H. (2020). COVID-19 worries and behavior changes in older and younger men and women. *The Journals of Gerontology: Series B*. https://doi.org/10.1093/geronb/gbaa068, gbaa068.

Bawden, D. (2008). Origins and concepts of digital literacy. In *Vol. 30. Digital literacies: Concepts, policies and practices* (pp. 17–32).

Bleidorn, W., & Schwaba, T. (2018). Retirement is associated with change in self-esteem. *Psychology and Aging*, *33*, 586–594.

Börsch-Supan, A., & Schuth, M. (2014). Early retirement, mental health, and social networks. In *Discoveries in the economics of aging* (pp. 225–250). University of Chicago Press.

Bruine de Bruin, W. (2020). Age differences in COVID-19 risk perceptions and mental health: Evidence from a national US survey conducted in March 2020. *The Journals of Gerontology: Psychological Sciences*. https://doi.org/10.1093/geronb/gbaa074.

Carstensen, L. L. (2006). The influence of a sense of time on human development. *Science*, *312*, 1913–1915. https://doi.org/10.1126/science.1127488.

CDC COVID-19 Response Team. (2020). Severe outcomes among patients with coronavirus disease 2019 (COVID-19)—United States, February 12–March 16, 2020. *MMWR. Morbidity and Mortality Weekly Report*, *69*, 343–346.

Chappell, N. L., & Badger, M. (1989). Social isolation and well-being. *Journal of Gerontology*, *44*, S169–S176.

Charles, S. T. (2010). Strength and vulnerability integration: A model of emotional well-being across adulthood. *Psychological Bulletin*, *136*, 1068–1091.

Choi, S. D., Guo, L., Kang, D., & Xiong, S. (2017). Exergame technology and interactive interventions for elderly fall prevention: A systematic literature review. *Applied Ergonomics*, *65*, 570–581. https://doi.org/10.1016/j.apergo.2016.10.013.

Ciboh, R. (2017). An exploratory study of older adults' social media use and social capital in Nigeria. *Athens Journal of Mass Media and Communications*, *3*, 149–165.

Collom, E. (2008). Engagement of the elderly in time banking: The potential for social capital generation in an aging society. *Journal of Aging & Social Policy*, *20*, 414–436. https://doi.org/10.1080/08959420802186282.

Comas-Herrera, A., Zalakaín, J., Litwin, C., Hsu, A. T., Lane, N., & Fernández, J. L. (2020). *Mortality associated with COVID-19 outbreaks in care homes: Early international evidence*. LTC-covid.org, International Long-Term Care Policy Network.

Cornwell, E. Y., & Waite, L. J. (2009). Social disconnectedness, perceived isolation, and health among older adults. *Journal of Health and Social Behavior*, *50*, 31–48. https://doi.org/10.1177/002214650905000103.

Counsell, S. R., Callahan, C. M., Tu, W., Stump, T. E., & Arling, G. W. (2009). Cost analysis of the geriatric resources for assessment and Care of Elders care management intervention.

Journal of the American Geriatrics Society, 57, 1420–1426. https://doi.org/10.1111/j.1532-5415.2009.02383.x.

De Leo, D., Vichi, M., Kolves, K., & Pompili, M. (2020). Late life suicide in Italy, 1980–2015. *Aging Clinical and Experimental Research, 32*, 465–474.

Dhungel, B., Sugai, M. K., & Gilmour, S. (2019). Trends in suicide mortality by method from 1979 to 2016 in Japan. *International Journal of Environmental Research and Public Health, 16*, 1794. https://doi.org/10.3390/ijerph16101794.

Dunbar, R. I. (2016). Do online social media cut through the constraints that limit the size of offline social networks? *Royal Society Open Science, 3*, 150292. https://doi.org/10.1098/rsos.150292.

Emerson, K. G. (2020). Coping with being cooped up: Social distancing during COVID-19 among 60+ in the United States. *Pan American Journal of Public Health, 44*. https://doi.org/10.26633/RPSP.2020.81, e81.

Fiske, A., Wetherell, J. L., & Gatz, M. (2009). Depression in older adults. *Annual Review of Clinical Psychology, 5*, 363–389. https://doi.org/10.1146/annurev.clinpsy.032408.153621.

Gao, J., Zheng, P., Jia, Y., Chen, H., Mao, Y., Chen, S., et al. (2020). Mental health problems and social media exposure during COVID-19 outbreak. *PLoS One, 15*. https://doi.org/10.1371/journal.pone.0231924, e0231924.

Gould, C. E., & Hantke, N. C. (2020). Promoting technology and virtual visits to improve older adult mental health in the face of COVID-19. *The American Journal of Geriatric Psychiatry, 28*, 889–890.

Grady, C. L., & Craik, F. I. (2000). Changes in memory processing with age. *Current Opinion in Neurobiology, 10*, 224–231.

Greenfield, E. A., & Marks, N. F. (2004). Formal volunteering as a protective factor for older adults' psychological well-being. *The Journals of Gerontology Series B: Psychological Sciences and Social Sciences, 59*, S258–S264. Retrieved from: https://doi.org/10.1093/geronb/59.5.S258.

Hartt, M. (2020). COVID-19: A lonely pandemic. *Cities & Health*, 1–3. https://doi.org/10.1080/23748834.2020.1788770.

Heisel, M. J., Neufeld, E., & Flett, G. L. (2016). Reasons for living, meaning in life, and suicide ideation: Investigating the roles of key positive psychological factors in reducing suicide risk in community-residing older adults. *Aging & Mental Health, 20*, 195–207.

Holmes, E. A., O'Connor, R. C., Perry, V. H., Tracey, I., Wessely, S., Arseneault, L., et al. (2020). Multidisciplinary research priorities for the COVID-19 pandemic: A call for action for mental health science. *The Lancet Psychiatry, 7*, 547–560. https://doi.org/10.1016/S2215-0366(20)30168-1.

Hu, Z., Song, C., Xu, C., Jin, G., Chen, Y., Xu, X., et al. (2020). Clinical characteristics of 24 asymptomatic infections with COVID-19 screened among close contacts in Nanjing, China. *Science China. Life Sciences, 63*, 706–711. https://doi.org/10.1007/s11427-020-1661-4.

Khalaila, R., & Vitman-Schorr, A. (2018). Internet use, social networks, loneliness, and quality of life among adults aged 50 and older: Mediating and moderating effects. *Quality of Life Research, 27*, 479–489.

Kivi, M., Hansson, I., & Bjälkebring, P. (2020). Up and about: Older adults' wellbeing during the COVID-19 pandemic in a Swedish longitudinal study. *The Journals of Gerontology: Series B*. https://doi.org/10.1093/geronb/gbaa084, gbaa084.

Lenhart, A. (2009). *Adults and social network websites*. Washington, DC: Pew Internet & American Life Project. Retrieved from: http://pewinternet.org/Reports=2009=Adults-and-Social-Network-Websites.aspx.

Levy, B. (2009). Stereotype embodiment: A psychosocial approach to aging. *Current Directions in Psychological Science, 18*, 332–336.

Liu, L., Gou, Z., & Zuo, J. (2016). Social support mediates loneliness and depression in elderly people. *Journal of Health Psychology*, *21*, 750–758.

Losada-Baltar, A., Jiménez-Gonzalo, L., Gallego-Alberto, L., Pedroso-Chaparro, M. D. S., Fernandes-Pires, J., & Márquez-González, M. (2020). "We're staying at home". Association of self-perceptions of aging, personal and family resources and loneliness with psychological distress during the lock-down period of COVID-19. *The Journals of Gerontology: Series B*. https://doi.org/10.1093/geronb/gbaa048, gbaa048.

Mækelæ, M. J., Reggev, N., Dutra, N., Tamayo, R. M., Silva-Sobrinho, R. A., Klevjer, K., et al. (2020). Perceived efficacy of COVID-19 restrictions, reactions and their impact on mental health during the early phase of the outbreak in six countries. *Royal Society Open Science*, *7*(8), 200644.

McLaren, S., Gomez, R., Gill, P., & Chesler, J. (2015). Marital status and suicidal ideation among Australian older adults: The mediating role of sense of belonging. *International Psychogeriatrics*, *27*, 145–154.

Momeni, M., Hariri, N., Nobahar, M., & Noshinfard, F. (2018). Barriers and challenges experienced by seniors in using online social networks: A phenomenological study. *Middle East Journal of Rehabilitation and Health*, *5*. https://doi.org/10.5812/mejrh.65310.

Myhre, J. W., Mehl, M. R., & Glisky, E. L. (2017). Cognitive benefits of online social networking for healthy older adults. *The Journals of Gerontology: Series B*, *72*, 752–760. https://doi.org/10.1093/geronb/gbw025.

Pachana, N. A., Beattie, E., Byrne, G. J., & Brodaty, H. (2020). COVID-19 and psychogeriatrics: The view from Australia. *International Psychogeriatrics*, 1–20. https://doi.org/10.1017/S1041610220000885.

Phillips, J. A. (2014). A changing epidemiology of suicide? The influence of birth cohorts on suicide rates in the United States. *Social Science & Medicine*, *114C*, 151–160. https://doi.org/10.1016/j.socscimed.2014.05.038.

Pinquart, M. (2002a). Creating and maintaining purpose in life in old age: A meta-analysis. *Ageing International*, *27*, 90–114.

Pinquart, M. (2002b). Good news about the effects of bad old-age stereotypes. *Experimental Aging Research*, *28*(3), 317–336. https://doi.org/10.1080/03610730290080353.

Pinquart, M., & Sorensen, S. (2001). Influences on loneliness in older adults: A meta-analysis. *Basic and Applied Social Psychology*, *23*, 245–266. https://doi.org/10.1207/S15324834BASP2304_2.

Rook, K. S. (1984). Research on social support, loneliness, and social isolation: Toward an integration. *Review of Personality & Social Psychology*, *5*, 239–264.

Şar, A. H., Göktürk, G. Y., Tura, G., & Kazaz, N. (2012). Is the internet use an effective method to cope with elderly loneliness and decrease loneliness symptom? *Procedia-Social and Behavioral Sciences*, *55*, 1053–1059. https://doi.org/10.1016/j.sbspro.2012.09.597.

Seifert, A., Cotten, S. R., & Xie, B. (2020). A double burden of exclusion? Digital and social exclusion of older adults in times of COVID-19. *The Journals of Gerontology: Series B*. https://doi.org/10.1093/geronb/gbaa098, gbaa098.

Shrira, A., Hoffman, Y., Bodner, E., & Palgi, Y. (2020). COVID-19 related loneliness and psychiatric symptoms among older adults: The buffering role of subjective age. *The American Journal of Geriatric Psychiatry*. https://doi.org/10.1016/j.jagp.2020.05.018.

Sinclair, T. J., & Grieve, R. (2017). Facebook as a source of social connectedness in older adults. *Computers in Human Behavior*, *66*, 363–369. https://doi.org/10.1016/j.chb.2016.10.003.

Smith, A. (2014). *Older adults and technology use: Usage and adoption* (pp. 1–7). Pew Research: Internet Project.

Stanley, M., Moyle, W., Ballantyne, A., Jaworski, K., Corlis, M., Oxlade, D., et al. (2010). 'Nowadays you don't even see your neighbours': Loneliness in the everyday lives of older Australians. *Health & Social Care in the Community*, *18*, 407–414.

Sum, S., Mathews, R. M., Pourghasem, M., & Hughes, I. (2009). Internet use as a predictor of sense of community in older people. *Cyber Psychology & Behavior*, *12*, 235–239.

Teo, A. R., Markwardt, S., & Hinton, L. (2019). Using Skype to beat the blues: Longitudinal data from a national representative sample. *The American Journal of Geriatric Psychiatry*, *27*, 254–262.

Thomas, J., et al. (2017). *Measuring Australia's digital divide: The Australian digital inclusion index 2017*. Melbourne: RMIT University.

Topa, G., & Valero, E. (2017). Preparing for retirement: How self-efficacy and resource threats contribute to retirees' satisfaction, depression, and losses. *European Journal of Work and Organizational Psychology*, *26*, 811–827.

Van Orden, K. A., Cukrowicz, K. C., Witte, T. K., & Joiner, T. E., Jr. (2012). Thwarted belongingness and perceived burdensomeness: Construct validity and psychometric properties of the interpersonal needs questionnaire. *Psychological Assessment*, *24*, 197–215. https://doi.org/10.1037/a0025358.

Vanderhorst, R. K., & McLaren, S. (2005). Social relationships as predictors of depression and suicidal ideation in older adults. *Aging & Mental Health*, *9*, 517–525. https://doi.org/10.1080/13607860500193062.

Vogel, E. A., Rose, J. P., Roberts, L. R., & Eckles, K. (2014). Social comparison, social media, and self-esteem. *Psychology of Popular Media Culture*, *3*, 206–222. https://doi.org/10.1037/ppm0000047.

Wand, A. P. F., Zhong, B. L., Chiu, H. F. K., Draper, B., & De Leo, D. (2020). Covid-19: The implications for suicide in older adults. *International Psychogeriatrics*, 1–16. https://doi.org/10.1017/S1041610220000770.

Wilber, K. H., & Reynolds, S. L. (1997). Introducing a framework for defining financial abuse of the elderly. *Journal of Elder Abuse & Neglect*, *8*, 61–80.

World Health Organization. (2018). *Ageing and health*. Retrieved 10 May 2019, from: https://www.who.int/news-room/fact-sheets/detail/ageing-and-health.

World Health Organization. (2020). https://covid19.who.int [Accessed 8 July, 2020].

Wu, B. (2020). Social isolation and loneliness among older adults in the context of COVID-19: A global challenge. *Global Health Research and Policy*, *5*, 1–3. https://doi.org/10.1186/s41256-020-00154-3.

Chapter 8

Social isolation as a laboratory model of depression

Gunes Unal
Behavioral Neuroscience Laboratory, Department of Psychology, Boğaziçi University, Istanbul, Turkey

Introduction: Social isolation as a laboratory model of depression

Chronic social isolation in humans, whether self-imposed or enforced, appears as a striking environmental condition that can be compared to the absence of basic physiological needs such as water, food, or sleep. Social isolation refers to a significantly diminished number of interpersonal interactions or a complete lack of any interaction. An adult person goes through an average of 12 social interactions per day according to a 2018 study on a comprehensive American sample (Zhaoyang, Sliwinski, Martire, & Smyth, 2018). These refer to in-person interactions that may take place in the household, workplace, or public space. Modern life contains several elaborate types of interpersonal interaction (Goffman, 1990). Social interactions are not only central to human life, but constitute the daily routine for several other species.

This chapter starts with a global definition of sociality, the tendency to engage in social interactions. I discuss how the negative effects of social isolation for an animal depend on the degree of sociality of that species. After reviewing the species-specific responses to isolation, I differentiate self-imposed isolation from enforced social isolation. The latter has been experienced by millions of people across the globe during the COVID-19 pandemic. It has also been utilized as a laboratory model of chronic stress for nonhuman primates and rodents. I review the behavioral and physiological effects of social isolation, and discuss the wide-range use of isolation as a laboratory model of depression.

In Maslow's famous model of human motivation, the five-stage hierarchy of needs, social needs such as love and belongingness occupy the middle (third) level (Maslow, 1943, 1954). According to this theory, the absence of social interaction cannot to be compared to the deficiency of physiological needs such as water, food, and sleep in terms of its immediate effects. The long-term effects of chronic social isolation, in contrast, can be devastating. Interpersonal

Mental Health Effects of COVID-19. https://doi.org/10.1016/B978-0-12-824289-6.00005-2

interaction occupies a core part in the human sociality as detailed later. Hence, the complete lack of it for a long period of time, as in solitary confinement, is associated with cognitive decline and several psychopathologies.

In order to appreciate the psychobiological significance of social interaction in humans, one does not need to observe the severe consequences of chronic (total) social isolation, as the early monkey studies revealed with precision (Harlow, Dodsworth, & Harlow, 1965). Irrespective of the actual level of isolation an individual experiences, the perception of social isolation is sufficient to produce serious negative results (Cacioppo & Hawkley, 2009). The relationship between loneliness, defined as the distress emerging from lack of a desired level of social interaction or connection, and health is well established in the literature (Heinrich & Gullone, 2006; House, Landis, & Umberson, 1988). Meta-analyses indicate a strong correlation between loneliness and cancer (Deckx, van den Akker, & Buntinx, 2014), cardiovascular disease (Valtorta, Kanaan, Gilbody, Ronzi, & Hanratty, 2016), dementia (Kuiper et al., 2015), psychosis (Michalska da Rocha, Rhodes, Vasilopoulou, & Hutton, 2018), and of course, depression (Erzen & Çikrikci, 2018). Recent work focused on loneliness as a major outcome of the COVID-19 pandemic and associated psychopathologies (Giallonardo et al., 2020; Killgore, Cloonan, Taylor, & Dailey, 2020; Tull et al., 2020). With these data at hand, loneliness, that is mere perception of social isolation, emerges as a risk factor for mortality (Holt-Lunstad, Smith, Baker, Harris, & Stephenson, 2015; Holt-Lunstad, Smith, & Layton, 2010).

The aforementioned research on humans, whether utilizing a longitudinal design, clinical correlations, or meta-analysis, reveals little about the physiological and neurological consequences of social isolation. These often require laboratory work with animal models. Then the question is species specificity of the versatile negative effects of actual or perceived social isolation. Species specificity refers to characteristic biological properties or behaviors of a species. These include any kind of feature that distinguishes one species from another. Different animals can show different types or levels of response to social isolation as part of their species-specific properties. Sociality, the biological tendency to associate with conspecifics, defines the species-specific meaning and outcomes of social isolation (Eisenberg, 1966). For this reason, how depressed an individual organism will be following a long period of social isolation depends on the *normal* social behavior of that organism. Linking the detailed biological findings of animal isolation studies to the correlational data from clinical research depends on the cross-species commonalities of social isolation as well as the distinctive features of human sociality.

Sociality and the meaning of isolation

The COVID-19 pandemic forced millions of people across the globe to self-isolate for the first time in their lives, creating a novel and devastating feeling of boredom. This global experience reminded us the centrality of social interaction in our lives. Being a key notion for human beings, we often consider other animals to share our strong need for social interaction. As such, we have an anthropomorphic tendency (Epley, Waytz, & Cacioppo, 2007) with regards to the sociality and isolation of other animals. How terrible must it be for all those animals that are kept in social isolation by humans either as pets or zoo residents? This question, naïve as it may seem, constitutes a key subject in ethology. Human beings are *social animals* that possess a strong need for social interaction and, thus, a high level of sociality. Still, the highest degree of sociality, known as eusociality (Wilson, 1971), is often observed in certain types of insects like the termites, ants, bees, and wasps (Sherman, Lacey, Reeve, & Keller, 1995). The criteria to be considered eusocial include living in large groups, having a collective care for babies, and possessing a division of labor in reproduction (i.e., not allowing every member to reproduce) (Wilson, 1971). Other insects, and yet other animals, would be categorized as presocial, quasisocial, subsocial, or parasocial based on how much an individual organism tends to associate with conspecifics (Costa, 2018). This rather complex scientific terminology of sociality emerges as a result of the variability of social behavior and different degrees of sociality in the animal kingdom (Costa & Fitzgerald, 1996; Dew, Tierney, & Schwarz, 2016).

Careful observation of other animals indicates that not all animals are as gregarious as humans (Alcock, 2001). The aforementioned question on pitying a caged animal may be flawed, that is irrelevant, depending on the species (Lorenz, 2002). For human beings, the answer is obvious and would not require a global trend in self-isolation due to a pandemic. Solitary confinement is a substantially severe type of imprisonment with several psychopathological effects in the long term (Grassian, 1983; Grassian & Friedman, 1986). While the highly social nature of human beings is well established, there is still a debate on the exact degree of their sociality and whether they can be considered eusocial, possessing the highest level of social organization observed in nature (Foster & Ratnieks, 2005; Wilson & Hölldobler, 2005).

The degree of sociality of a species is assessed by observation of social behavior under normal conditions and is a reflection of the evolutionary, that is *biological*, need for sociality. Social behaviors, by definition, have evolved to provide a better chance for survival, just like other forms of animal behavior, emotions, and instincts (Bailey & Moore, 2018; Nowak, 2006; Rubenstein & Abbot, 2017). The *psychological* need for sociality, however, may not easily be understood under normal conditions within the habitat of a species. Social isolation constitutes the paradigm for testing this kind of mental need for sociality. The metabolic, physiological, and psychological effects of long-term enforced social isolation vary between different species, and these negative effects do not show a simple, linear correlation between the degree of sociality (Bailey & Moore, 2018).

With regards to interspecies differences in social behavior and the need for sociality, it must be remembered that *social stress*, the type of stress emerging in the presence of an unfamiliar conspecific, can be as distressing as social isolation. This phenomenon, also observed/assessed in humans (Kirschbaum, Pirke, & Hellhammer, 1993), develops with the opposite environmental conditions. The presence, as opposed to absence, of social interaction may also be a source of significant distress (Masis-Calvo et al., 2018; Tamashiro, Nguyen, & Sakai, 2005). Confrontation studies that introduce an animal to a new cage with unknown same-sex conspecifics to induce social stress have documented the versatile negative effects in guinea pigs (Sachser & Lick, 1989) as well as rats and mice (Koolhaas, de Boer, Buwalda, & Meerlo, 2016; Koolhaas, De Boer, De Rutter, Meerlo, & Sgoifo, 1997). Like the distress created by chronic social isolation, social stress can induce pathological alterations in several biological processes including immune functions (Bartolomucci, 2007; Takahashi, Flanigan, McEwen, & Russo, 2018).

Laboratory rodents and humans share numerous common features in relation to sociality. In both species, a relatively long-term isolation period is associated with cognitive decline and different health problems (Kappeler, Cremer, & Nunn, 2015). This chapter reviews the validity and reliability of social isolation as a laboratory model of depression in relation to its effects in humans, a subject of study which attracted substantial attention with the COVID-19 pandemic.

Defining social isolation

The classical definition of social isolation refers to the absence of sensory stimuli from conspecifics. These could include visual stimuli such as one's image, auditory or acoustic cues such as spoken language or species-specific alarm signals, tactile, and olfactory stimuli (Kim & Kirkpatrick, 1996). This objective definition is sufficient when there is no external social stimulus. It does not, however, incorporate the interspecies differences in the degree of sociality. As described before, certain animals show, and require, substantially more social interaction than others.

For some species, a complete absence of social stimuli is not needed to create (the perception of) social isolation. Differences in social behavior and the differential stress responses to isolation across the animal kingdom require an overarching definition that can account for all species. As an alternative to the classical definition based on the mere frequency of socially relevant sensory stimuli, social isolation was proposed to be calculated with an index of social interaction incorporating the population parameters (Bailey & Moore, 2018). According to this functional theory, social isolation must be assessed by comparing an individual's social interaction to an ideal, that is optimal, level of social interaction within a population (Bailey & Moore, 2018). This framework defines social interaction in relation to the evolutionary or ecological *fitness* of the organism, describing how well an individual adapts to its environment (Hawkley & Capitanio, 2015).

It is known that the same idea holds true for human beings. Social isolation cannot be defined merely based on how much time an individual spends avoiding conspecifics, that is the deviation from mean frequency of interaction within the population. Social isolation, as a by-product of evolution, has an impact on fitness traits, which leads to the interindividual variation in seeking isolation (Hawkley & Capitanio, 2015). The psychological effects of isolation vary across people even following long-term solitary confinement (Grassian, 1983; Grassian & Friedman, 1986).

Social isolation can be enforced by an external force or self-imposed by the organism. The former constitutes a potent laboratory model of despair for several animals. In the lab, isolation of an animal is enforced by the experimenter, as governments or local authorities enforced people to self-isolate during the COVID-19 pandemic. Self-imposed isolation, in which the organism isolates itself without any external order or force, is also designated as social isolation. Why would an organism, human, or other animal would want to self-isolate? The answer, once again, relies in our evolutionary heritage.

Social isolation is a natural process emerging as a consequence of evolutionary needs. It has been inherited, like many other physiological and psychological features, through generations of interaction with conspecifics as well the surrounding environment (Bailey & Moore, 2018; Nowak, 2006). Social isolation is not only a product, but also a determinant of evolutionary dynamics via natural selection. Animals that are isolated from their conspecifics influence evolution in several ways. Social isolation inhibits evolution by decreasing the chances for sexual selection (see Judge, 2010). It may also lead to cryptic genetic variation, a latent form of genetic variation that is expressed under abnormal conditions (Paaby & Rockman, 2014). This, in contrast, would potentiate evolution by providing a rapid evolutionary change (Bailey & Moore, 2018). The strong desire for solitude and self-imposed long-term isolation in humans, as observed in certain hermits and other recluses, should be evaluated with this evolutionary perspective (see Boyd, Rubin, & Wessely, 2012).

Self-imposed/voluntary vs. enforced isolation

Doing something voluntarily and being forced to do the same thing often lead to different psychological effects, even when the action is highly desirable (Lewes, 1877). This difference between voluntary and involuntary activity is well studied in the laboratory for motor actions by using running wheels. Voluntary and forced treadmill running in rodents have different physiological effects especially in relation to the recovery after hemorrhagic stroke (Auriat, Grams, Yan, & Colbourne, 2006; Hayes et al., 2008; Ke, Yip, Li, Zheng, & Tong, 2011; Sato et al., 2020). This does not mean that forced exercise does no good or is always less effective than voluntary locomotor activity. While both were reported to be equally effective in attenuating cognitive impairment in an animal model of vascular dementia (Lin et al., 2015), forced, but not voluntary, exercise was found to reduce infarct volume in another study (Hayes et al., 2008). These results do not directly translate to other forms of activity or state. Locomotor activity has substantial ameliorative effects on health (Dunn, Trivedi, Kampert, Clark, & Chambliss, 2005; Niemann, Godde, Staudinger, & Voelcker-Rehage, 2014), which can merely shadow the potential negative effects rising from the forced nature of an involuntary task. Studies that identify the negative effects of forced running, however, can reflect the physiological outcome of the involuntariness component. The different physiological outcomes of voluntary and involuntary forms of a seemingly mechanical activity, that is exercise, can be useful to understand the differential effects of enforced vs. voluntary isolation.

To my knowledge, there is no laboratory model to test the specific physiological effects of the "voluntary" dimension of self-isolation in terms of its physiological effects, as typical laboratory rodents would not normally choose to be isolated like most humans. The differential psychological effects of voluntary vs. involuntary isolation cannot be revealed either. It is important to remember that voluntary self-isolation is very rare in human beings, as compared to other mammals (Eisenberg, 1966).

The Novel Coronavirus Disease (COVID-19), declared a pandemic by the World Health Organization in March 2020, constitutes the most novel and recent example of enforced human isolation. The so-called self-isolation during this worldwide incident would not occur without the official warnings and emergency regulations of the involved authorities. Self-isolation as a personal precaution may appear as an autonomous decision if not enforced by a ruling authority. However, these decisions are still enforced by the environment, the pandemic, and cannot be compared to the aforementioned forms of monastic living that constitute self-chosen social isolation (Boyd et al., 2012). Social isolation of humans can not only be categorized as enforced as in solitary confinement or self-chosen, but observed with different levels of intention, as it became clear during COVID-19 (Farooq, Laato, & Islam, 2020). Furthermore, perceived social isolation, that is a strong feeling of loneliness, also leads to varying levels of hormonal and neuronal alterations (Cacioppo, Cacioppo, Capitanio, & Cole, 2015; Cacioppo, Capitanio, & Cacioppo, 2014). The motivation for reclusion can be medical (i.e., quarantine) as observed in 2020, political or religious with varying degree of intentionality (Boyd et al., 2012).

The behavioral effects of social isolation

The classical monkey social isolation study by Harlow et al. (1965) showed that 3 months of total social isolation or a prolonged period of semi-isolation in newborn monkeys is sufficient to produce highly fearful or aggressive behaviors, which were termed by the authors as "social damage." These animals were isolated during the *critical period* for developing social behavior (Scott, 1958). Strikingly, two out of six monkeys in the 3-month total isolation group developed anorexia, a severe loss of appetite, following termination of isolation, and one animal died for refusing to eat. Early social isolation studies in monkeys revealed several other negative consequences, including emergence of severe psychopathologies, including abnormal fear responses, hyperaggression (Mitchell, 1968; Suomi, Harlow, & Kimball, 1971). Similar observations of abnormal affective behavior, described as *isolation syndrome*, were also observed in rats (Hatch et al., 1965; Hatch, Wiberg, Balazs, & Grice, 1963).

This research gave rise to utilization of social isolation as a general psychopathology model. In different studies, the effects of various social isolation paradigms have been associated with schizophrenia (Geyer, Wilkinson, Humby, & Robbins, 1993; Wilkinson et al., 1994), hyperactivity and attention deficit hyperactive disorder (ADHD) (Einon & Morgan, 1978; Gentsch, Lichtsteiner, Frischknecht, Feer, & Siegfried, 1988; Matsumoto, Fujiwara, Araki, & Yabe, 2019), autism (Burrows et al., 2017; Matsumoto et al., 2019), alcoholism (Roske, Baeger, Frenzel, & Oehme, 1994), drug abuse (Jones, Marsden, & Robbins, 1990), and anxiety (Weiss, Pryce, Jongen-Rêlo, Nanz-Bahr, & Feldon, 2004; Zorzo, Méndez-López, Méndez, & Arias, 2019). Rodent isolation was then proposed as a model for anxiety (Parker & Morinan, 1986).

Another particular psychopathology, depression, also attracted significant scientific attention in relation to social isolation. With its versatile behavioral outcomes on various cognitive and affective tasks, social isolation became a widespread laboratory model of depression (Jesberger & Richardson, 1985). Its consequences were found to be comparable to the behavioral despair induced in the forced swim test (Jaffe, De Frias, & Ibarra, 1993), the gold standard rodent model of clinical depression (Unal & Canbeyli, 2019). Unlike the majority of neuroscientific research, the relationship between social isolation and depression-like behavior in rodents was also tested and confirmed in female animals (Martin & Brown, 2010). Furthermore, in a mouse study, even a 12-h isolation paradigm led to behavioral despair in the forced swim test (Takatsu-Coleman et al., 2013), indicating acute social isolation as a separate despair model emerging via distinct neuronal and hormonal mechanisms (Shahar-Gold, Gur, & Wagner, 2013).

In addition to its affective outcomes, social isolation in the laboratory led to observable cognitive consequences. Isolated rearing in monkeys leads to diminished performance in learning tasks that involve object recognition and discrimination (Sánchez, Hearn, Do, Rilling, & Herndon, 1998). Later research in rodents revealed impaired spatial working memory (Zorzo et al., 2019) and reversal learning performance, indicating cognitive rigidity and deficits in rule learning (Jones, Marsden, & Robbins, 1991). Similar results were observed in humans with substantially fewer social connections, even when they are not in a state of total isolation. Gerontological studies revealed that elderly people with few social contacts are more likely to display global cognitive decline (Ellwardt, Van Tilburg, & Aartsen, 2015; Lee & Kim, 2016). In line with the laboratory findings, social isolation in elderly people was correlated with impairments in working memory (McGue & Christensen, 2007). Hippocampus-dependent episodic memory performance was also impaired in socially isolated seniors (Klaming, Annese, Veltman, & Comijs, 2017; Mousavi-Nasab, Kormi-Nouri, & Nilsson, 2014). These results are not surprising as the strong association between cognitive competence, which refers to creative thinking and problem solving skills, and depression is well established by clinical (Channon, Baker, & Robertson, 1993), correlational (Burt, Zembar, & Niederehe, 1995), functional imaging (Eugène, Joormann, Cooney, Atlas, & Gotlib, 2010), and animal studies (Atesyakar, Canbeyli, & Unal, 2020). Indeed, a cognitive model of depression has been developed by Beck (1967) more than 50 years ago (also see Beck, 2008).

Reversing the devastating effects of social isolation, especially the apparent depressed state, emerged as the next major research question since the early monkey isolation studies. Imipramine, a tricyclic antidepressant (TCA), was proved useful (Suomi, Seaman, Lewis, DeLizio, & McKinney Jr, 1978). Interestingly, the most successful attempt was to use other (healthy) monkeys, designated therapist monkeys as a form of rehabilitation (Suomi, Harlow, & McKinney, 1972). Later research in rodents found several other antidepressants, including fluoxetine, to be effective in isolation-induced despair (Martin & Brown, 2010). The therapeutic effects of antidepressants on the isolation-led behavioral despair in animals strengthen the face validity of social isolation as a laboratory model of clinical depression.

The physiological effects of social isolation

The versatile psychological effects of social isolation point to pathological alterations in several systems of the body. Research revealed long-term isolation to cause substantial changes in neuroendocrine and immune functions in addition to its neuroanatomical and neurophysiological effects, leading to dysfunction in different neuronal circuits/pathways. Not surprisingly, many of these systems that are summarized as follows are also involved in the pathophysiology of depression (Krishnan & Nestler, 2008; Nestler et al., 2002). In this regard, one particular correlation is noteworthy to mention: clinical depression has been associated with higher mortality rates by several studies (Machado et al., 2018). Similarly, increased mortality, derived from long-term correlation studies, do not only emerge as a result of social isolation, but also loneliness (Holt-Lunstad et al., 2010; Steptoe, Shankar, Demakakos, & Wardle, 2013).

Disrupted immune functions are well-documented consequences of social isolation (Bartolomucci, 2007). Human social isolation and loneliness lead to heightened inflammatory responses (Cole et al., 2007; Steptoe, Owen, Kunz-Ebrecht, & Brydon, 2004). These are accompanied with different metabolic, neuroendocrine, and cardiovascular problems (Caspi, Harrington, Moffitt, Milne, & Poulton, 2006; Steptoe et al., 2004). Postweaning isolation in rats leads to HPA axis hyperfunction, observed as substantially elevated levels of ACTH and corticosterone in response to stress in male rats (Weiss et al., 2004) and impairs glucocorticoid-mediated negative feedback in response to acute stress (Boero et al., 2018). Furthermore, altered glucocorticoid levels in social isolation are correlated with the coping strategy (see Unal & Canbeyli, 2019) in the forced swim test (Vargas, Junco, Gomez, & Lajud, 2016). The association between HPA axis reactivity and depression is also observed in humans: loneliness is positively correlated with increased HPA axis function (Doane & Adam, 2010; Nowland, Robinson, Bradley, Summers, & Qualter, 2018). Interestingly, similar to the aforementioned rodent study on the differential relationship between isolation-led glucocorticoid levels and coping strategy in the forced swim test (Vargas et al., 2016), HPA axis activation in humans is differentially correlated with different types of depression. Clinically high levels of CRH are observed in atypical depression, whereas a down-regulated HPA axis activity and a resultant deficiency in CRH underlie melancholic depression (Gold & Chrousos, 2002).

Dysfunction of the HPA axis is accompanied by disruptions in the oxidative/nitrosative stress pathway (Filipović, Todorović, Bernardi, & Gass, 2017; Gądek-Michalska, Tadeusz, Bugajski, & Bugajski, 2019). In addition to dysfunction in neuronal pathways, a number of region-specific neuroanatomical alterations were discovered in animal models of isolation. Studies that incorporate social deprivation in monkeys revealed decreased dendritic arborization in Layer IV neurons of the motor cortex (Struble & Riesen, 1978) and Purkinje cells of the cerebellum (Floeter & Greenough, 1979). These early results, however, may also reflect the neuronal consequences of decreased locomotor activity rather than a lack of social interaction. Subsequent research in rodents pinpointed to another cortical region, the prefrontal cortex, as the foremost neuroanatomical target of isolation. Mice placed in postweaning isolation for 2 to 8 weeks in different studies showed significantly decreased myelin thickness in the prefrontal cortex due to oligodendrocyte dysfunction (Liu et al., 2012; Makinodan, Rosen, Ito, & Corfas, 2012). Morphological and other cellular changes were also observed in astrocytes (Sun et al., 2017) and principal neurons (i.e., pyramidal cells) (Yamamuro et al., 2018) of the prefrontal cortex.

Cellular level alterations in the prefrontal cortex are accompanied by pathological changes in its synaptic inputs, especially the mesocortical dopaminergic pathway (Blanc et al., 1980). Dopaminergic neurons that constitute the so-called *reward pathway* of the mammalian brain respond to social isolation (Matthews et al., 2016). Significantly lower levels of dopamine immunoreactivity were revealed in the neocortex and striatum of monkeys reared in total isolation for 9 months. No such difference was observed in the amygdala, the bed nucleus of the stria terminalis and basal forebrain, pointing to a selective reduction in dopaminergic innervation of the cortico-striatal circuitry (Martin, Spicer, Lewis, Gluck, & Cork, 1991). Later microdialysis studies in rats showed that long-term social isolation following weaning (postnatal day 21) led to several synaptic alterations in the dopaminergic system of the striatum (Hall et al., 1998) and the medial prefrontal cortex (Leng, Feldon, & Ferger, 2004). A more recent electrophysiological study showed that isolated rearing in rats led to an heightened dopamine terminal function in ex vivo slice recordings (Yorgason et al., 2016). Psychostimulant potency in the striatum was enhanced by social isolation in the same study, pinpointing to the potential neuronal link between isolation-induced depression and drug abuse (Yorgason et al., 2016). Social isolation of rats during their adolescent transition period (postnatal day 23 to 77) was sufficient to decrease dopamine D2 receptor expression in the prefrontal cortex (Fitzgerald, Mackie, & Pickel, 2013).

Pathological alterations in the dopaminergic system were also discovered following acute social isolation. Dopaminergic neurons of the dorsal raphe nucleus were discovered to be sensitive to acute isolation in mice (Matthews et al., 2016). Not surprisingly, increased synaptic dopamine levels have been observed during introduction of conspecifics at the end of an isolation period (Robinson, Heien, & Wightman, 2002). These studies altogether identify disrupted dopaminergic innervation of the prefrontal cortex, as a major component of isolation pathophysiology. Since dysfunction of the dopaminergic system constitutes a key factor in the etiology of clinical depression and underlies psychomotor symptoms of the disease (Unal & Canbeyli, 2019), the mesocortical pathway emerges as a key link between social isolation and depression.

Conclusion: The uniquely human aspect of social isolation

This chapter reviewed the basic evolutionary, psychological, and physiological aspects of social isolation, and its wide-range use as a laboratory model of depression. Some of these features are shared by several species while others cannot be generalized. Some animals including giant pandas, polar bears, jaguars, and blue whales are generally solitary, displaying true self-isolation in their habitat. As such, social isolation would not constitute a despair model for them. Nobel laureate ethologist Konrad Lorenz spent a lifetime observing and comparing social interactions of different species, expressing that the "state of mind, common to human prisoners, called boredom" (p. 54, Lorenz, 2002) is not a common feature of the animal kingdom, but shared by some monkeys, apes, and parrots, against our anthropological tendency to attribute our own drives and emotions to other animals. Boredom is the key emotion and state behind the effects of social isolation. It is not unique to human beings, but appears to be a fundamental human experience, as much as depression is a complex human psychopathology.

As surveyed in this chapter, numerous equivalent findings from clinical and longitudinal human studies as well as the laboratory work on other animals revealed social isolation as a major cause of depression. The use of social isolation in other animals as a despair model would depend on their regular sociality, that is to say how much boredom isolation would create. Rhesus monkeys and common laboratory rodents that share several biological and psychological properties with humans suffer similarly from long-term isolation. Social isolation, in this respect, is a solid model of depression for animals that are similar to humans in terms of their need for interaction with conspecifics. The devastating psychological consequences of COVID-19 precautions affected millions of people across the globe, reminding us of our deep urge for social interaction. It is likely that many humans will develop, or already have developed, depression as a result of the enforced social isolation procedures. Several new lines of research are currently investigating the effects of COVID-19 on mood and anxiety disorders, and related psychological phenomena (see Castelli, Di Tella, Benfante, & Romeo, 2020; Fofana et al., 2020; Giallonardo et al., 2020; Killgore et al., 2020; Tang et al., 2020; Tu, He, & Zhou, 2020; Tull et al., 2020). Future research may differentiate the role of social isolation from other psychological effects of COVID-19 (i.e., pandemic stress/fear) in postpandemic psychopathologies. Considering the psychosocial (Barbalet, 1999; Vodanovich & Kass, 1990) and cultural factors (Brissett & Snow, 1993) linking sociality and boredom in human life, and the recent isolation experience of the COVID-19 pandemic, social isolation emerges as a *human* model of depression more than anything.

References

Alcock, J. (2001). *Animal behavior: An evolutionary approach* (7th ed.). Sunderland, MA, USA: Sinauer Associates.

Atesyakar, N., Canbeyli, R., & Unal, G. (2020). Low cognitive competence as a vulnerability factor for behavioral despair in rats. *Behavioural Processes, 174*. https://doi.org/10.1016/j.beproc.2020.104103, 104103.

Auriat, A. M., Grams, J. D., Yan, R. H., & Colbourne, F. (2006). Forced exercise does not improve recovery after hemorrhagic stroke in rats. *Brain Research, 1109*(1), 183–191. https://doi.org/10.1016/j.brainres.2006.06.035.

Bailey, N. W., & Moore, A. J. (2018). Evolutionary consequences of social isolation. *Trends in Ecology & Evolution, 33*(8), 595–607. https://doi.org/10.1016/j.tree.2018.05.008.

Barbalet, J. M. (1999). Boredom and social meaning. *The British Journal of Sociology, 50*(4), 631–646. https://doi.org/10.1111/j.1468-4446.1999.00631.x.

Bartolomucci, A. (2007). Social stress, immune functions and disease in rodents. *Frontiers in Neuroendocrinology, 28*(1), 28–49. https://doi.org/10.1016/j.yfrne.2007.02.001.

Beck, A. T. (1967). *Depression: Clinical, experimental, and theoretical aspects*. Hoeber Medical Division, Harper & Row.

Beck, A. T. (2008). The evolution of the cognitive model of depression and its neurobiological correlates. *American Journal of Psychiatry, 165*(8), 969–977.

Blanc, G., Hervé, D., Simon, H., Lisoprawski, A., Glowinski, J., & Tassin, J. P. (1980). Response to stress of mesocortico-frontal dopaminergic neurones in rats after long-term isolation. *Nature*. https://doi.org/10.1038/284265a0.

Boero, G., Pisu, M. G., Biggio, F., Muredda, L., Carta, G., Banni, S., et al. (2018). Impaired glucocorticoid-mediated HPA axis negative feedback induced by juvenile social isolation in male rats. *Neuropharmacology, 133*, 242–253. https://doi.org/10.1016/j.neuropharm.2018.01.045.

Boyd, I., Rubin, G., & Wessely, S. (2012). Taking refuge from modernity: 21st century hermits. *Journal of the Royal Society of Medicine, 105*(12), 523–529. https://doi.org/10.1258/jrsm.2012.120060.

Brissett, D., & Snow, R. P. (1993). Boredom: Where the future isn't. *Symbolic Interaction*, *16*(3), 237–256. https://doi.org/10.1525/si.1993.16.3.237.

Burrows, E. L., Eastwood, A. F., May, C., Kolbe, S. C., Hill, T., McLachlan, N. M., et al. (2017). Social isolation alters social and mating behavior in the R451C neuroligin mouse model of autism. *Neural Plasticity*, *2017*, 8361290. https://doi.org/10.1155/2017/8361290.

Burt, D. B., Zembar, M. J., & Niederehe, G. (1995). Depression and memory impairment: A meta-analysis of the association, its pattern, and specificity. *Psychological Bulletin*. https://doi.org/10.1037/0033-2909.117.2.285.

Cacioppo, J. T., Cacioppo, S., Capitanio, J. P., & Cole, S. W. (2015). The neuroendocrinology of social isolation. *Annual Review of Psychology*, *66*(1), 733–767. https://doi.org/10.1146/annurev-psych-010814-015240.

Cacioppo, J. T., & Hawkley, L. C. (2009). Perceived social isolation and cognition. *Trends in Cognitive Sciences*, *13*(10), 447–454. https://doi.org/10.1016/j.tics.2009.06.005.

Cacioppo, S., Capitanio, J. P., & Cacioppo, J. T. (2014). Toward a neurology of loneliness. *Psychological Bulletin*, *140*(6), 1464–1504. https://doi.org/10.1037/a0037618.

Caspi, A., Harrington, H., Moffitt, T. E., Milne, B. J., & Poulton, R. (2006). Socially isolated children 20 years later: Risk of cardiovascular disease. *Archives of Pediatrics & Adolescent Medicine*, *160*(8), 805–811. https://doi.org/10.1001/archpedi.160.8.805.

Castelli, L., Di Tella, M., Benfante, A., & Romeo, A. (2020). The spread of COVID-19 in the Italian population: Anxiety, depression, and post-traumatic stress symptoms. *Canadian Journal of Psychiatry. Revue Canadienne de Psychiatrie*. https://doi.org/10.1177/0706743720938598, 706743720938598.

Channon, S., Baker, J. E., & Robertson, M. M. (1993). Working memory in clinical depression: An experimental study. *Psychological Medicine*, *23*(1), 87–91. https://doi.org/10.1017/s0033291700038873.

Cole, S. W., Hawkley, L. C., Arevalo, J. M., Sung, C. Y., Rose, R. M., & Cacioppo, J. T. (2007). Social regulation of gene expression in human leukocytes. *Genome Biology*, *8*(9), R189. https://doi.org/10.1186/gb-2007-8-9-r189.

Costa, J. T. (2018). The other insect societies: Overview and new directions. *Current Opinion in Insect Science*, *28*, 40–49. https://doi.org/10.1016/j.cois.2018.04.008.

Costa, J. T., & Fitzgerald, T. D. (1996). Developments in social terminology: Semantic battles in a conceptual war. *Trends in Ecology & Evolution*, *11*(7), 285–289. https://doi.org/10.1016/0169-5347(96)10035-5.

Deckx, L., van den Akker, M., & Buntinx, F. (2014). Risk factors for loneliness in patients with cancer: A systematic literature review and meta-analysis. *European Journal of Oncology Nursing*, *18*(5), 466–477. https://doi.org/10.1016/j.ejon.2014.05.002.

Dew, R. M., Tierney, S. M., & Schwarz, M. P. (2016). Social evolution and casteless societies: Needs for new terminology and a new evolutionary focus. *Insectes Sociaux*, *63*(1), 5–14. https://doi.org/10.1007/s00040-015-0435-1.

Doane, L. D., & Adam, E. K. (2010). Loneliness and cortisol: Momentary, day-to-day, and trait associations. *Psychoneuroendocrinology*, *35*(3), 430–441. https://doi.org/10.1016/j.psyneuen.2009.08.005.

Dunn, A. L., Trivedi, M. H., Kampert, J. B., Clark, C. G., & Chambliss, H. O. (2005). Exercise treatment for depression: Efficacy and dose response. *American Journal of Preventive Medicine*, *28*(1), 1–8. https://doi.org/10.1016/j.amepre.2004.09.003.

Einon, D. F., & Morgan, M. J. (1978). Early isolation produces enduring hyperactivity in the rat, but no effect upon spontaneous alternation. *The Quarterly Journal of Experimental Psychology*. https://doi.org/10.1080/14640747808400663.

Eisenberg, J. F. (1966). *The social organization of mammals/J.F. Eisenberg*. Berlin: Walter de Gruyter.

Ellwardt, L., Van Tilburg, T. G., & Aartsen, M. J. (2015). The mix matters: Complex personal networks relate to higher cognitive functioning in old age. *Social Science & Medicine, 125*, 107–115. https://doi.org/10.1016/j.socscimed.2014.05.007.

Epley, N., Waytz, A., & Cacioppo, J. T. (2007). On seeing human: A three-factor theory of anthropomorphism. *Psychological Review*. https://doi.org/10.1037/0033-295X.114.4.864. Epley, Nicholas: University of Chicago, 5807 South Woodlawn Avenue, Chicago, IL, US, 60637, epley@chicagogsb.edu: American Psychological Association.

Erzen, E., & Çikrikci, Ö. (2018). The effect of loneliness on depression: A meta-analysis. *International Journal of Social Psychiatry, 64*(5), 427–435. https://doi.org/10.1177/0020764018776349.

Eugène, F., Joormann, J., Cooney, R. E., Atlas, L. Y., & Gotlib, I. H. (2010). Neural correlates of inhibitory deficits in depression. *Psychiatry Research: Neuroimaging, 181*(1), 30–35. https://doi.org/10.1016/j.pscychresns.2009.07.010.

Farooq, A., Laato, S., & Islam, A. K. M. N. (2020). Impact of online information on self-isolation intention during the COVID-19 pandemic: Cross-sectional study. *Journal of Medical Internet Research, 22*(5), e19128. https://doi.org/10.2196/19128.

Filipović, D., Todorović, N., Bernardi, R. E., & Gass, P. (2017). Oxidative and nitrosative stress pathways in the brain of socially isolated adult male rats demonstrating depressive- and anxiety-like symptoms. *Brain Structure and Function, 222*(1), 1–20. https://doi.org/10.1007/s00429-016-1218-9.

Fitzgerald, M. L., Mackie, K., & Pickel, V. M. (2013). The impact of adolescent social isolation on dopamine D2 and cannabinoid CB1 receptors in the adult rat prefrontal cortex. *Neuroscience, 235*, 40–50. https://doi.org/10.1016/j.neuroscience.2013.01.021.

Floeter, M. K., & Greenough, W. T. (1979). Cerebellar plasticity: Modification of Purkinje cell structure by differential rearing in monkeys. *Science, 206*(4415), 227–229. https://doi.org/10.1126/science.113873.

Fofana, N. K., Latif, F., Sarfraz, S., Bilal, Bashir, M. F., & Komal, B. (2020). Fear and agony of the pandemic leading to stress and mental illness: An emerging crisis in the novel coronavirus (COVID-19) outbreak. *Psychiatry Research*. https://doi.org/10.1016/j.psychres.2020.113230. Ireland.

Foster, K. R., & Ratnieks, F. L. W. (2005). A new eusocial vertebrate? *Trends in Ecology & Evolution, 20*(7), 363–364. https://doi.org/10.1016/j.tree.2005.05.005.

Gądek-Michalska, A., Tadeusz, J., Bugajski, A., & Bugajski, J. (2019). Chronic isolation stress affects subsequent crowding stress-induced brain nitric oxide synthase (NOS) isoforms and hypothalamic-pituitary-adrenal (HPA) Axis responses. *Neurotoxicity Research, 36*(3), 523–539. https://doi.org/10.1007/s12640-019-00067-1.

Gentsch, C., Lichtsteiner, M., Frischknecht, H.-R., Feer, H., & Siegfried, B. (1988). Isolation-induced locomotor hyperactivity and hypoalgesia in rats are prevented by handling and reversed by resocialization. *Physiology & Behavior, 43*(1), 13–16. https://doi.org/10.1016/0031-9384(88)90091-1.

Geyer, M. A., Wilkinson, L. S., Humby, T., & Robbins, T. W. (1993). Isolation rearing of rats produces a deficit in prepulse inhibition of acoustic startle similar to that in schizophrenia. *Biological Psychiatry, 34*(6), 361–372. https://doi.org/10.1016/0006-3223(93)90180-L.

Giallonardo, V., Sampogna, G., Del Vecchio, V., Luciano, M., Albert, U., Carmassi, C., et al. (2020). The impact of quarantine and physical distancing following COVID-19 on mental health: Study protocol of a multicentric Italian population trial. *Frontiers in Psychiatry, 11*, 533. https://doi.org/10.3389/fpsyt.2020.00533.

Goffman, E. (1990). *The presentation of self in everyday life*. Doubleday.

Gold, P. W., & Chrousos, G. P. (2002). Organization of the stress system and its dysregulation in melancholic and atypical depression: High vs low CRH/NE states. *Molecular Psychiatry*, *7*(3), 254–275. https://doi.org/10.1038/sj.mp.4001032.

Grassian, S. (1983). Psychopathological effects of solitary confinement. *The American Journal of Psychiatry*, *140*(11), 1450–1454. https://doi.org/10.1176/ajp.140.11.1450.

Grassian, S., & Friedman, N. (1986). Effects of sensory deprivation in psychiatric seclusion and solitary confinement. *International Journal of Law and Psychiatry*, *8*(1), 49–65. https://doi.org/10.1016/0160-2527(86)90083-x.

Hall, F. S., Wilkinson, L. S., Humby, T., Inglis, W., Kendall, D. A., Marsden, C. A., et al. (1998). Isolation rearing in rats: Pre- and postsynaptic changes in striatal dopaminergic systems. *Pharmacology Biochemistry and Behavior*, *59*(4), 859–872. https://doi.org/10.1016/S0091-3057(97)00510-8.

Harlow, H. F., Dodsworth, R. O., & Harlow, M. K. (1965). Total social isolation in monkeys. *Proceedings of the National Academy of Sciences*, *54*(1), 90 LP–97. https://doi.org/10.1073/pnas.54.1.90.

Hatch, A., Wiberg, G. S., Balazs, T., & Grice, H. C. (1963). Long-term isolation stress in rats. *Science*, *142*(3591), 507. https://doi.org/10.1126/science.142.3591.507.

Hatch, A. M., Wiberg, G. S., Zawidzka, Z., Cann, M., Airth, J. M., & Grice, H. C. (1965). Isolation syndrome in the rat. *Toxicology and Applied Pharmacology*, *7*(5), 737–745. https://doi.org/10.1016/0041-008X(65)90132-8.

Hawkley, L. C., & Capitanio, J. P. (2015). Perceived social isolation, evolutionary fitness and health outcomes: A lifespan approach. *Philosophical Transactions of the Royal Society of London. Series B, Biological Sciences*, *370*(1669). https://doi.org/10.1098/rstb.2014.0114, 20140114.

Hayes, K., Sprague, S., Guo, M., Davis, W., Friedman, A., Kumar, A., et al. (2008). Forced, not voluntary, exercise effectively induces neuroprotection in stroke. *Acta Neuropathologica*, *115*(3), 289–296. https://doi.org/10.1007/s00401-008-0340-z.

Heinrich, L. M., & Gullone, E. (2006). The clinical significance of loneliness: A literature review. *Clinical Psychology Review*, *26*(6), 695–718. https://doi.org/10.1016/j.cpr.2006.04.002.

Holt-Lunstad, J., Smith, T. B., Baker, M., Harris, T., & Stephenson, D. (2015). Loneliness and social isolation as risk factors for mortality: A meta-analytic review. *Perspectives on Psychological Science*, *10*(2), 227–237. https://doi.org/10.1177/1745691614568352.

Holt-Lunstad, J., Smith, T. B., & Layton, J. B. (2010). Social relationships and mortality risk: A meta-analytic review. *PLoS Medicine*, *7*(7). https://doi.org/10.1371/journal.pmed.1000316, e1000316.

House, J. S., Landis, K. R., & Umberson, D. (1988). Social relationships and health. *Science*, *241*(4865), 540–545. https://doi.org/10.1126/science.3399889.

Jaffe, E. H., De Frias, V., & Ibarra, C. (1993). Changes in basal and stimulated release of endogenous serotonin from different nuclei of rats subjected to two models of depression. *Neuroscience Letters*, *162*(1), 157–160. https://doi.org/10.1016/0304-3940(93)90584-8.

Jesberger, J. A., & Richardson, J. S. (1985). Animal models of depression: Parallels and correlates to severe depression in humans. *Biological Psychiatry*, *20*(7), 764–784. https://doi.org/10.1016/0006-3223(85)90156-8.

Jones, G. H., Marsden, C. A., & Robbins, T. W. (1990). Increased sensitivity to amphetamine and reward-related stimuli following social isolation in rats: Possible disruption of dopamine-dependent mechanisms of the nucleus accumbens. *Psychopharmacology*, *102*(3), 364–372. https://doi.org/10.1007/BF02244105.

Jones, G. H., Marsden, C. A., & Robbins, T. W. (1991). Behavioural rigidity and rule-learning deficits following isolation-rearing in the rat: Neurochemical correlates. *Behavioural Brain Research, 43*(1), 35–50. https://doi.org/10.1016/S0166-4328(05)80050-6.

Judge, K. A. (2010). Female social experience affects the shape of sexual selection on males. *Evolutionary Ecology Research, 12*(3), 389–402.

Kappeler, P. M., Cremer, S., & Nunn, C. L. (2015). Sociality and health: Impacts of sociality on disease susceptibility and transmission in animal and human societies. *Philosophical Transactions of the Royal Society, B: Biological Sciences, 370*(1669). https://doi.org/10.1098/rstb.2014.0116, 20140116.

Ke, Z., Yip, S. P., Li, L., Zheng, X.-X., & Tong, K.-Y. (2011). The effects of voluntary, involuntary, and forced exercises on brain-derived neurotrophic factor and motor function recovery: A rat brain ischemia model. *PLoS One, 6*(2), e16643. https://doi.org/10.1371/journal.pone.0016643.

Killgore, W. D. S., Cloonan, S. A., Taylor, E. C., & Dailey, N. S. (2020, May). Loneliness: A signature mental health concern in the era of COVID-19. *Psychiatry Research.* https://doi.org/10.1016/j.psychres.2020.113117.

Kim, J. W., & Kirkpatrick, B. (1996). Social isolation in animal models of relevance to neuropsychiatric disorders. *Biological Psychiatry, 40*(9), 918–922. https://doi.org/10.1016/0006-3223(95)00546-3.

Kirschbaum, C., Pirke, K.-M., & Hellhammer, D. H. (1993). The "Trier social stress test"—A tool for investigating psychobiological stress responses in a laboratory setting. *Neuropsychobiology, 28*(1–2), 76–81. https://doi.org/10.1159/000119004.

Klaming, R., Annese, J., Veltman, D. J., & Comijs, H. C. (2017). Episodic memory function is affected by lifestyle factors: A 14-year follow-up study in an elderly population. *Aging, Neuropsychology, and Cognition, 24*(5), 528–542.

Koolhaas, J. M., de Boer, S. F., Buwalda, B., & Meerlo, P. (2016). Social stress models in rodents: Towards enhanced validity. *Neurobiology of Stress, 6*, 104–112. https://doi.org/10.1016/j.ynstr.2016.09.003.

Koolhaas, J. M., De Boer, S. F., De Rutter, A. J., Meerlo, P., & Sgoifo, A. (1997). Social stress in rats and mice. *Acta Physiologica Scandinavica. Supplementum, 640*, 69–72.

Krishnan, V., & Nestler, E. J. (2008). The molecular neurobiology of depression. *Nature, 455*(7215), 894–902. https://doi.org/10.1038/nature07455.

Kuiper, J. S., Zuidersma, M., Oude Voshaar, R. C., Zuidema, S. U., van den Heuvel, E. R., Stolk, R. P., et al. (2015). Social relationships and risk of dementia: A systematic review and meta-analysis of longitudinal cohort studies. *Ageing Research Reviews, 22*, 39–57. https://doi.org/10.1016/j.arr.2015.04.006.

Lee, S. H., & Kim, Y. B. (2016). Which type of social activities may reduce cognitive decline in the elderly?: A longitudinal population-based study. *BMC Geriatrics, 16*(1), 165.

Leng, A., Feldon, J., & Ferger, B. (2004). Long-term social isolation and medial prefrontal cortex: Dopaminergic and cholinergic neurotransmission. *Pharmacology Biochemistry and Behavior, 77*(2), 371–379. https://doi.org/10.1016/j.pbb.2003.11.011.

Lewes, G. H. (1877). Voluntary and involuntary actions. In *The physical basis of mind*. Boston, MA, USA: James R Osgood and Company. https://doi.org/10.1037/12769-018.

Lin, Y., Lu, X., Dong, J., He, X., Yan, T., Liang, H., et al. (2015). Involuntary, forced and voluntary exercises equally attenuate neurocognitive deficits in vascular dementia by the BDNF–pCREB mediated pathway. *Neurochemical Research, 40*(9), 1839–1848. https://doi.org/10.1007/s11064-015-1673-3.

Liu, J., Dietz, K., DeLoyht, J. M., Pedre, X., Kelkar, D., Kaur, J., et al. (2012). Impaired adult myelination in the prefrontal cortex of socially isolated mice. *Nature Neuroscience*, *15*(12), 1621–1623. https://doi.org/10.1038/nn.3263.

Lorenz, K. (2002). *King Solomon's ring: New light on animal ways*. London: Routledge.

Machado, M. O., Veronese, N., Sanches, M., Stubbs, B., Koyanagi, A., Thompson, T., et al. (2018). The association of depression and all-cause and cause-specific mortality: An umbrella review of systematic reviews and meta-analyses. *BMC Medicine*, *16*(1), 112. https://doi.org/10.1186/s12916-018-1101-z.

Makinodan, M., Rosen, K. M., Ito, S., & Corfas, G. (2012). A critical period for social experience–dependent oligodendrocyte maturation and myelination. *Science*, *337*(6100), 1357–1360. https://doi.org/10.1126/science.1220845.

Martin, A. L., & Brown, R. E. (2010). The lonely mouse: Verification of a separation-induced model of depression in female mice. *Behavioural Brain Research*, *207*(1), 196–207. https://doi.org/10.1016/j.bbr.2009.10.006.

Martin, L. J., Spicer, D. M., Lewis, M. H., Gluck, J. P., & Cork, L. C. (1991). Social deprivation of infant rhesus monkeys alters the chemoarchitecture of the brain: I. Subcortical regions. *Journal of Neuroscience*, *11*(11), 3344–3358. Retrieved from: https://www.scopus.com/inward/record.uri?eid=2-s2.0-0025840188&partnerID=40&md5=b4065f4526fcbe694733eb041c9879f2.

Masis-Calvo, M., Schmidtner, A. K., de Moura Oliveira, V. E., Grossmann, C. P., de Jong, T. R., & Neumann, I. D. (2018). Animal models of social stress: The dark side of social interactions. *Stress (Amsterdam, Netherlands)*, *21*(5), 417–432. https://doi.org/10.1080/10253890.2018.1462327.

Maslow, A. H. (1943). A theory of human motivation. *Psychological Review*, *50*(4), 370–396. https://doi.org/10.1037/h0054346.

Maslow, A. H. (1954). *Motivation and personality*. Oxford, England: Harpers.

Matsumoto, K., Fujiwara, H., Araki, R., & Yabe, T. (2019). Post-weaning social isolation of mice: A putative animal model of developmental disorders. *Journal of Pharmacological Sciences*, *141*(3), 111–118. https://doi.org/10.1016/j.jphs.2019.10.002.

Matthews, G. A., Nieh, E. H., Vander Weele, C. M., Halbert, S. A., Pradhan, R. V., Yosafat, A. S., et al. (2016). Dorsal raphe dopamine neurons represent the experience of social isolation. *Cell*, *164*(4), 617–631. https://doi.org/10.1016/j.cell.2015.12.040.

McGue, M., & Christensen, K. (2007). Social activity and healthy aging: A study of aging Danish twins. *Twin Research and Human Genetics*, *10*(2), 255–265.

Michalska da Rocha, B., Rhodes, S., Vasilopoulou, E., & Hutton, P. (2018). Loneliness in psychosis: A meta-analytical review. *Schizophrenia Bulletin*, *44*(1), 114–125. https://doi.org/10.1093/schbul/sbx036.

Mitchell, G. D. (1968). Persistent behavior pathology in rhesus monkeys following early social isolation. *Folia Primatologica*, *8*(2), 132–147. https://doi.org/10.1159/000155140.

Mousavi-Nasab, S., Kormi-Nouri, R., & Nilsson, L. (2014). Examination of the bidirectional influences of leisure activity and memory in old people: A dissociative effect on episodic memory. *British Journal of Psychology*, *105*(3), 382–398.

Nestler, E. J., Barrot, M., DiLeone, R. J., Eisch, A. J., Gold, S. J., & Monteggia, L. M. (2002). Neurobiology of depression. *Neuron*, *34*(1), 13–25. https://doi.org/10.1016/S0896-6273(02)00653-0.

Niemann, C., Godde, B., Staudinger, U. M., & Voelcker-Rehage, C. (2014). Exercise-induced changes in basal ganglia volume and cognition in older adults. *Neuroscience*, *281*, 147–163. https://doi.org/10.1016/j.neuroscience.2014.09.033.

Nowak, M. A. (2006). Five rules for the evolution of cooperation. *Science*, *314*(5805), 1560–1563. https://doi.org/10.1126/science.1133755.

Nowland, R., Robinson, S. J., Bradley, B. F., Summers, V., & Qualter, P. (2018). Loneliness, HPA stress reactivity and social threat sensitivity: Analyzing naturalistic social challenges. *Scandinavian Journal of Psychology*, *59*(5), 540–546. https://doi.org/10.1111/sjop.12461.

Paaby, A. B., & Rockman, M. V. (2014). Cryptic genetic variation: evolution's hidden substrate. *Nature Reviews Genetics*, *15*(4), 247–258. https://doi.org/10.1038/nrg3688.

Parker, V., & Morinan, A. (1986). The socially-isolated rat as a model for anxiety. *Neuropharmacology*. https://doi.org/10.1016/0028-3908(86)90224-8.

Robinson, D. L., Heien, M. L. A. V., & Wightman, R. M. (2002). Frequency of dopamine concentration transients increases in dorsal and ventral striatum of male rats during introduction of conspecifics. *The Journal of Neuroscience*, *22*(23), 10477–10486. https://doi.org/10.1523/JNEUROSCI.22-23-10477.2002.

Roske, I., Baeger, I., Frenzel, R., & Oehme, P. (1994). Does a relationship exist between the quality of stress and the motivation to ingest alcohol? *Alcohol*, *11*(2), 113–124. https://doi.org/10.1016/0741-8329(94)90052-3.

Rubenstein, D. R., & Abbot, P. (2017). *Comparative social evolution*. Cambridge University Press.

Sachser, N., & Lick, C. (1989). Social stress in guinea pigs. *Physiology & Behavior*, *46*(2), 137–144. https://doi.org/10.1016/0031-9384(89)90246-1.

Sánchez, M. M., Hearn, E. F., Do, D., Rilling, J. K., & Herndon, J. G. (1998). Differential rearing affects corpus callosum size and cognitive function of rhesus monkeys. *Brain Research*, *812*(1), 38–49. https://doi.org/10.1016/S0006-8993(98)00857-9.

Sato, C., Tanji, K., Shimoyama, S., Chiba, M., Mikami, M., Koeda, S., et al. (2020). Effects of voluntary and forced exercises on motor function recovery in intracerebral hemorrhage rats. *Neuroreport*, *31*(2). Retrieved from: https://journals.lww.com/neuroreport/Fulltext/2020/01020/Effects_of_voluntary_and_forced_exercises_on_motor.15.aspx.

Scott, J. P. (1958). Critical periods in the development of social behavior in puppies. *Psychosomatic Medicine*, *20*(1). Retrieved from: https://journals.lww.com/psychosomaticmedicine/Fulltext/1958/01000/Critical_Periods_in_the_Development_of_Social.5.aspx.

Shahar-Gold, H., Gur, R., & Wagner, S. (2013). Rapid and reversible impairments of short-and long-term social recognition memory are caused by acute isolation of adult rats via distinct mechanisms. *PLoS One*, *8*(5).

Sherman, P., Lacey, E., Reeve, H., & Keller, L. (1995). The eusociality continuum. *Behavioral Ecology*, *6*. https://doi.org/10.1093/beheco/6.1.102.

Steptoe, A., Owen, N., Kunz-Ebrecht, S. R., & Brydon, L. (2004). Loneliness and neuroendocrine, cardiovascular, and inflammatory stress responses in middle-aged men and women. *Psychoneuroendocrinology*, *29*(5), 593–611. https://doi.org/10.1016/S0306-4530(03)00086-6.

Steptoe, A., Shankar, A., Demakakos, P., & Wardle, J. (2013). Social isolation, loneliness, and all-cause mortality in older men and women. *Proceedings of the National Academy of Sciences*, *110*(15), 5797 LP–5801. https://doi.org/10.1073/pnas.1219686110.

Struble, R. G., & Riesen, A. H. (1978). Changes in cortical dendritic branching subsequent to partial social isolation in stumptailed monkeys. *Developmental Psychobiology*, *11*(5), 479–486. https://doi.org/10.1002/dev.420110511.

Sun, L., Min, L., Zhou, H., Li, M., Shao, F., & Wang, W. (2017). Adolescent social isolation affects schizophrenia-like behavior and astrocyte biomarkers in the PFC of adult rats. *Behavioural Brain Research*, *333*, 258–266. https://doi.org/10.1016/j.bbr.2017.07.011.

Suomi, S. J., Harlow, H. F., & Kimball, S. D. (1971). Behavioral effects of prolonged partial social isolation in the rhesus monkey. *Psychological Reports*, *29*(3_suppl), 1171–1177. https://doi.org/10.2466/pr0.1971.29.3f.1171.

Suomi, S. J., Harlow, H. F., & McKinney, W. T. (1972). Monkey psychiatrists. *American Journal of Psychiatry*, *128*(8), 927–932. https://doi.org/10.1176/ajp.128.8.927.

Suomi, S. J., Seaman, S. F., Lewis, J. K., DeLizio, R. D., & McKinney, W. T., Jr. (1978). Effects of imipramine treatment of separation-induced social disorders in rhesus monkeys. *Archives of General Psychiatry*, *35*(3), 321–325. https://doi.org/10.1001/archpsyc.1978.01770270071006.

Takahashi, A., Flanigan, M. E., McEwen, B. S., & Russo, S. J. (2018). Aggression, social stress, and the immune system in humans and animal models. *Frontiers in Behavioral Neuroscience*, *12*, 56. https://doi.org/10.3389/fnbeh.2018.00056.

Takatsu-Coleman, A. L., Patti, C. L., Zanin, K. A., Zager, A., Carvalho, R. C., Borçoi, A. R., et al. (2013). Short-term social isolation induces depressive-like behaviour and reinstates the retrieval of an aversive task: Mood-congruent memory in male mice? *Journal of Psychiatry & Neuroscience*, *38*(4), 259–268. https://doi.org/10.1503/jpn.120050.

Tamashiro, K. L. K., Nguyen, M. M. N., & Sakai, R. R. (2005). Social stress: From rodents to primates. *Frontiers in Neuroendocrinology*, *26*(1), 27–40. https://doi.org/10.1016/j.yfrne.2005.03.001.

Tang, F., Liang, J., Zhang, H., Kelifa, M. M., He, Q., & Wang, P. (2020). COVID-19 related depression and anxiety among quarantined respondents. *Psychology & Health*, 1–15. https://doi.org/10.1080/08870446.2020.1782410.

Tu, Z.-H., He, J.-W., & Zhou, N. (2020). Sleep quality and mood symptoms in conscripted frontline nurse in Wuhan, China during COVID-19 outbreak: A cross-sectional study. *Medicine*, *99*(26), e20769. https://doi.org/10.1097/MD.0000000000020769.

Tull, M. T., Edmonds, K. A., Scamaldo, K. M., Richmond, J. R., Rose, J. P., & Gratz, K. L. (2020). Psychological outcomes associated with stay-at-home orders and the perceived impact of COVID-19 on daily life. *Psychiatry Research*, *289*. https://doi.org/10.1016/j.psychres.2020.113098, 113098.

Unal, G., & Canbeyli, R. (2019). Psychomotor retardation in depression: A critical measure of the forced swim test. *Behavioural Brain Research*, *372*. https://doi.org/10.1016/j.bbr.2019.112047, 112047.

Valtorta, N. K., Kanaan, M., Gilbody, S., Ronzi, S., & Hanratty, B. (2016). Loneliness and social isolation as risk factors for coronary heart disease and stroke: Systematic review and meta-analysis of longitudinal observational studies. *Heart (British Cardiac Society)*, *102*(13), 1009–1016. https://doi.org/10.1136/heartjnl-2015-308790.

Vargas, J., Junco, M., Gomez, C., & Lajud, N. (2016). Early life stress increases metabolic risk, HPA Axis reactivity, and depressive-like behavior when combined with postweaning social isolation in rats. *PLoS One*, *11*(9), e0162665. https://doi.org/10.1371/journal.pone.0162665.

Vodanovich, S. J., & Kass, S. J. (1990). A factor analytic study of the boredom proneness scale. *Journal of Personality Assessment*, *55*(1–2), 115–123. https://doi.org/10.1080/00223891.1990.9674051.

Weiss, I. C., Pryce, C. R., Jongen-Rêlo, A. L., Nanz-Bahr, N. I., & Feldon, J. (2004). Effect of social isolation on stress-related behavioural and neuroendocrine state in the rat. *Behavioural Brain Research*, *152*(2), 279–295. https://doi.org/10.1016/j.bbr.2003.10.015.

Wilkinson, L. S., Killcross, S. S., Humby, T., Hall, F. S., Geyer, M. A., & Robbins, T. W. (1994). Social isolation in the rat produces developmentally specific deficits in prepulse inhibition of the acoustic startle response without disrupting latent inhibition. *Neuropsychopharmacology*, *10*(1), 61–72. https://doi.org/10.1038/npp.1994.8.

Wilson, E. O. (1971). *The insect societies*. The Insect Societies.

Wilson, E. O., & Hölldobler, B. (2005). Eusociality: Origin and consequences. *Proceedings of the National Academy of Sciences of the United States of America*, *102*(38), 13367–13371. https://doi.org/10.1073/pnas.0505858102.

Yamamuro, K., Yoshino, H., Ogawa, Y., Makinodan, M., Toritsuka, M., Yamashita, M., et al. (2018). Social isolation during the critical period reduces synaptic and intrinsic excitability of a subtype of pyramidal cell in mouse prefrontal cortex. *Cerebral Cortex (New York, N.Y.: 1991)*, *28*(3), 998–1010. https://doi.org/10.1093/cercor/bhx010.

Yorgason, J. T., Calipari, E. S., Ferris, M. J., Karkhanis, A. N., Fordahl, S. C., Weiner, J. L., et al. (2016). Social isolation rearing increases dopamine uptake and psychostimulant potency in the striatum. *Neuropharmacology*, *101*, 471–479. https://doi.org/10.1016/j.neuropharm.2015.10.025.

Zhaoyang, R., Sliwinski, M. J., Martire, L. M., & Smyth, J. M. (2018). Age differences in adults' daily social interactions: An ecological momentary assessment study. *Psychology and Aging*, *33*(4), 607–618. https://doi.org/10.1037/pag0000242.

Zorzo, C., Méndez-López, M., Méndez, M., & Arias, J. L. (2019). Adult social isolation leads to anxiety and spatial memory impairment: Brain activity pattern of COx and c-Fos. *Behavioural Brain Research*, *365*(February), 170–177. https://doi.org/10.1016/j.bbr.2019.03.011.

Chapter 9

Increased hallucinations in patients with Alzheimer's disease during the Covid-19 lockdown: A presentation of two cases

Mohamad El Haj[a,b,c] and Frank Larøi[d,e,f]

[a]*Laboratoire de Psychologie des Pays de la Loire (LPPL–EA 4638), Nantes Université, University of Angers, Nantes, France,* [b]*Unité de Gériatrie, Centre Hospitalier de Tourcoing, Tourcoing, France,* [c]*Institut Universitaire de France, Paris, France,* [d]*Department of Biological and Medical Psychology, University of Bergen, Bergen, Norway,* [e]*Norwegian Center of Excellence for Mental Disorders Research, University of Oslo, Oslo, Norway,* [f]*Psychology and Neuroscience of Cognition Research Unit, University of Liège, Liège, Belgium*

Because of their cognitive and functional impairments, patients with dementia are particularly vulnerable during crises, and this has been especially true during the coronavirus (Covid-19) pandemic. While Covid-19 has significantly turned our daily lives upside down, this impact is significantly pronounced in patients with dementia, especially those living in nursing homes. Residents of nursing homes have a significant risk of Covid-19 infection. To cope with infection and to limit its spread among residents, nursing homes in France (in addition to nursing homes in Europe and North America) have been obliged to prohibit physical contact between residents and families and friends and, in several cases, even between residents or between residents and caregivers. In France, lockdown in retirement homes was first announced on March 17th 2020. While the lockdown served to prevent infections, nursing homes were forced to separate residents physically from the outside world and to drastically reduce their activities. This lockdown was partially lifted on April 27th 2020 as residents were then allowed to receive visitations from one or two family members under strict conditions (e.g., short visits and only once per week). From May 11th, these social restrictions were further alleviated in some nursing homes, for instance, residents were allowed two, but short, visits per week and some wellbeing activities (e.g., hairdressing) were allowed. Because these restrictions are likely to come at a cost to residents and their wellbeing and mental health, we present two cases of patients with Alzheimer's disease (AD) who live

Mental Health Effects of COVID-19. https://doi.org/10.1016/B978-0-12-824289-6.00004-0

in a nursing home during the Covid-19 crisis. We show how these two patients have demonstrated an increase in hallucinations during the lockdown period.

A brief introduction of literature on hallucinations in AD is required before presenting the study case. While at the cognitive level, AD is mainly characterized by memory decline (McKhann et al., 2011), the disease is also characterized by psychiatric symptoms such as hallucinations (El Haj et al., 2019; El Haj et al., 2017). The prevalence of hallucinations in AD can range from 4% to 76% (median 23%) (Bassiony & Lyketsos, 2003), and the occurrence of hallucinations can be observed in patients with moderate or advanced AD (Linszen et al., 2018). Hallucinations in AD are mainly visual and auditory but olfactory, somatic, and tactile hallucinations can sometimes be observed (El Haj et al., 2017). Regardless of their modality, hallucinations are associated with greater cognitive impairment and a more rapidly deteriorating course in AD (Weamer et al., 2009). At the behavioral level, hallucinations in AD can lead to aggressive behavior (Aarsland, Cummings, Yenner, & Miller, 1996), verbal outbursts (Lerner et al., 1994), and functional decline (Haupt, Kurz, & Janner, 2000; Scarmeas et al., 2005). In turn, aggressive behavior and functional decline, due to hallucinations, often lead to stress, depression, and a high level of burden of care in caregivers (Ornstein et al., 2013; Rocca et al., 2010).

Furthermore, it is reasonable to suppose that particular conditions, such as those during the Covid-19 lockdown, may increase the occurrence of hallucinations in AD patients who are residents in nursing homes. This increased occurrence of hallucinations can occur because of a number of different elements, such as decreased daily activities, social distancing, and lack of physical contact with family members during the lockdown. We thus present two cases of patients with moderate AD who had already reported hallucinations prior the Covid-19 crisis, and where an increase in the occurrence of hallucinations was observed during the lockdown.

The two cases

We present two cases, Mrs. L and Mrs. C. The first case (Mrs. L) is 78 years of age, has had 8 years of formal education, is right-handed, and is a native French speaker. The second case (Mrs. C) is 85 years of age, has had 9 years of formal education, is right-handed, and is a native French speaker. Both patients have been living in a nursing home in the region of Nantes (France). The amnestic AD diagnosis was established (6 years ago for Mrs. L and 8 years ago for Mrs. C) based on NINCDS-ADRDA diagnostic criteria (McKhann et al., 2011). Prior to the crisis, on March 5th 2020, their hallucinations and cognitive ability were evaluated as part of an ongoing research project on the general relationship between hallucinations and cognition. The cognitive evaluation included an evaluation of general cognitive functioning, episodic memory, and working memory. General cognitive functioning was evaluated with the Mini Mental State Examination (Folstein, Folstein, & McHugh, 1975) on which Mrs.

L obtained a score of 13/30 points and Mrs. C obtained a score of 15/30 points. Episodic memory was evaluated with the Grober and Buschke task (Grober & Buschke, 1987), where they were asked to retrieve as many of the previously exposed 16 words as possible for 2 min. Mrs. L retrieved three words and Mrs. L retrieved four words. Working memory was evaluated with forward and backward spans on which the two cases were invited to repeat a string of single digits in the same order (i.e., forward span) or in the inverse order (i.e., backward span). Mrs. L did not retain more than three numbers on both the forward and backward spans, while Mrs. C did not retain more than four numbers on the forward spans and three numbers on the backward spans.

Hallucination assessment and results

We invited the caregiver (i.e., the nurse in charge of the ward) of Mrs. L and Mrs. C to evaluate their hallucinations on April 25th 2020. More specifically, we invited the caregiver to rate the following three items: "*The patient sees objects or animals even though there is nothing there*," "*The patient is troubled by hearing voices in her head*," "*The patient declares that she hears a voice speaking aloud*." These three items were used in previous studies involving hallucinations in AD (El Haj, Gallouj, Dehon, Roche, & Laroi, 2018; El Haj, Jardri, Laroi, & Antoine, 2016; El Haj, Laroi, Gely-Nargeot, & Raffard, 2015). The three items were assessed, during a phone interview, by the caregiver with the help of a five-point Likert scale ranging from zero ("certainly does not apply to her") to four ("certainly applies to her"). The maximum score was thus 12 points. Scores on the hallucination assessment for Mrs. L and Mrs. C were, respectively, nine and eight points. We compared this score to the scores obtained on March 5th 2020 when hallucinations of the two cases were rated by the same caregiver. The hallucination scores on March 5th 2020 for Mrs. L and Mrs. C were, respectively, six and five points. Thus the hallucination scores for Mrs. L and Mrs. C increased by three points from March 5th 2020 (before the lockdown) to April 25th 2020 (during the lockdown). In other words, the score of Mrs. L and Mrs. C increased, respectively, by 24% and 25% compared with before the lockdown.

Discussion

The two cases presented here demonstrated an increase in the occurrence of hallucinations during, compared to before, the Covid-19 lockdown. This increase can be attributed to several factors such as social distancing, as implemented by the nursing home in which the two cases are living. Social distancing and isolation may lead to spatiotemporal orientation, anxiety, and increasing somatic discomfort which may lead to stress reaction and hallucinations. The nursing home where the two cases resided (as did other facilities on a national level) implemented strict social distancing measures and drastic changes in the daily life of the residents from March 16th 2020 to April 25th 2020. Nonessential activities and services (e.g., hairdressers) were restricted, including basic social activities such as communal dining. Residents were invited not to leave their wards; however, when they did so, they were asked to keep a safe distance from other residents in order to avoid contracting the virus. Critically, residents were not allowed to have any physical contact with their family members and friends. In the case of Mrs. L, her daughter used to visit her once per week before the lockdown, but was not able to visit her during the lockdown. Regarding Mrs. C, her two sons used to visit her once to twice per week before the lockdown, but were not able to visit her during the lockdown. In addition, due to their cognitive decline, as observed on the cognitive evaluation, both Mrs. C and Mrs. L were not able to use the current technology (e.g., Skype) to get in touch with their children or grandchildren. The only contact occurred by phone.

While the (physical) social restrictions, as implemented by nursing homes, may be deemed necessary in order to avoid Covid-19 infections, these restrictions are likely to come at a cost to residents in retirement homes by affecting their mental health. The decrease in social activities in the facilities and the decrease in physical contact with family members may increase loneliness, itself leading to hallucinations. This assumption can be supported by research demonstrating how hallucinations in patients with AD can be associated with loneliness (El Haj et al., 2016). To compensate for boredom and emptiness, as this is associated with loneliness, patients with AD may generate internal stimuli to fulfill their need to communicate (El Haj et al., 2016). In other words, hallucinations in patients with AD can be regarded as a compensatory mechanism that aims to fulfill their communicatory needs (El Haj et al., 2016). These hallucinations can also be attributed to confusion or diminished orientation in time. Because of the lack of visits and social activities, patients can get bored and feel time passing very slowly. Patients can therefore generate hallucinations to fill this temporal emptiness. While this assumption is clinically appealing, it should be considered with some caution as our study did not include an evaluation of time perception.

The assumption that social restrictions, as implemented during the Covid-19 crisis, may affect the mental health of patients with AD can be supported by two recent studies. The first study included patients living in retirement homes and the second study included patients living in their own homes. In the first study (El Haj, Altintas, Chapelet, Kapogiannis, & Gallouj, 2020), patients with mild AD living in retirement homes were invited to rate their depression and anxiety during and before the Covid-19 crisis. Participants reported higher depression and anxiety during than before the Covid-19 crisis. The increased distress was attributed to the isolation of the residents and/or to the drastic changes in their daily life and to the care they receive in the retirement homes during the crisis. The effect of confinement on mental health of patients with AD was also reported by a study demonstrating increased neuropsychiatric symptoms in patients with AD who were confined in their own homes during the Covid-19 crisis (Boutoleau-Bretonnière et al., 2020). In this study, caregivers were invited to report whether patients experienced increased neuropsychiatric symptoms during the confinement and, if it was the case, to rate this increase. Results demonstrated increased neuropsychiatric symptoms only in patients with advanced AD and this increased symptomatology significantly correlated with the duration of confinement.

To summarize, while the lockdown in retirement homes during the Covid-19 crisis is necessary in order to prevent infection, this lockdown may negatively impact the wellbeing and mental health of residents. The decrease in daily activities and social contact during the lockdown, as well as the physical separation of residents from loved ones, may lead to confusion, despair, and loneliness. Ultimately, the lockdown may increase hallucinations in residents, at least in those who were already experiencing hallucination prior to the lockdown. Research on a large scale is required to further investigate the effects of Covid-19 lockdown on hallucinations in patients with dementia living in nursing homes.

Conflict of interest

The author declares no conflict of interest.

References

Aarsland, D., Cummings, J. L., Yenner, G., & Miller, B. (1996). Relationship of aggressive behavior to other neuropsychiatric symptoms in patients with Alzheimer's disease. *The American Journal of Psychiatry*, *153*(2), 243–247. https://doi.org/10.1176/ajp.153.2.243.

Bassiony, M. M., & Lyketsos, C. G. (2003). Delusions and hallucinations in Alzheimer's disease: Review of the brain decade. *Psychosomatics*, *44*(5), 388–401. https://doi.org/10.1176/appi.psy.44.5.388.

Boutoleau-Bretonnière, C., Pouclet-Courtemanche, H., Gillet, A., Bernard, A., Deruet, A. L., Gouraud, I., et al. (2020). The effects of confinement on neuropsychiatric symptoms in Alzheimer's disease during the COVID-19 crisis. *Journal of Alzheimer's Disease*, *76*(1), 41–47. https://doi.org/10.3233/jad-200604.

El Haj, M., Altintas, E., Chapelet, G., Kapogiannis, D., & Gallouj, K. (2020). High depression and anxiety in people with Alzheimer's disease living in retirement homes during the Covid-19 crisis. *Psychiatry Research*, *291*, 113294. https://doi.org/10.1016/j.psychres.2020.113294.

El Haj, M., Badcock, J. C., Jardri, R., Larøi, F., Roche, J., Sommer, I. E., et al. (2019). A look into hallucinations: The relationship between visual imagery and hallucinations in Alzheimer's disease. *Cognitive Neuropsychiatry*, *24*(4), 275–283. https://doi.org/10.1080/13546805.2019.1632180.

El Haj, M., Gallouj, K., Dehon, H., Roche, J., & Laroi, F. (2018). Hallucinations in Alzheimer's disease: Failure to suppress irrelevant memories. *Cognitive Neuropsychiatry*, *23*(3), 142–153. https://doi.org/10.1080/13546805.2018.1443062.

El Haj, M., Jardri, R., Laroi, F., & Antoine, P. (2016). Hallucinations, loneliness, and social isolation in Alzheimer's disease. *Cognitive Neuropsychiatry*, *21*(1), 1–13. https://doi.org/10.1080/13546805.2015.1121139.

El Haj, M., Laroi, F., Gely-Nargeot, M. C., & Raffard, S. (2015). Inhibitory deterioration may contribute to hallucinations in Alzheimer's disease. *Cognitive Neuropsychiatry*, *20*(4), 281–295. https://doi.org/10.1080/13546805.2015.1023392.

El Haj, M., Roche, J., Jardri, R., Kapogiannis, D., Gallouj, K., & Antoine, P. (2017). Clinical and neurocognitive aspects of hallucinations in Alzheimer's disease. *Neuroscience and Biobehavioral Reviews*, *83*, 713–720. https://doi.org/10.1016/j.neubiorev.2017.02.021.

Folstein, M. F., Folstein, S. E., & McHugh, P. R. (1975). "Mini-mental state". A practical method for grading the cognitive state of patients for the clinician. *Journal of Psychiatric Research*, *12*(3), 189–198.

Grober, E., & Buschke, H. (1987). Genuine memory deficits in dementia. *Developmental Neuropsychology*, *3*(1), 13–36.

Haupt, M., Kurz, A., & Janner, M. (2000). A 2-year follow-up of behavioural and psychological symptoms in Alzheimer's disease. *Dementia and Geriatric Cognitive Disorders*, *11*(3), 147–152. https://doi.org/10.1159/000017228.

Lerner, A. J., Koss, E., Patterson, M. B., Ownby, R. L., Hedera, P., Friedland, R. P., et al. (1994). Concomitants of visual hallucinations in Alzheimer's disease. *Neurology*, *44*(3 Pt 1), 523–527.

Linszen, M. M. J., Lemstra, A. W., Dauwan, M., Brouwer, R. M., Scheltens, P., & Sommer, I. E. C. (2018). Understanding hallucinations in probable Alzheimer's disease: Very low prevalence rates in a tertiary memory clinic. *Alzheimer's & Dementia: Diagnosis, Assessment & Disease Monitoring*. https://doi.org/10.1016/j.dadm.2018.03.005.

McKhann, G., Knopman, D. S., Chertkow, H., Hyman, B. T., Jack, C. R., Jr., Kawas, C. H., et al. (2011). The diagnosis of dementia due to Alzheimer's disease: Recommendations from the National Institute on Aging-Alzheimer's Association workgroups on diagnostic guidelines for Alzheimer's disease. *Alzheimers Dement*, *7*(3), 263–269. https://doi.org/10.1016/j.jalz.2011.03.005.

Ornstein, K., Gaugler, J. E., Devanand, D. P., Scarmeas, N., Zhu, C., & Stern, Y. (2013). The differential impact of unique behavioral and psychological symptoms for the dementia caregiver: How and why do patients' individual symptom clusters impact caregiver depressive symptoms? *The American Journal of Geriatric Psychiatry*, *21*(12), 1277–1286. https://doi.org/10.1016/j.jagp.2013.01.062.

Rocca, P., Leotta, D., Liffredo, C., Mingrone, C., Sigaudo, M., Capellero, B., et al. (2010). Neuropsychiatric symptoms underlying caregiver stress and insight in Alzheimer's disease. *Dementia and Geriatric Cognitive Disorders*, *30*(1), 57–63. https://doi.org/10.1159/000315513.

Scarmeas, N., Brandt, J., Albert, M., Hadjigeorgiou, G., Papadimitriou, A., Dubois, B., et al. (2005). Delusions and hallucinations are associated with worse outcome in Alzheimer disease. *Archives of Neurology*, *62*(10), 1601–1608. https://doi.org/10.1001/archneur.62.10.1601.

Weamer, E. A., Emanuel, J. E., Varon, D., Miyahara, S., Wilkosz, P. A., Lopez, O. L., et al. (2009). The relationship of excess cognitive impairment in MCI and early Alzheimer's disease to the subsequent emergence of psychosis. *International Psychogeriatrics*, *21*(1), 78–85. https://doi.org/10.1017/S1041610208007734.

Chapter 10

Eating disorders during a coronavirus pandemic

Samantha Hayes and Evelyn Smith
School of Psychology, Western Sydney University, Penrith, NSW, Australia

Introduction

The novel coronavirus SARS-CoV-2 (COVID-19) rapidly evolved into a global pandemic since initial cases were documented in Wuhan, China (Davis et al., 2020; Todisco & Donini, 2020). With no current treatment or vaccine for COVID-19 (as of October 2020), the looming threat has significantly transformed the healthcare system (Cooper et al., 2020; Wood et al., 2020). Subsequent efforts to reduce the spread have dramatically altered daily life and led to a deterioration in mental and physical health (Cooper et al., 2020; Fernandez-Aranda et al., 2020; Rodgers et al., 2020). Restrictions to abate the rate of infection have resulted in the implementation of social distancing and self-quarantine measures (Ammar et al., 2020; Zachary et al., 2020). During the COVID-19 pandemic, social gatherings have been largely prohibited, fitness centers were closed, working from home was encouraged, and grocery stores saw frenzied bulk purchasing and empty shelves, and in some places, travel was banned (Ammar et al., 2020; Cooper et al., 2020). These dramatic changes to normal daily life, physical activity, and access to basic necessities have resulted in unprecedented stress, sensationalized broadcast of traumatic health messages, increased concerns over access and development of mental health disorders (Ammar et al., 2020; Cooper et al., 2020; Zachary et al., 2020). Adaptive coping mechanisms and access to support services have been limited during this unique time period (Cooper et al., 2020). During the COVID-19 crisis, it is believed that individuals with eating disorders may be disproportionately impacted with symptoms being exacerbated; however, there is also greater risk of healthy individuals developing eating disorders due to increased unstructured routine, limited physical activity opportunities, and higher rates of anxiety (Fernandez-Aranda et al., 2020). Eating disorders are primarily characterized as psychiatric disturbances of body weight and shape (American Psychiatric Association, 2013) and are the deadliest psychiatric mental illnesses (Arcelus, Mitchell, Wales, & Nielsen, 2011). Therefore it is important to consider the

Mental Health Effects of COVID-19. https://doi.org/10.1016/B978-0-12-824289-6.00002-7

impact of COVID-19 on individuals with eating disorders, and the clinical implications during this global pandemic. In this chapter, we would outline the evidence of the impact on COVID-19 on individuals with eating disorders, including the media, food access, exercise limitations, family dynamics, and social isolation. We will also outline the clinical implications of COVID-19 and how treatment expectations and delivery has changed.

Eating disorders

It is possible that the present circumstances of COVID-19 may precipitate or exacerbate the onset of eating disorder pathology for many individuals due to the ever-changing nature of daily life (Cooper et al., 2020; Rodgers et al., 2020). For example, a preliminary survey found that within the first 2 weeks of lockdown in Spain, 38% of patients with eating disorders reported an increase in their eating disorder symptoms and 56.2% reported an increase in anxiety (Fernandez-Aranda et al., 2020). The COLLATE study, comprised of 5469 participants (180 with eating disorders), which examines the effects of COVID-19 on mental health, found that there was an increase in dieting and binge eating in the general population, but a decrease in exercise. However, those who already have an eating disorder had an increase in food restriction, binge eating, purging, and exercise (Phillipou et al., 2020). A large study of individuals with eating disorders, 511 from the US and 510 from the Netherlands, revealed that those with anorexia nervosa reported an increase in dieting, fear of not being able to find the food for the meal plan, higher anxiety, and overall impact on their mental health due to COVID-19. However, individuals also reported greater connection with family, more time for self-care, and higher motivation to recover (Termorshuizen et al., 2020). This highlights a need for the development of tailored interventions that supports these individuals' needs during this global pandemic.

Multiple pathways have been identified that may aggravate eating disorder symptoms among this vulnerable group who are already characterized by a decreased physiological resilience (Rodgers et al., 2020; Todisco & Donini, 2020). Diminished immune function due to malnutrition is often a consequence of eating disorders, making individuals with eating disorders more susceptible to contracting COVID-19 (Todisco & Donini, 2020), and thus considered an "at risk" group. For example, patients with eating disorders are already placed at a higher physical risk of developing comorbid conditions due to the frailty in individuals with anorexia nervosa and bulimia nervosa suffering metabolic imbalances, while those with binge eating disorder also have an increased risk of cardiovascular conditions (Fernandez-Aranda et al., 2020).

The increased health concerns associated with the current global pandemic may perpetuate the development of orthorexia nervosa, defined by excessive restriction of eating patterns driven by concerns over the quality of food and health concerns (Rodgers et al., 2020). Individuals may adopt restrictive dietary patterns over health concerns of poor-quality food and to protect themselves from contracting COVID-19 (Rodgers et al., 2020). Other individuals may also develop unhealthy restrictive eating habits in an attempt to consume only foods that are suggestive of improving your immunity (Rodgers et al., 2020).

Eating disorder symptomatology

It is evident that during COVID-19 and the consequent home confinements, there has been a significant increase in unhealthy eating behaviors. One study found that 22% of the sampled adults reported gaining weight during social isolation (Zachary et al., 2020). Changes to daily routine can significantly impact eating behaviors, physical activities, and sleep. The current push to stay indoors, increased unstructured time, and stress associated with the pandemic can result in lack of sleep, snacking, eating in response to stress or negative emotions, and decreased physical activity often linked to weight gain (Zachary et al., 2020). Another study found that adults reported significantly more episodes of feeling out of control while eating, increased snacking between meals, increase late-night snacking, and significantly higher number of main meals (Ammar et al., 2020). Therefore disordered eating behaviors during COVID-19 have not been limited to those with a previous diagnosis of an eating disorder. The development of unhealthy eating behaviors could be attributed to eating in response to stress, anxiety, or boredom (Ammar et al., 2020). Greater difficulties with emotion regulation due to home confinement may trigger eating disorder symptoms as a means to cope, including binge eating, purging, and dietary restraint (Fernandez-Aranda et al., 2020). The absence of clear routines can also alter mealtimes and impair clear separation of home and work space, which may increase risk of eating disorder behaviors such as snacking, grazing, and overconsumption (Rodgers et al., 2020).

The global pandemic is also believed to increase other unhealthy eating patterns. The unprecedented and unpredictable nature of the current crisis may result in individuals striving for control and thus engage in more restrictive eating behaviors (Todisco & Donini, 2020). Alternatively, engaging in binge or emotional eating may result in greater implementation of compensatory behaviors (e.g. excessive exercise or purging) in order to manage the associated emotion regulation (Todisco & Donini, 2020). One study found that during self-quarantine, 52% of participants ate more in response to stress, 73% increased eating when bored, and 65% reported snacking after dinner (Zachary et al., 2020). It was also reported that 22% of the sample reported gaining between 5 and 10 pounds (Zachary et al., 2020). Therefore disordered eating patterns may be increased during the pandemic and may include increases in binge eating, purging, dietary restraint, disinhibited/mindless eating, and emotional eating (Rodgers et al., 2020).

Mental health

COVID-19 has been associated with the adverse development of mental health conditions and significantly exacerbates eating disorder symptomology. The rampant spread of sensationalized reporting and misinformation about coronavirus is associated with an increase in health anxiety and a significant deterioration of mental health (Cooper et al., 2020). The onset of COVID-19 crisis has created global stress over the health of society (Cooper et al., 2020). The fear of virus contamination, especially in individuals with disordered eating who already may have associated health-related concerns, has resulted in increased health anxiety and obsessive-compulsive behaviors in attempts to cope (Clark Bryan et al., 2020; Davis et al., 2020). Self-isolation and social distancing may result in increased experiences of depression, loneliness, sadness, posttraumatic disorder, and insomnia which may exacerbate eating disorder symptoms (Todisco & Donini, 2020; Wood et al., 2020; Zachary et al., 2020).

Patients with anorexia nervosa reported that the sudden lack of routine and inability to engage in their usual activities prompted feelings of restlessness, fear of uncertainty, and even lack of motivation to engage in recovery (Clark Bryan et al., 2020). They also reported feeling dependent on their eating disorder or engaging in more obsessive-compulsive behaviors such as excessive handwashing for a sense of reassurance and control (Clark Bryan et al., 2020). However, individuals with eating disorders may feel more equipped to manage their condition if they experience a decrease in social anxiety associated with social distancing and self-isolation (Cooper et al., 2020).

The global pandemic has resulted in increased financial, social, and occupational stress, which significantly impacts mental health and is associated with greater onset, maintenance, and relapse of eating disorder pathology (Cooper et al., 2020). Those who contract COVID-19 are also at a high risk of developing eating disorders due to heightened psychological distress and eating dysregulation (Cooper et al., 2020). There may also be increased experience of comorbid posttraumatic stress within these patients (Shah, Sachdeva, & Johnston, 2020). Fear of contagion and health anxiety may also increase restrictive eating patterns as individuals fear leaving their house to purchase groceries (Rodgers et al., 2020).

Impact of the media on eating disorders

Social distancing and self-isolation led to an increase in media consumption and the use of social media (Cooper et al., 2020; Rodgers et al., 2020). Increased media attention during lockdown presents new eating and body image concerns (Clark Bryan et al., 2020). During lockdown, social media has displayed increased fatphobic messages surrounding diet and exercise with media sparking fear of weight gain alluding to the possibility of gaining the "Quarantine 15," the 15 pounds weight gain during self-isolation (Cooper et al., 2020; Shah et al., 2020). The media is also reporting that there is a significant risk of hospitalization and the need of ventilation of individuals with a higher body weight infected with COVID-19 (Cooper et al., 2020). Fear of weight gain and weight stigma promoted on social media can increase stress during times of crisis (Cooper et al., 2020; Rodgers et al., 2020; Todisco & Donini, 2020). Individuals are often praised and glorified on social media for their motivation and perseverance to engage in healthy eating and regular exercise during COVID-19, which perpetuates thin ideals within society and could be detrimental to vulnerable individuals with eating disorders (Fernandez-Aranda et al., 2020). The internalization of negative weight-related stereotypes and thin ideals can result in harmful implications on an individual's effective control over their eating behaviors (Todisco & Donini, 2020). It should be encouraged for these individuals to limit media consumption and altering the type of media consumed to mitigate the potential harm of these negative messages on social media (Cooper et al., 2020).

The current global pandemic has resulted in greater use of video calls as a means of communication. This presents a new concern, especially for individuals with anorexia nervosa, as the use of video calls may lead to heightened awareness of their physical appearance (Fernandez-Aranda et al., 2020; Rodgers et al., 2020). Increased preoccupation with physical appearance along with the constant influence of the thin ideals on social media could prompt higher levels of self-criticism and consequential increase in eating disorder symptoms or be harmful to recovery (Fernandez-Aranda et al., 2020). Patients with anorexia nervosa who were engaged in treatment during COVID-19 reported having to modify what was visible on their social media accounts and attempted to focus on positive, recovery focused messages, while others believed it was safer not to use video calls to eliminate the potential triggers associated with it (Fernandez-Aranda et al., 2020).

Exercise limitations

The global pandemic of COVID-19 resulted in lockdown restrictions and the closure of fitness centers (Clark Bryan et al., 2020). A study found that the number of days per week and minutes per day in which individuals engaged in vigorous or moderate intensity physical activity significantly reduced during home confinement compared to before COVID-19 (Ammar et al., 2020). This paper also reported that participants engaged in significantly less walking per day and significantly more sitting per day during COVID-19 (Ammar et al., 2020). It concluded that despite greater access to online exercise classes, individuals were not able to engage in the same amount of exercise during the global pandemic (Ammar et al., 2020). These changes to access to physical activities could produce concerns about health, fitness, and body image during confinement and might serve as precipitating factor for the development of eating disorders (Fernandez-Aranda et al., 2020). These unprecedented times have also been associated with feelings of restlessness, especially within those individuals with eating disorders that may be engaging in exercise as a means to reduce negative emotions and anxiety (Clark Bryan et al., 2020; Cooper et al., 2020). One study found that individuals with eating disorders reported struggling with controlling the urge to engage in more exercise due to lack of other activities to engage in to prevent boredom (Clark Bryan et al., 2020). Alternatively, inability to exercise normally can increase distress associated with heightened weight and shape concerns and result in alternative coping methods or contribute to adopting other unhealthy compensatory behaviors such as greater dietary restraint or purging (Cooper et al., 2020).

Food access

During the outbreak of COVID-19, grocery stores hosted unprecedented purchasing frenzies and food hoarding often resulting in empty shelves, food shortages, long lines of panicked shoppers, and purchasing restrictions (Clark Bryan et al., 2020; Rodriguez-Perez et al., 2020). The current pandemic also created financial pressures which led to the closure of food suppliers and interrupted supply distribution (Ammar et al., 2020; Rodgers et al., 2020). Not only does this place a strain on normal food-related behaviors, but it also severely impacts individuals with eating disorders (Ammar et al., 2020). It bares considerable concern for individuals that are already excessively limiting their food intake as it may impair the "safe" routine foods that they do consume (Rodgers et al., 2020). It is evident that the changes associated with COVID-19 may present new food-related triggers during lockdown (Clark Bryan et al., 2020). One study reported that individuals who significantly restricted their food intake may restrict their food intake further as they believe that less food was required when staying at home (Clark Bryan et al., 2020). Patients with anorexia nervosa may also have increased feelings of guilt when purchasing food during periods of food scarcity as well as when consuming their recommended high-calorie diets (Shah et al., 2020).

Alternatively, food scarcity may heighten fear and encourage stocking up on food (Rodgers et al., 2020). With larger amounts of food in the house it can increase the likelihood of snacking or binge eating episodes (Rodgers et al., 2020). Irrespective of a previous eating disorder diagnosis, the changes to food access may create alternating periods of food abundance resulting in overconsumption with or without compensatory behaviors, followed by periods of food scarcity linked to dietary restraint and fasting (Cooper et al., 2020). These patterns are more commonly associated with binge eating disorder and bulimia nervosa. These unprecedented changes to access to basic necessities can be associated with increased food preoccupation, rigid eating rituals, binge eating, and body image concerns (Cooper et al., 2020). It is assumed that with more time at home individuals will also have more time to cook and organize meals; however, it can also be associated with frequent snacking and mindless overconsumption of energy-dense foods (Rodriguez-Perez et al., 2020).

Roles and family dynamics

The restrictions associated with the development of COVID-19 created new arrangements within the home environment. During the COVID-19 pandemic, family members were working from home, all children were out of school, and there was a significant reduction in personal space, autonomy, and freedom (Clark Bryan et al., 2020). Carers of individuals with anorexia nervosa reported that the sudden transition of family dynamics created added pressure and expectation on themselves to be able to care for the entire household equally (Clark Bryan et al., 2020; Fernandez-Aranda et al., 2020). Individuals with anorexia nervosa also reported exacerbated negative emotions with constant family contact due to feeling more dependent on more individuals within their house for support (Fernandez-Aranda et al., 2020; Todisco & Donini, 2020).

The stress of confinement may result in maladaptive emotional reactions from family members and can lead to greater emotional distress within the house and thus trigger eating disorder symptomology or reduce the impact of treatment for individuals with an eating disorder (Fernandez-Aranda et al., 2020). It has been reported that routine and structure is crucial for the recovery of individuals with an eating disorder and thus COVID-19 has significantly impaired these factors. Coping with change and boredom often results in increased eating disorder preoccupation and thus carers have reported their role in support and management of symptoms has increased within their patients' lives during COVID-19 (Fernandez-Aranda et al., 2020).

Social isolation and decreased social support

Work and school provide structure and routine within everyday life; however, these have been significantly altered during the coronavirus pandemic (Davis et al., 2020). Social restrictions have enforced social distancing and in some cases self-isolation (Cooper et al., 2020). This has resulted in significant changes to socializing, employment, education, and access to services (Clark Bryan et al., 2020). The global pandemic has resulted in a significant barrier for social support, making vulnerable individuals more susceptible to engaging in maladaptive coping strategies (Rodgers et al., 2020). These restrictions have led to increased experiences of isolation and loneliness, which may be exaggerated in individuals living alone or who already feel segregated due to a condition such as those with anorexia nervosa (Fernandez-Aranda et al., 2020). Social support is often seen as a buffer for the development of eating disorder pathology and with reduced social contact individuals may engage in more emotion-related eating behaviors (Cooper et al., 2020; Rodgers et al., 2020). People are generally accustomed to social interactions and support; thus this rapid reduction in social support is bound to result in less psychological well-being and the adaption of maladaptive coping strategies such as disordered eating (Todisco & Donini, 2020).

Clinical implications

The COVID-19 pandemic has significantly challenged clinicians and forced them to rapidly alter their services to provide high-quality care while meeting restrictions and attempting to meet public health needs (Barney, Buckelew, Mesheriakova, & Raymond-Flesch, 2020). The clinical implications of the changes to "treatment as usual" for individuals with eating disorders are significant. Individuals with eating disorders are often medically monitored with regular weight assessments, vital sign checks, dietary histories, electrolyte monitoring, and specialist collaboration (Barney et al., 2020). However, during COVID-19 this medical monitoring and standard treatment might have been significantly adapted in order to be able to be conducted at home. This might have resulted in family members being taught how to take blind weight measures at home, utilizing external clinics to collect vital signs, and having parents and patients participating in telehealth using separate devices to facilitate confidential discussions (Barney et al., 2020). These changes away from face-to-face contact to telehealth were deemed necessary to protect both patients and healthcare staff (Clark Bryan et al., 2020).

Note that changes due to the COVID-19 pandemic have not been all negative. Some individuals with anorexia nervosa reported that the changed service provisions resulted in a higher standard of support compared to normal circumstances and allowed new opportunities for family members to participate in their treatment (Clark Bryan et al., 2020). The clinical implications of this shift away from face-to-face therapy for majority of patients provided increased collaboration and creativity to develop new approaches for managing the eating disorder and the challenges associated with COVID-19, encouraging patients to feel more included and boosting their self-efficacy (Clark Bryan et al., 2020).

Due to the severity of COVID-19 and the ease of transmission, only urgent visits and inpatient treatment settings have been utilized for individuals with severe eating disorders (Fernandez-Aranda et al., 2020). It is important to highlight individuals with eating disorders often have poor insight into their illness, delay help-seeking, and have difficulties communicating their needs (Fernandez-Aranda et al., 2020). In order to provide ongoing care and manage the implications of COVID-19 on individuals with eating disorders, it is vital to establish a strong foundation of teamwork, understand the impact of mental health, increase the use of technology, develop appropriate task shifting within the support network, and encourage self-care (Davis et al., 2020; Fernandez-Aranda et al., 2020).

Inpatient

Healthcare services are stretched during the global pandemic with a number of services having to be altered in order to accommodate the unprecedented strain of the coronavirus pandemic. Patients with severe eating disorders still have the option to be admitted as an inpatient for treatment; however, the team of practitioners will be significantly altered and reduced to ensure the safety of the patient and staff (Fernandez-Aranda et al., 2020). Multidisciplinary clinical meetings have been significantly reduced and information is often communicated through encrypted texts, emails, or phone calls (Davis et al., 2020). This clinic also reported changes from group meal supervision to individual meal supervision, and only one visitor is allowed (Davis et al., 2020; Gordon & Gatzman, 2020). The major concern during COVID-19 is that patients with severe eating disorders may go undiagnosed or delay starting treatment resulting in the worsening of symptoms, thus the need to have accessible inpatient clinics still operating (Fernandez-Aranda et al., 2020).

Outpatient

In order to minimize nonurgent hospitalization, outpatient practices have maintained some face-to-face appointments, especially for early treatment stage patients or new patients with suspected eating disorders (Davis et al., 2020). Face-to-face appointments for patients with stable weights have been spaced out or changed to telehealth consultations (Davis et al., 2020). It was reported, however, that if there was suspicion for medical deterioration, patients are asked to attend a face-to-face session at an outpatient clinic to be medically monitored (Barney et al., 2020).

Telehealth

Telehealth is the live communication between the patient and provider through the use of audio or video equipment (Barney et al., 2020). Since the beginning of COVID-19, some psychology clinics completely transitioned to telehealth consultations for the safety of both patient and practitioner. While this was not possible for all clinics, the clinics that did transition reported that the number of patients who engaged in telehealth treatment was consistent with the number of patients who engaged in face-to-face treatment the year prior (Barney et al., 2020). Preliminary evidence suggests that treatment for eating disorders via telehealth can be successful (Waller et al., 2020; Wood et al., 2020).

However, the implementation of telehealth has created new problems of privacy, confidentiality, and access (Barney et al., 2020; Wood et al., 2020). The ability to conduct treatment from the comfort of the patients' home may also have reduced the financial burden of traveling to and from the specialized clinics and thus minimizing risk of transmission of COVID-19 (Barney et al., 2020). However, for telehealth to be an efficient mode of treatment, both practitioner and patient must have access to a quiet and private environment as well as a phone or laptop that was able to support this form of communication (Barney et al., 2020). Successful participation in telehealth requires stable internet/reception and a level of health literacy and therefore may be impaired by race, socioeconomic status, age, and literacy levels (Rodgers et al., 2020; Todisco & Donini, 2020; Wood et al., 2020). A concern of changing to telehealth was that individuals from a lower socioeconomic status may not be able to access an electronic device or have the privacy to be able to talk freely (Barney et al., 2020). There is a chance that telehealth also limited the practitioner's comfort with making clinical decisions without being able to conduct a physical examination of the patient (Barney et al., 2020; Wood et al., 2020).

The implementation of telehealth consultations requires task shifting with family members or carers often being required to complete tasks that were previously completed by the practitioner, including calibrating home scales, taking blind weights, documenting vital signs, and providing the data to the team

(Barney et al., 2020; Cooper et al., 2020). Additionally, continuing to engage patients and provide regular care to patients with eating disorders has required the implementation of telehealth-based intervention procedures for the safety of both patient and practitioner (Cooper et al., 2020). Cognitive behavioral therapy, family-based treatment, and parent-based prevention all have evidence-based support for use via telehealth with the interventions being able to continue with weight monitoring, family meals, and exposure experiences, even during a global pandemic (Cooper et al., 2020). Additional challenges in treating individuals with eating disorders via telehealth methods are bound to occur; however; it may also create new opportunities to develop more efficient interventions and treatment modes (Wood et al., 2020). The severity of symptoms may not be accurately identified and treatment may not be as effective for all patients via telehealth; however, it also presents a unique opportunity to provide support and intervention to a greater number of patients and ensure that they do not feel as isolated during this global pandemic.

In the context of family-based therapy (FBT) with adolescents with anorexia nervosa, Matheson, Bohon, and Lock (2020) report that when using telehealth, patients might feel less connected and accountable. Other common issues of doing FBT for anorexia nervosa are comprehensively outlined by Matheson et al. (2020) and Walsh and McNicholas (2020), including medical monitoring, weight checking, rapport building, patient one-on-one check-in, setting the intense scene and family meals, and managing in-session behaviors.

Guided self-help

Social distancing and self-isolation have also encouraged some individuals with eating disorders to be proactive toward their treatment and engage in guided self-help interventions (Clark Bryan et al., 2020). Self-help interventions are all based on evidence-based interventions and should be encouraged if usual treatment is not available during COVID-19. One study found that over half the individuals with anorexia nervosa interviewed reported increased attempts to self-manage their eating disorder recovery (Clark Bryan et al., 2020). Due to the increased barriers of access, cost, stigma, and scarcity of eating disorder intervention during COVID-19, patients with anorexia nervosa have proactively sought out alternative practical self-help interventions, which usually encourage self-monitoring, psychoeducation, urge surfing, and problem solving (Cooper et al., 2020).

Technology may be beneficial for maintaining appropriate physical activity, recovery-focused self-monitoring food intake, adaptive coping behaviors, and social support (Ammar et al., 2020; Cooper et al., 2020). It may streamline communication, encourage self-monitoring and self-regulation, while also reducing the feelings of social isolation and in turn reducing the likelihood of engaging in disordered eating behaviors in order to cope (Cooper et al., 2020). It is important that clinicians guide individuals with eating disorders to the recovery-focused apps when appropriate (Cooper et al., 2020). Similarly, some patients with eating disorders may require extra support during this pandemic, which could be provided through the use of clinically appropriate emails and text messages to complement the provided services (Cooper et al., 2020).

Conclusion

It is evident that COVID-19 has impacted on the way we treat eating disorders. It has also exacerbated eating disorder symptoms and coping mechanisms in those with or without a previously diagnosed eating disorder. It is important to consider potential modifications to assessment and treatment, while realizing that treatment for this vulnerable population is essential.

References

American Psychiatric Association. (2013). *Diagnostic and statistical manual of mental disorders* (5th edition). Arlington, VA: American Psychiatric Association.

Ammar, A., Brach, M., Trabelsi, K., Chtourou, H., Boukhris, O., Masmoudi, L., et al. (2020). Effects of COVID-19 home confinement on eating behaviour and physical activity: Results of the ECLB-COVID19 international online survey. *Nutrients*, *12*(6), 28. https://doi.org/10.3390/nu12061583.

Arcelus, J., Mitchell, A. J., Wales, W., & Nielsen, S. (2011). Mortality rates in patients with anorexia nervosa and other eating disorders - A meta-analysis of 36 studies. *Archives of General Psychiatry*, *68*(7), 724–731. https://doi.org/10.1001/archgenpsychiatry.2011.74.

Barney, A., Buckelew, S., Mesheriakova, V., & Raymond-Flesch, M. (2020). The COVID-19 pandemic and rapid implementation of adolescent and young adult telemedicine: Challenges and opportunities for innovation. *The Journal of Adolescent Health*. https://doi.org/10.1016/j.jadohealth.2020.05.006.

Clark Bryan, D., Macdonald, P., Ambwani, S., Cardi, V., Rowlands, K., Willmott, D., et al. (2020). Exploring the ways in which COVID-19 and lockdown has affected the lives of adult patients with anorexia nervosa and their carers. *European Eating Disorders Review*, *09*, 09. https://doi.org/10.1002/erv.2762.

Cooper, M., Reilly, E. E., Siegel, J. A., Coniglio, K., Sadeh-Sharvit, S., Pisetsky, E. M., et al. (2020). Eating disorders during the COVID-19 pandemic and quarantine: An overview of risks and recommendations for treatment and early intervention. *Eating Disorders*, 1–23. https://doi.org/10.1080/10640266.2020.1790271.

Davis, C., Ng, K. C., Oh, J. Y., Baeg, A., Rajasegaran, K., & Chew, C. S. E. (2020). Caring for children and adolescents with eating disorders in the current coronavirus 19 pandemic: A Singapore perspective. *The Journal of Adolescent Health*, *67*(1), 131–134. https://doi.org/10.1016/j.jadohealth.2020.03.037.

Fernandez-Aranda, F., Casas, M., Claes, L., Bryan, D. C., Favaro, A., Granero, R., et al. (2020). COVID-19 and implications for eating disorders. *European Eating Disorders Review*, *28*(3), 239–245. https://doi.org/10.1002/erv.2738.

Gordon, C., & Gatzman, D. (2020). Lessons learned in caring for adolescents with eating disorders: The Singapore experience. *Journal of Adolescent Health*, *67*, 5e6.

Matheson, B., Bohon, C., & Lock, J. (2020). Family-based treatment via videoconference: Clinical recommendations for treatment providers during COVID-19 and beyond. *International Journal of Eating Disorders*, *53*, 1142–1154.

Phillipou, A., Meyer, D., Neill, E., Jan, E., Lin, W., Van Rheenen, T., et al. (2020). Eating and exercise behaviors in eating disorders and the general population during the COVID-19 pandemic in Australia: Initial results from the COLLATE project. *International Journal of Eating Disorders*, *53*, 1158–1165.

Rodgers, R. F., Lombardo, C., Cerolini, S., Franko, D. L., Omori, M., Fuller-Tyszkiewicz, M., et al. (2020). The impact of the COVID-19 pandemic on eating disorder risk and symptoms. *The International Journal of Eating Disorders*, *53*(7), 1166–1170. https://doi.org/10.1002/eat.23318.

Rodriguez-Perez, C., Molina-Montes, E., Verardo, V., Artacho, R., Garcia-Villanova, B., Guerra-Hernandez, E. J., et al. (2020). Changes in dietary behaviours during the COVID-19 outbreak confinement in the Spanish COVIDiet study. *Nutrients*, *12*(6), 10. https://doi.org/10.3390/nu12061730.

Shah, M., Sachdeva, M., & Johnston, H. (2020). Eating disorders in the age of COVID-19. *Psychiatry Research*, *290*. https://doi.org/10.1016/j.psychres.2020.113122, 113122.

Termorshuizen, J. D., et al. (2020). Early impact of COVID-19 on individuals with eating disorders: A survey of ~1000 individuals in the United States and the Netherlands. Version 2 *medRxiv*. https://doi.org/10.1101/2020.05.28.20116301.

Todisco, P., & Donini, L. M. (2020). Eating disorders and obesity (ED&O) in the COVID-19 storm. *Eating and Weight Disorders*, *01*, 01. https://doi.org/10.1007/s40519-020-00938-z.

Waller, G., et al. (2020). Cognitive-behavioral therapy in the time of coronavirus: Clinician tips for working with eating disorders via telehealth when face-to-face meetings are not possible. *International Journal of Eating Disorders*, *53*, 1132–1141.

Walsh, O., & McNicholas, F. (2020). Assessment and management of anorexia nervosa during COVID-19. *Irish Journal of Psychological Medicine*. https://doi.org/10.1017/ipm.2020.60.

Wood, S. M., White, K., Peebles, R., Pickel, J., Alausa, M., Mehringer, J., et al. (2020). Outcomes of a rapid adolescent telehealth scale-up during the COVID-19 pandemic. *The Journal of Adolescent Health*, *28*, 28. https://doi.org/10.1016/j.jadohealth.2020.05.025.

Zachary, Z., Brianna, F., Brianna, L., Garrett, P., Jade, W., Alyssa, D., et al. (2020). Self-quarantine and weight gain related risk factors during the COVID-19 pandemic. *Obesity Research & Clinical Practice*, *14*(3), 210–216. https://doi.org/10.1016/j.orcp.2020.05.004.

Chapter 11

Obsessive-compulsive disorder during and after Covid-19 pandemic

Anıl Şafak Kaçar[a,b]

[a]*Graduate School of Health Sciences, Koç University, Istanbul, Turkey,* [b]*Koc University Research Center for Translational Medicine (KUTTAM), Istanbul, Turkey*

Introduction

The World Health Organization (WHO) declared Coronavirus Disease (Covid-19) a public health emergency of international concern at the end of January 2020 and declared it as a pandemic by March 11, 2020 (Baddeley, 1992; WHO, 2020). Since there is no known vaccine or treatment for this novel infectious disease, in order to minimize the detrimental effects of the Covid-19 pandemic, the Centers for Disease Control and Prevention (CDC) recommends measures such as frequent handwashing and maintaining social distance (CDC, 2020). These recommended measures are necessary and indispensable to reduce the rate of spread of the Covid-19 outbreak. However, these measures are expected to lead to an increase in the incidence of many psychiatric illnesses (Galea, Merchant, & Lurie, 2020). Obsessive-compulsive disorder (OCD) is one of such diseases. There is a similarity between OCD symptoms and the measures to be taken against the Covid-19 outbreak. For example, OCD patients with contamination obsession and cleaning/washing compulsion have frequent and prolonged handwashing behavior. Same behaviors regarding handwashing are expected from the general population as a preventive measure against the Covid-19 pandemic. During the Covid-19 pandemic, an increase in the severity of symptoms can be expected in some of the patients diagnosed with OCD. The case reports of relapsing OCD patients during the Covid-19 pandemic have already been reported (French & Lyne, 2020; Kumar & Somani, 2020). This chapter will cover the general features of OCD and the effect of Covid-19 pandemic on patients with OCD. This chapter will also advocate that there will be an increase in OCD prevalence incited by Covid-19 pandemic.

Obsessive-compulsive disorder

OCD is one of the most debilitating psychiatric disorders impairing affected individual's quality of life enormously (Subramaniam, Soh, Vaingankar,

Mental Health Effects of COVID-19. https://doi.org/10.1016/B978-0-12-824289-6.00009-X

Picco, & Chong, 2013). It affects approximately 1.3% of general population at some point during their lifetime (Fawcett, Power, & Fawcett, 2020). The age of onset has bimodal distribution suggesting early onset and late-onset OCD subgroups (Taylor, 2011). The average age of onset of the early onset OCD subgroup is 11 years old (range: 6–16 years), while the average age of onset of late-onset OCD subgroup is around 23 years old (range: 18–50 years) (Bloch, 2017). The early onset OCD group is associated with greater proportion of males, greater overall OCD symptom severity, and greater prevalence of OCD among first-degree relatives when compared to the late-onset OCD group, greater risk of comorbid tic disorders which consist of sudden, recurrent, nonrhythmic motor movement or vocalizations (American Psychiatric Association, 2013; Taylor, 2011).

The core clinical features of OCD include, as the name implies, obsessions and compulsions (American Psychiatric Association, 2013). Obsessions are intrusive thoughts, images or urges that evoke anxiety, discomfort, or doubt (Penzel, 2017). The discomfort associated with obsessions can be extreme, and the desire to alleviate these aversive feelings is compelling (Penzel, 2017). Compulsions, the other component of the disorder, are mental or behavioral acts that are hard to be abstained from performing (Penzel, 2017). They often must be performed by following specific set of rules and/or constant series of steps (Penzel, 2017). Compulsions with these features are commonly referred to as rituals. When patients with OCD diagnosis engage with ritualistic behaviors, they follow a specific sequence of actions which may need to be repeated a certain number of times. In the typical case of OCD, compulsions are performed to alleviate discomfort caused by obsessions. Thus performing compulsions to achieve relief also provides negative reinforcement (removal of aversive state) which causes repetition of the same compulsive behavior when the discomfort associated with obsessions is emerged (Abramovitch & McKay, 2016). In some cases, if any "error" made during the performance of a ritual, then all steps must be repeated from the beginning. Additionally, the relief provided by the compulsive acts is only partial and intermittent, which means that compulsive acts will not fully reduce the anxiety and will not provide a long-term relief. Moreover, as compulsions are mostly performed in ritualistic or in particular ways, it is very possible that patients will not be satisfied with the way they performed the compulsive act and will likely to stick in the repeating cycle of the compulsive ritual. Patients with OCD diagnosis have hard time to break the loop of obsessions and compulsions. This causes significant discomfort for patients, consumption of time, and impairment in quality of life.

The clinical picture depicted previously is only a simple description of OCD which does not fit every single patient. For some patients, there is a clear and reasonable association between obsessions and compulsions, such as those patients may wash their hands repeatedly whenever they feel that their hands are dirty. But in other patients, this relationship between obsessions and compulsions may seem arbitrary (Penzel, 2017). For example, they may need to say a specific phrase repeatedly in order to prevent any possibility of harm to their loved ones. In the former case, there is a reasonable association between the feeling of dirty hands and handwashing behavior; however, in the latter example, there is no reasonable association between preventing harm to patient's loved ones and repeatedly saying a phrase. Moreover, the content of obsessions and compulsive acts varies between patients, thus no single case can truly be representative of OCD. The symptom profile among OCD patients has a very diverse range, therefore the dimensional approach suggests that there are at least four different symptom dimensions for OCD, namely cleaning (contamination obsessions and cleaning compulsion), symmetry (symmetry obsessions and repeating ordering, and counting compulsion), forbidden or taboo thoughts (for example, sexual, religious, or aggressive obsessions and related compulsions), and harm (for example, fears of harm to oneself or others and checking compulsions) (American Psychiatric Association, 2013; Mataix-Cols, do Rosario-Campos, & Leckman, 2005).

The significant portion of patients with OCD diagnosis has an insight about their disorder. Those patients who have good insight think that their compulsive acts are excessive and unnecessary when compared to the threat associated with the obsessive thoughts. For example, they know that there is no additional preventive benefit of their checking behavior hot stove repeatedly against the risk of fire. The insight associated with OCD is not a temporarily stable feature of the disorder. OCD patients may have insight about their symptoms at some point of their life, and then they may lose this insight. Patients with higher insight bother less with the content of their obsessions, feel less anxiety, and their life is less dominated with compulsive acts than patients with lower insight (Penzel, 2017). OCD patients with higher insight may reattribute the discomfort caused by obsessions as one of the symptoms of their disorder and they can refrain from performing the compulsive acts.

The current neurobiological understanding of OCD implies the hyperactivity of cortico-striato-thalamo-cortical pathways (Milad & Rauch, 2012). The mechanism underlying this hyperactivity is proposed in relation to serotonergic dysfunction (Dougherty et al., 2018). The decrease in the serotonin level disturbs its inhibitory role in striatum, thalamus, and cortical areas, and results with the hyperactivation of cortico-striato-thalamo-cortical loops (Dougherty et al., 2018). The neural structures involved in the pathophysiology of OCD are particularly indicated as caudate nucleus, dorsal anterior cingulate cortex, and orbitofrontal cortex (Dougherty et al., 2018). These brain areas are found to be abnormally active at rest and with symptom provocation (Dougherty et al., 2018). It is possible to counteract the decrease in serotonin level with selective serotonin reuptake inhibitors (SSRI). With this initial SSRI treatment, only 40%–60% of patients with OCD diagnosis achieve partial response (Pallanti & Quercioli, 2006). The gold standard psychological treatment of OCD is exposure and response prevention (ERP) (Storch, Schneider, Guzick, McKay, & Goodman, 2020). With this technique, OCD patients are gradually and systematically exposed to triggers which evoke obsessive-compulsive symptoms while refraining from compulsive or avoidance behaviors is expected.

How to decide excessive behavior during the Covid-19 pandemic?

As previously mentioned, compulsive acts are mostly performed to alleviate the discomfort caused by obsessions. One of the features of compulsive acts is being excessive when compared to the risk associated with not performing compulsive acts. For example, if a patient has contamination obsession and cleaning compulsion, the duration and/or frequency of cleaning behavior must be out of proportion to the risk of being contaminated with a germ to be called as compulsion. During the Covid-19 pandemic, the line between excessive and necessary cleaning behavior is blurred. Thus how to decide excessive behavior which aims to prevent getting or transmitting coronavirus infection is a debatable question. This difficulty is not limited to cleaning behavior. OCD patients may stay at their homes as an avoidance behavior in order not to have any risk of getting infected. Although staying at home is recommended to reduce the rate of transmission of Covid-19, OCD patients may stay in their homes even in essential situations.

Frequent handwashing for 20 seconds is recommended to prevent the dissemination of infection. Celebrities and public figures prepared and published in social media several videos to present how to wash hands properly. During the Covid-19 pandemic, frequent handwashing behavior became normalized. All these recommendations and campaigns may lead to repeated, stereotypical, and timed handwashing behavior in the general population who may have obsessive-compulsive behavior tendencies. While categorizing a frequent handwashing behavior as compulsion or adaptive response to ongoing risk of getting infection, the degree of protection produced by these rituals must be carefully compared with the interference of these rituals in daily lives of the individuals (Silva, Shavitt, & Costa, 2020). Patients with OCD diagnosis should not be encouraged to outgrow their adaptive responses to ongoing risk of getting infection. However, it must be remembered that CDC recommendations are sufficient to reduce the risk of getting and transmitting infection. Washing hands longer than 20 seconds or with stronger disinfectants other than regular soaps will not reduce the risk of getting infection further (Shafran, Coughtrey, & Whittal, 2020). The handwashing behavior is recommended only in response to external contact when the person comes back home from outside or has contact with an item which comes from outside of the home. Importantly, if there is no external contact, there is no need for handwashing in cases of anxiety or fears of potential contamination. Currently, clinicians intuitively decide based on these notes, but there is a need for a clearer diagnostic threshold to differentiate the adaptive behavior to avoid infection from the compulsive behavior which is excessive compared to the risk of infection.

Effect of Covid-19 pandemic on OCD patients

The coronavirus pandemic has serious detrimental effects on the mental health of many individuals (Galea et al., 2020). It made governments take extensive measures to reduce the harmful impact of the virus. As a result, people had to stay at home for weeks without any social interactions and external activities. Many people could not see their families and friends for long periods of time. Even if they could, they were advised to be no closer than 1.5 m. Frequently washing hands and wearing masks became a must in daily lives during the Covid-19 pandemic. People were afraid of not being able to reach the indispensable items; thus, markets were looted. During this stressful period, many mental health problems, such as depressive symptoms, emerged even in the population with no known psychiatric disorder (Brooks et al., 2020). This effect was doubtlessly more severe for people who had OCD, considering the fact that OCD patients are "experts by nature" in attempting to prevent harmful incidents through enacting compulsive acts (Fineberg et al., 2020). Many protective behaviors against Covid-19 pandemic resemble the compulsive acts of patients with OCD diagnosis and are likely to substitute a cognitive justification for their symptoms. For instance, frequent handwashing is a well-known symptom of OCD and the necessity to frequently wash hands during the pandemic might further reinforce this behavior for many patients with OCD diagnosis. Celebrities, public figures, and other authorities published videos on how to wash hands on social media and television. As people with the diagnosis of OCD already wash their hands in ritualistic ways (Banerjee, 2020), the social media campaigns likely play a supportive role for this symptom. Similarly, the danger of going out of home might be validated for OCD people who cannot go out with the fear of getting infected.

Cognitive distortions pertinent to OCD disorder are expected to have a significant role in making the already affected individuals more vulnerable for the effects of the pandemic (Pozza, Mucci, & Marazziti, 2020). One of those cognitive distortions is intolerance of uncertainty which is the tendency to interpret ambiguous situations as threatening (Garami et al., 2017). Intolerance of uncertainty implies transdiagnostic set of maladaptive beliefs (Mahoney & McEvoy, 2012). People with intolerance of uncertainty suffer from inability to cope with ambiguity or unpredictability (Garami et al., 2017). Covid-19 is an unknown disease in terms of its effects, and considering the "intolerance of uncertainty" nature of OCD, people suffering from this disorder are more likely to get influenced by the risks the virus has created. This cognitive distortion might manifest itself as excessive and repeated reviewing of news about the Covid-19 in order to decrease the uncertainty associated with the related pandemic. Similarly, children might show excessive and repeated reassurance seeking to deal with the anxiety of uncertainty. People with OCD diagnosis might also have cognitive distortions, such as overvalued ideas about their responsibility in harmful incidences (Foa, Sacks, Tolin, Prezworski, & Amir, 2002). For instance, they might have excessive fear of transmitting infection to their beloved ones. Their threat estimation is also higher than people with no OCD diagnosis (Steketee, Frost, & Cohen, 1998). Most of the people infected by Covid-19 recover from the disease with mild symptoms; however, patients with OCD diagnosis might overestimate the already serious outcomes of the virus (Shafran et al., 2020).

As previously mentioned, the presentation of OCD disorder is very diverse. In order to conceptualize OCD, categorical symptom dimensions are necessary. Fear of contamination and cleaning/washing compulsions is one of the most common symptom dimensions affecting about 50% of patients (Mataix-Cols et al., 2002). Patients who are in this symptom dimension frequently wash their hands, take showers, and clean their homes. Moreover, avoidance behaviors, such as not going out of home in order not to get contaminated, are observed in 80% of OCD patients (Rajkumar, 2020). These symptoms might easily be precipitated by the coronavirus pandemic. Another symptom dimension associated with OCD is associated with the fears of harming oneself or others (American Psychiatric Association, 2013). Patients in this symptom dimension might not differentiate their thoughts and actions. For instance, the thought of harming someone might result in tremendous anxiety. Patients in this symptom dimension might disturb themselves with compulsive acts in order to halt such thoughts or they might take compulsive preventions against the risk of actualization of these thoughts. This cognitive pattern might manifest itself as excessive fear of transmitting infection and taking excessive preventive measures not to infect others. Additionally, they might repeatedly check their temperature to be sure about their infection status. These two symptom dimensions arguably represent the most vulnerable group of OCD patients. However, this does not imply that patients in other symptom dimensions will not be affected during this very stressful pandemic period. The nature of their preoccupations might alter their phenotype and the focus of their preoccupations (Fontenelle & Miguel, 2020). Patients from other symptom dimensions might start to show symptoms from these dimensions during pandemic according to their tendencies. Although the symptom dimensions of patients with OCD diagnosis have temporal stability over the course of the disorder, it is possible to observe alterations in the symptom dimensions (Rufer, Grothusen, Maß, Peter, & Hand, 2005).

The Covid-19 pandemic also might be suggested to have a disruptive influence on the psychotherapy process of patients with OCD diagnosis. As briefly mentioned before, Exposure and Response Prevention (ERP) is the gold standard psychological intervention for OCD patients. During this intervention, OCD patients are expected to refrain from compulsive acts or avoidance behaviors after exposure of triggers that evoke obsessive-compulsive symptoms. Considering that OCD patients struggle to resist the discomfort caused by not performing their compulsions such as handwashing, pandemic conditions even make it harder for them to follow these steps, because many sources (such as press, social media) reinforce the compulsions of OCD patients as mentioned before. Moreover, during the psychotherapy process, insightfulness plays a major role. During ERP, patients will reattribute the cause of their discomfort induced by obsessions as a symptom of their disorder, then they try to refrain from compulsive acts. This process is easier if they have insight about their disorder. The pandemic conditions might negatively affect the insightfulness of OCR patients. Some patients have told their clinicians they were "right all along," as everybody looks like them during Covid-19 pandemic (Fineberg et al., 2020). It is possible to argue that protection recommendations can reinforce the irrational beliefs of OCD patients more if they have poor insight.

A case report presented a deterioration in the symptoms of a patient with relatively well-controlled OCD after the media reports of the emergence of Covid-19 (French & Lyne, 2020). In this case, the main dimension of obsessions was related to the fear of contamination before and after the pandemic. The patient's compulsive rituals were intensified during the pandemic. The time consumed for handwashing and cleaning compulsions reached to several hours per day. Another case report presented a relapsing case during the Covid-19 pandemic (Kumar & Somani, 2020). Similar to the previous case report, the fear of getting infected was intensified with watching programs on television and reading/watching messages on social media platforms. The patient started to avoid meeting people and to wash his hands excessively. In another study, the Yale-Brown Obsessive-Compulsive Scale (YBOCS) was applied to patients with OCD before and 6 weeks after quarantine (Davide et al., 2020). The measurement before the quarantine was taken at the end of the therapeutic intervention. YBOCS scores both in obsession and compulsion subscales were statistically significantly increased during quarantine when compared to prequarantine assessment. 13.33% of the study population who are remitted before quarantine returned to clinically significant OCD status (Davide et al., 2020). In this study, the unavoidable lack of control group of patients unexposed to quarantine rendered impossible to eliminate the possible confound of lack of psychiatric visits during quarantine (Davide et al., 2020). A similar study was conducted with children in Turkey. Children's Yale-Brown Obsessive-Compulsive Scale (CY-BOCS) was applied to children and adolescents with OCD diagnosis before and during Covid-19 pandemic (Tanir et al., 2020). The significant increase in the scores of contamination obsession and cleaning/washing compulsion subscales was detected. More than half of the study subjects reported an increase in the severity of OCD symptoms. This proportion is found to be more than 30% of the study population among children and adolescents with OCD diagnosis (Tanir et al., 2020). Another study reported that more than one-third of the study population has clinical worsening of OCD symptoms (Benatti et al., 2020). These patients had both an increase in the severity of preexisting symptoms and emergence of new obsessions and compulsions. The experience of suicidal ideation is also found to be more common among the patients who have an increase in OCD symptoms during the Covid-19 pandemic than the group of patients without an increase in OCD symptoms.

Some studies present some risk and protective factors associated with the increase in OCD symptoms of patients during pandemic. For instance, living with a relative in the same house during the quarantine is found as a risk factor for YBOCS score increase (Davide et al., 2020). According to the same study, having contamination-related symptoms before quarantine was also a risk factor for exacerbation of OCD symptoms (Davide et al., 2020). Patients who could work/study remotely during the quarantine had significantly less worsening on the severity of OCD symptoms (Davide et al., 2020). On the other hand, the diagnosis of Covid-19 in someone familiar has been detected as a predictor of the increase in CY-BOCS scores among children and adolescents with OCD diagnosis (Tanir et al., 2020). Additionally, the duration of OCD diagnosis is found to be a risk factor for increase in OCD symptoms among child and adolescent patients during pandemic (Tanir et al., 2020). The fear of Covid-19 was also a predictor of OCD scores among adolescents (Secer & Ulas, 2020).

International College of Obsessive Compulsive Spectrum Disorders (ICOCS) and the Obsessive-Compulsive and Related Disorders Research Network of the European College of Neuropsychopharmacology (OCRN) have published a consensus statement as a guidance for the management of OCD during the Covid-19 pandemic (Fineberg et al., 2020). Firstly, a compassionate and calming approach is recommended for the experts who are working with the OCD population during the pandemic. Additionally, the consensus statement indicated that careful history taking is important in order to segregate rational or exaggerated reactions to the Covid-19 pandemic from exacerbation of obsessive-compulsive symptomatology. Patients having contamination obsession and cleaning or washing compulsion in the past may reexperience these symptoms during the Covid-19 pandemic. However, it is also important not to assume that all OCD patients will excessively be concerned about Covid-19 and have worsening in their symptoms. It is also important to be careful about the comorbid conditions (such as anxiety disorders, depression, or bipolar disorder) that might worsen with stress induced by the pandemic. Furthermore, the risk of suicide must be assessed and considered carefully. Access to treatment services got limited during the Covid-19 pandemic because of the governmental measures; however, in some cases, it is critical to be in close contact with physicians, especially for the patients who have high risk for suicide. In those cases, telemedicine should be applied when necessary and appropriate. Another suggestion in the consensus statement implies that psychoeducation and giving information about the known risks and impact of Covid-19 is very important. Adequate information helps OCD patients to manage stress associated with the uncertainty about Covid-19. However, excessive information seeking might trigger more anxiety associated with the pandemic. The time consumed to follow news and developments about coronavirus must be assessed carefully. Some patients might be spending hours to search the internet and watch TV in order not to miss any news and get reassurance. The exposure to news about the Covid-19 pandemic must be limited especially in child and adolescent OCD groups to decrease symptom deterioration (Tanir et al., 2020). Reliable sources must be recommended to avoid misinformation. As a treatment approach, pharmacotherapy has been shown as the first option for OCD patients with contamination obsessions during Covid-19 pandemics (Fineberg et al., 2020). In some cases, CBT with exposure and response prevention might be considered as an additional treatment option. However, it needs to be adapted to the pandemic conditions. For instance, instead of recommending not washing hands after exposure, it is important to tailor CBT regarding the CDC guidance as handwashing for 20 seconds with soap.

Expected increase in OCD prevalence

The number of individuals affected by OCD is expected to be increased during and after the Covid-19 pandemic (Fontenelle & Miguel, 2020). The first signs of this increase can be seen in the study of Tian and colleagues. Obsessive-Compulsive (OC) scores, collected during the first weeks of pandemic (January 31–February 2, 2020) measured by Symptom Checklist (SCL-90), were found have increased in the general population (Tian et al., 2020). In addition to OC scores, interpersonal sensitivity and phobia scores were also increased in the general population during the pandemic compared with the previous norm study (Jin, Wu, & Zhang, 1986). Although an increase in scores is not specific to OC in this study, it is possible to suggest that an increase in OCD prevalence is more likely than other mental health disorders, considering the similarity of the symptomatology of OCD and the measures against the virus (e.g., washing hand excessively). For individuals who are genetically predisposed to develop OCD but with no clinical diagnosis yet, the pandemic might be a strong environmental trigger. For instance, first-degree relatives of patients with OCD diagnosis are within the risk group of this stressful period of pandemic to develop OCD. Furthermore, the prevalence of individuals who have a subthreshold OC symptoms is higher than the prevalence of OCD patients in the general population (Ruscio, Stein, Chiu, & Kessler, 2010) and these individuals, who are close to the clinical threshold, are very likely to become full-blown OCD patients as a result of the environmental triggering nature of Covid-19 pandemic (Pozza et al., 2020). In sum, individuals who have a tendency for OCD symptomatology are likely to receive the diagnosis of OCD as a result of the environmental triggers during the pandemic; however, research should investigate if the Covid-19 pandemic can also trigger OCD symptoms in individuals who are not at risk of developing OCD (Fig. 1).

Healthcare professionals constitute a high-risk group for OCD development during and after Covid-19 pandemic (Pozza et al., 2020). They are exposed to contamination risk more than many parts of the society. Additionally, they experience traumatic incidents like deaths of infected patients and colleagues at a higher rate than before. They are also likely to have higher feelings of responsibility about transmitting the disease to their loved ones. One study compared

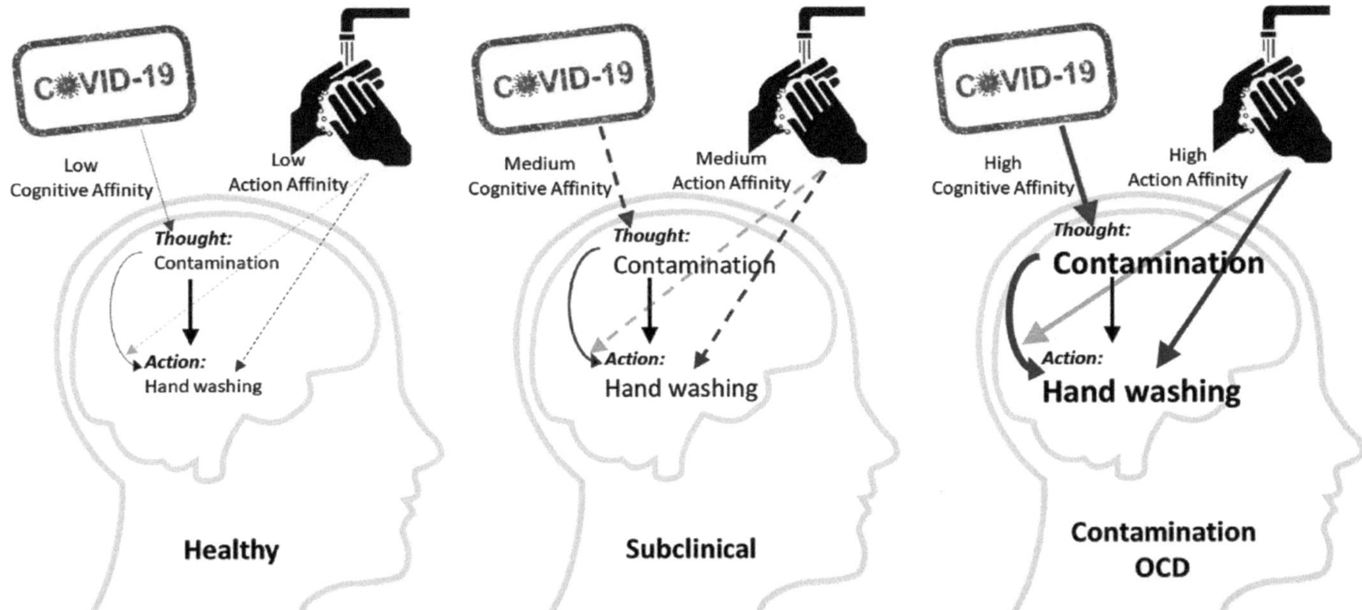

FIG. 1 The effect of Covid-19 pandemic on individuals with different levels of contamination obsession and cleaning compulsion tendencies. During the pandemic, the fear of getting Covid-19 spread along with the infection itself. This fear related with Covid-19 may feed the obsessions about contamination of both individuals with subclinical obsessive-compulsive symptoms and OCD patients. The preventive measures against the Covid-19 were recommended repeatedly on television and social media. For individuals with subclinical obsessive-compulsive symptoms and OCD patients, these indispensable announcements about the preventive measures may substitute cognitive justification for the enactment of compulsive behaviors (such as handwashing).

medical healthcare workers and nonmedical healthcare workers in terms of the mental health symptoms emerged during pandemic (Zhang et al., 2020). Medical healthcare workers had higher OC scores measured using the SCL-90-R than nonmedical healthcare workers. Living in rural areas (where medical conditions are worse), being at risk of contact with Covid-19 patients in hospitals, and having organic diseases were found to be risk factors for increased obsessive-compulsive symptoms for medical healthcare workers in the same study. Another study compared mental health symptoms of medical personnel dealing with coronavirus infection with the results of a norm study (Xing, Sun, Xu, Geng, & Li, 2020). They found that medical personnel had higher OC, phobia, and anxiety scores measured by SCL-90 scores.

Considering the aforementioned risks of increase in the prevalence of OCD, it is crucial to identify the early signs of OC symptoms, especially in the groups who are thought to be within the risk group of OCD. Early intervention and prevention strategies can play a vital role in prevention of the exacerbation of OCD. Psychoeducation can be considered as one of the most important preventive interventions (Pfefferbaum & North, 2020). Informing the society about Covid-19 adequately might help stress management of individuals who have intolerance of uncertainty and OCD tendency. Considering the negative effects of excessive and inappropriate information seeking on the development of OCD symptomatology, it is important to recommend reliable sources of information to follow. Additionally, having an active social network even remotely has beneficial effects on reducing distress, therefore keeping the social network active as much as possible must be recommended as a preventive mechanism (Brooks et al., 2020).

Conclusions

The Covid-19 pandemic caused an abrupt change in our daily lives. We spend more time at home than we did before the pandemic. When we need to go outside, we wear a face mask. We wash our hands more frequently than before. In addition to those changes, we have the fear of getting and transmitting the coronavirus. The increase in the incidence of psychiatric disorders is expected during this stressful period. As one of those psychiatric disorders, OCD comes to the forefront with its similar symptoms with the measures taken against the Covid-19. This similarity also appears as a challenge for the diagnostic criteria and it is very hard to differentiate disease-driven excessive accommodation to pandemic from necessary measures of cleaning and handwashing. A subgroup of patients with the diagnosis of OCD has already been preoccupied with the contamination risk, thus, they are very vulnerable to the threatening atmosphere of pandemic. The limited literature about the clinical presentation of OCD patients during the Covid-19 pandemic indicates the clinical exacerbation of patients with OCD diagnosis during the pandemic. Additionally, the obsessive thoughts of patients with OCD diagnosis are now supported by societal spread of messages. The increase in the prevalence of OCD diagnosis can also be expected during and after the pandemic. For individuals with subthreshold obsessive-compulsive symptoms, the pandemic period can constitute an environmental risk factor to develop full-blown OCD (Pozza et al., 2020). It is very important to provide adequate information about Covid-19 to society in order to diminish the triggering effect of this stressful period of pandemic. The importance of frequent handwashing, wearing mask, and keeping social distance to reduce the rate of the spread of the Covid-19 cannot be overlooked. While disseminating these preventive measures, it must be remembered that the additional precautions will not provide more benefit against the pandemic.

Acknowledgments

The author gratefully acknowledges use of the services and facilities of the Koç University Research Center for Translational Medicine (KUTTAM), funded by the Presidency of Turkey, Presidency of Strategy and Budget. The content is solely the responsibility of the authors and does not necessarily represent the official views of the Presidency of Strategy and Budget.

References

Abramovitch, A., & McKay, D. (2016). Behavioral impulsivity in obsessive–compulsive disorder. *Journal of Behavioral Addictions*, *5*(3), 395–397.

American Psychiatric Association. (2013). *Diagnostic and statistical manual of mental disorders (DSM-5®)* (5th ed.). Washington, DC: American Psychiatric Pub.

Baddeley, A. (1992). Working memory. *Science*, *255*(5044), 556–559.

Banerjee, D. D. (2020). The other side of COVID-19: Impact on obsessive compulsive disorder (OCD) and hoarding. *Psychiatry Research*, *288*, 112966. https://doi.org/10.1016/j.psychres.2020.112966.

Benatti, B., Albert, U., Maina, G., Fiorillo, A., Celebre, L., Girone, N., … Dell'Osso, B. (2020). What happened to patients with obsessive compulsive disorder during the COVID-19 pandemic? A multicentre report from tertiary clinics in northern Italy. *Frontiers in Psychiatry*, *11*. https://doi.org/10.3389/fpsyt.2020.00720.

Bloch, M. H. (2017). Natural history and long-term outcome of OCD. In C. Pittenger (Ed.), *Obsessive-compulsive disorder: Phenomenology, pathophysiology, and treatment* Oxford University Press.

Brooks, S. K., Webster, R. K., Smith, L. E., Woodland, L., Wessely, S., Greenberg, N., & Rubin, G. J. (2020). The psychological impact of quarantine and how to reduce it: Rapid review of the evidence. *The Lancet*, *395*(10227), 912–920. https://doi.org/10.1016/s0140-6736(20)30460-8.

CDC. (2020). *How to protect yourself & others*.

Davide, P., Andrea, P., Martina, O., Andrea, E., Davide, D., & Mario, A. (2020). The impact of the COVID-19 pandemic on patients with OCD: Effects of contamination symptoms and remission state before the quarantine in a preliminary naturalistic study. *Psychiatry Research*, *291*, 113213. https://doi.org/10.1016/j.psychres.2020.113213.

Dougherty, D. D., Brennan, B. P., Stewart, S. E., Wilhelm, S., Widge, A. S., & Rauch, S. L. (2018). Neuroscientifically informed formulation and treatment planning for patients with obsessive-compulsive disorder. *JAMA Psychiatry*, *75*(10), 1081. https://doi.org/10.1001/jamapsychiatry.2018.0930.

Fawcett, E. J., Power, H., & Fawcett, J. M. (2020). Women are at greater risk of OCD than men: A meta-analytic review of OCD prevalence worldwide. *The Journal of Clinical Psychiatry*, *81*(4). https://doi.org/10.4088/JCP.19r13085.

Fineberg, N. A., Van Ameringen, M., Drummond, L., Hollander, E., Stein, D. J., Geller, D., … Dell'Osso, B. (2020). How to manage obsessive-compulsive disorder (OCD) under COVID-19: A clinician's guide from the International College of Obsessive Compulsive Spectrum Disorders (ICOCS) and the Obsessive-Compulsive and Related Disorders Research Network (OCRN) of the European College of Neuropsychopharmacology. *Comprehensive Psychiatry*, *100*, 152174. https://doi.org/10.1016/j.comppsych.2020.152174.

Foa, E. B., Sacks, M. B., Tolin, D. F., Prezworski, A., & Amir, N. (2002). Inflated perception of responsibility for harm in OCD patients with and without checking compulsions: A replication and extension. *Journal of Anxiety Disorders*, *16*(4), 443–453.

Fontenelle, L. F., & Miguel, E. C. (2020). The impact of COVID-19 in the diagnosis and treatment of obsessive-compulsive disorder. *Depression and Anxiety*. https://doi.org/10.1002/da.23037.

French, I., & Lyne, J. (2020). Acute exacerbation of OCD symptoms precipitated by media reports of COVID-19. *Irish Journal of Psychological Medicine*, 1–14. https://doi.org/10.1017/ipm.2020.61.

Galea, S., Merchant, R. M., & Lurie, N. (2020). The mental health consequences of COVID-19 and physical distancing. *JAMA Internal Medicine*, *180*(6), 817. https://doi.org/10.1001/jamainternmed.2020.1562.

Garami, J., Haber, P., Myers, C. E., Allen, M. T., Misiak, B., Frydecka, D., & Moustafa, A. A. (2017). Intolerance of uncertainty in opioid dependency–Relationship with trait anxiety and impulsivity. *PLoS One*, *12*(7), e0181955.

Jin, H., Wu, W., & Zhang, M. (1986). Preliminary analysis of SCL-90 assessment results of Chinese normal people. *Chinese Journal of Neurological and Psychiatric Diseases*, *12*(5), 260–263.

Kumar, A., & Somani, A. (2020). Dealing with Corona virus anxiety and OCD. *Asian Journal of Psychiatry*, *51*, 102053. https://doi.org/10.1016/j.ajp.2020.102053.

Mahoney, A. E., & McEvoy, P. M. (2012). A transdiagnostic examination of intolerance of uncertainty across anxiety and depressive disorders. *Cognitive Behaviour Therapy*, *41*(3), 212–222.

Mataix-Cols, D., do Rosario-Campos, M. C., & Leckman, J. F. (2005). A multidimensional model of obsessive-compulsive disorder. *American Journal of Psychiatry*, *162*(2), 228–238.

Mataix-Cols, D., Rauch, S. L., Baer, L., Eisen, J. L., Shera, D. M., Goodman, W. K., … Jenike, M. A. (2002). Symptom stability in adult obsessive-compulsive disorder: Data from a naturalistic two-year follow-up study. *American Journal of Psychiatry*, *159*(2), 263–268.

Milad, M. R., & Rauch, S. L. (2012). Obsessive-compulsive disorder: Beyond segregated cortico-striatal pathways. *Trends in Cognitive Sciences*, *16*(1), 43–51.

Pallanti, S., & Quercioli, L. (2006). Treatment-refractory obsessive-compulsive disorder: Methodological issues, operational definitions and therapeutic lines. *Progress in Neuro-Psychopharmacology and Biological Psychiatry*, *30*(3), 400–412.

Penzel, F. (2017). Clinical presentation of OCD. In C. Pittenger (Ed.), *Obsessive-compulsive disorder: Phenomenology, pathophysiology, and treatment* Oxford University Press.

Pfefferbaum, B., & North, C. S. (2020). Mental health and the Covid-19 pandemic. *New England Journal of Medicine*. https://doi.org/10.1056/nejmp2008017.

Pozza, A., Mucci, F., & Marazziti, D. (2020). Risk for pathological contamination fears at coronavirus time: Proposal of early intervention and prevention strategies. *Clinical Neuropsychiatry*, *17*(2), 100–102. https://doi.org/10.36131/Cn20200214.

Rajkumar, R. P. (2020). Contamination and infection: What the coronavirus pandemic could reveal about the evolutionary origins of obsessive-compulsive disorder. *Psychiatry Research*. https://doi.org/10.1016/j.psychres.2020.113062.

Rufer, M., Grothusen, A., Maß, R., Peter, H., & Hand, I. (2005). Temporal stability of symptom dimensions in adult patients with obsessive–compulsive disorder. *Journal of Affective Disorders*, *88*(1), 99–102. https://doi.org/10.1016/j.jad.2005.06.003.

Ruscio, A. M., Stein, D. J., Chiu, W. T., & Kessler, R. C. (2010). The epidemiology of obsessive-compulsive disorder in the National Comorbidity Survey Replication. *Molecular Psychiatry*, *15*(1), 53–63. https://doi.org/10.1038/mp.2008.94.

Secer, I., & Ulas, S. (2020). An investigation of the effect of COVID-19 on OCD in youth in the context of emotional reactivity, experiential avoidance, depression and anxiety. *International Journal of Mental Health and Addiction*. https://doi.org/10.1007/s11469-020-00322-z.

Shafran, R., Coughtrey, A., & Whittal, M. (2020). Recognising and addressing the impact of COVID-19 on obsessive-compulsive disorder. *Lancet Psychiatry*, *7*(7), 570–572. https://doi.org/10.1016/S2215-0366(20)30222-4.

Silva, R. M., Shavitt, R. G., & Costa, D. L. (2020). Obsessive-compulsive disorder during the COVID-19 pandemic. *Brazilian Journal of Psychiatry*. https://doi.org/10.1590/1516-4446-2020-1189.

Steketee, G., Frost, R. O., & Cohen, I. (1998). Beliefs in obsessive-compulsive disorder. *Journal of Anxiety Disorders*, *12*(6), 525–537.

Storch, E. A., Schneider, S. C., Guzick, A., McKay, D., & Goodman, W. K. (2020). Impact of COVID-19 on exposure and response prevention for obsessive-compulsive disorder: Present and post-pandemic considerations. *Psychiatry Research*, *292*, 113310. https://doi.org/10.1016/j.psychres.2020.113310.

Subramaniam, M., Soh, P., Vaingankar, J. A., Picco, L., & Chong, S. A. (2013). Quality of life in obsessive-compulsive disorder: Impact of the disorder and of treatment. *CNS Drugs*, *27*(5), 367–383. https://doi.org/10.1007/s40263-013-0056-z.

Tanir, Y., Karayagmurlu, A., Kaya, İ., Kaynar, T. B., Türkmen, G., Dambasan, B. N., … Coşkun, M. (2020). Exacerbation of obsessive compulsive disorder symptoms in children and adolescents during COVID-19 pandemic. *Psychiatry Research*, 113363. https://doi.org/10.1016/j.psychres.2020.113363.

Taylor, S. (2011). Early versus late onset obsessive–compulsive disorder: Evidence for distinct subtypes. *Clinical Psychology Review*, *31*(7), 1083–1100. https://doi.org/10.1016/j.cpr.2011.06.007.

Tian, F., Li, H., Tian, S., Yang, J., Shao, J., & Tian, C. (2020). Psychological symptoms of ordinary Chinese citizens based on SCL-90 during the level I emergency response to COVID-19. *Psychiatry Research*, *288*, 112992. https://doi.org/10.1016/j.psychres.2020.112992.

WHO. (2020). *Timeline: WHO's COVID-19 response*. Retrieved from https://www.who.int/emergencies/diseases/novel-coronavirus-2019/interactive-timeline.

Xing, J., Sun, N., Xu, J., Geng, S., & Li, Y. (2020). Study of the mental health status of medical personnel dealing with new coronavirus pneumonia. *PLoS One*, *15*(5), e0233145. https://doi.org/10.1371/journal.pone.0233145.

Zhang, W. R., Wang, K., Yin, L., Zhao, W. F., Xue, Q., Peng, M., … Wang, H. X. (2020). Mental health and psychosocial problems of medical health workers during the COVID-19 epidemic in China. *Psychotherapy and Psychosomatics*, *89*(4), 242–250. https://doi.org/10.1159/000507639.

Part II

Recent topics on impact of COVID-19 on health

Chapter 12

The role of nutrition in respiratory disease and COVID-19 management

Kingsley Kwadwo Asare Pereko[a], Enock Dugbatey Mensah[b], Victoria Akuorkor Acquaye[c], Christiana Nsiah-Asamoah[d], Flora Chadare[e], Freda Dzifa Intiful[f], Jacob Setorglo[g], Nancy Innocentia Ebu[h], and Alfred Dickson Dai-Kosi[i]

[a]*Department of Community Medicine, School of Medical Sciences, College of Health and Allied Sciences, University of Cape Coast, Cape Coast, Ghana,* [b]*Department of Biochemistry, School of Biological Sciences, College of Agricultural and Natural Sciences, University of Cape Coast, Cape Coast, Ghana,* [c]*Department of Psychological Medicine and Mental Health, School of Medical Sciences, College of Health and Allied Sciences, University of Cape Coast, Cape Coast, Ghana,* [d]*Department of Clinical Nutrition and Dietetics, School of Allied Health, College of Health and Allied Sciences, University of Cape Coast, Cape Coast, Ghana,* [e]*Laboratoire de Sciences et Technologie des Aliments et Bioressources et de Nutrition Humaine, Université Nationale d'Agriculture, Ketou, Benin,* [f]*Department of Dietetics, School of Biomedical and Allied Health Sciences, College of Health Sciences, University of Ghana, Korle-Bu, Ghana,* [g]*Department of Medical Biochemistry, School of Medical Sciences, College of Health and Allied Sciences, University of Cape Coast, Cape Coast, Ghana,* [h]*School of Mursing and Midwifery, College of Health and Allied Sciences, University of Cape Coast, Cape Coast, Ghana,* [i]*Department of Community and Preventive Dentistry, School of Medicine and Dentistry, University of Ghana, Legon, Ghana*

Introduction

The role of nutrition in immune development and disease recovery as well as the impact of infection on one's nutrition is widely known. However, many other evidences on this relationship are not conclusive most especially for emerging diseases such as corona virus disease (COVID-19). This chapter will review existing systematic reviews and meta-analysis literature on the subject of nutrition and infection with special emphasis on respiratory infection and COVID-19. The chapter will look at existing relationships between nutrition and respiratory infections, immunity and infection and patient recovery, nutrition and COVID-19, and the role of nutrition in infection control and management.

Mental Health Effects of COVID-19. https://doi.org/10.1016/B978-0-12-824289-6.00011-8

Background

The role of nutrition on the human defense system cannot be overemphasized as nutrition, diet, and nutritional status is an important determinant of the body's immunity. Existing evidence has established relationship between disease infectivity, mortality, and micronutrient deficiencies. Reviews of research over the past years on nutrition and immune function have suggested a dire consequence of nutritional deficiency on host immune response to disease infections. Malnutrition has been linked to immune function depression resulting in disease susceptibility (Naja & Hamadeh, 2020). Earlier studies by Maggini, Pierre, and Calder (2018) reported poor nutritional status as a leading cause of immune impairment. Thus adequate nutritional intake has been recommended as a potent intervention to restoring the body's immune function and resistance to infection.

Recent global reports on nutrition have indicated that malnutrition is among the major factors leading to an increase in death rate worldwide. The novel corona virus pandemic to a large extent has exposed our vulnerable food systems, as efforts in containing the spread of infection have resulted in food shortages globally. This consequently has exposed persons with underlying conditions and compromised immune state as a result of a poor nutritional status to disease infection (Global Nutrition Report, 2020).

This chapter is presented in three sections. The first section of the chapter discusses generally the role of nutrition/correlation between nutrition and immunity, infectious cycle, infectivity and disease recovery. The second section of the chapter deals with the association between nutrition and immunity against respiratory diseases, nutrition and infectivity of respiratory diseases and nutrition and recovery from respiratory illnesses. The final section of the chapter focuses on the role of nutrition in the development of the immune system against COVID-19, infectivity of COVID-19, recovery, optimizing nutrition for improved mental health during COVID-19, and management of COVID-19.

Nutrition and immunity

Nutrition has been reported to improve the body's resistance to infection aside modulating immune functions. Nutritional deficiency of certain micronutrients has been found to impair immune responses (Bhaskaram, 2001). Numerous micronutrients, including vitamins A, D, C, E, B6, and B12, folate, zinc, iron, copper, and selenium, are critically essential as they mutually support each other in the immune protection and response process (Gombart, Pierre, & Maggini, 2020). Jayawardena, Sooriyaarachchi, Chourdakis, Jeewandara, and Ranasinghe (2020) highlighted the importance of micronutrients, nutraceuticals, and probiotics to immunity against the COVID-19 pandemic. Poor nutritional status in Chronic Kidney Disease (CKD) patients was reported as a risk to weakened serologic response to Hepatitis B Vaccine (HBV). Patients with an improved nutritional status were better protected against viral infections in a recent study

(Calder, Carr, Gombart, & Eggersdorfer, 2020). In a systematic review to unravel the relationship between immune function and nutritional status among highly active antiretroviral therapy (HAART)-treated patients, it was observed that malnourished patients recorded early deaths due to poor immune function (Sicotte, Langlois, Aho, Ziegler, & Zunzunegui, 2014). Researchers assessed the correlation between parameters such as the composition of microbiota, feeding status, and immunity in a case-control study of Ecuadorian children with Autism Spectrum Disorder. Outcome of the study showed variations in feeding behavior, immune function, and microbiota composition (Zurita et al., 2020). Grueber, Gray, Morris, Stephen, and Senior (2018) identified certain inheritable immune characteristics in offspring that are dependent on the variation in parental nutritional intake. The study measured the outcome of maternal nutrition on child immune status by employing frameworks that defined dietary manipulations with respect to energy and macronutrient compositions. The alteration in maternal dietary intake was observed to affect child's immune function by decreasing the expression of certain inflammatory markers (Grueber et al., 2018).

With the emergence of the Corona virus pandemic, there have been reports that micronutrient interventions could possibly play a key role in patient recovery by improving immune function. Several research findings to a large extent have investigated the immune modulatory effect of vitamin D. Maalmi, Tangour, and Hamzaoui (2012) pointed out the role of vitamin D in the regulation of T cells in younger asthmatic patients. They observed that only 6 out of 39 asthmatic children enrolled for the study had adequate calcifediol levels whiles sufficient levels were found in the vast majority of healthy controls. Also, it was observed that 17 of the asthmatic patients expressed deficiency in serum vitamin D levels. Healthy participants, however, expressed no signs of serum vitamin D deficiency. The levels of Th1, Th2, and Th17 were found to correspond with the serum concentrations of calcifediol. There have been speculations over how critical lower vitamin D status may influence immune response to influenza vaccines administered in the elderly population. Lee et al. (2018) underscored no substantial link between the vitamin and its immunogenic influence on influenza vaccines. They however noted that specific influenza strains may present peculiarities, lower rate of protection in influenza A virus H3N2 and B strains in vitamin D-deficient patients compared with vitamin D-rich patients (Lee et al., 2018). Probiotics and prebiotics administration have been found to trigger immunogenic response to influenza vaccines in the elderly as the rate of seroprotection in influenza H1N1, H3N2, and B subtypes improved dramatically in subjects who took prebiotics or probiotics (Lei, Shih, & Liu, 2018). The administration of probiotics bacteria has been reported to reduce both upper and lower respiratory tract infections (Campbell, 2020). Probiotic strains could be employed to manipulate these microbiotas, offering new perspectives in the management of respiratory failures (Enaud et al., 2020). Mounting evidence supports a relationship between the gut and lungs, thus more studies to explore the potential role of probiotic in attenuating COVID-19 either through immunomodulatory actions on systemic inflammation or by direct association with the lungs have been recommended (Bottari, Castellone, & Neviani, 2020; Mak, Chan, & Ng, 2020).

A review of the role of vitamin C and some micronutrient supplementation in triggering changes in immune function in exercising athletes found two trials that backed the use of vitamin C as a preventive agent against Upper Respiratory Tract (URT) infections (Moreira et al., 2007).

In relation to URT infections, a review which included 82 eligible studies that considered the preventive role of vitamin C in immune clusters and in common cold reported that regular supplementation of vitamin C (1 to 2 g/day) reduces cold duration (by 8% in adults and in children by 14%) and the severity of common cold (Rondanelli et al., 2018). There is evidence that a high dose of intravenous vitamin C (HIVC) can inhibit numerous key components of cytokine storms which can eventually degrade the endothelium and alveolar membrane in clinical trials. These trials were conducted on patients with bacterial-induced sepsis and acute respiratory distress syndrome (ARDS) which are conditions that occur in severe critically ill COVID-19 patients (Liu, Zhu, Zhang, Li, & Peng, 2020). Findings from a meta-analysis of 29 controlled trials with 11,306 participants revealed that vitamin C administration shortened the period of being infected with URTIs (Hemilä & Chalker, 2019). In adults, the duration of infections was reduced by 8% and in children by 14% (Hemilä & Chalker, 2019). Considering the fact that critically ill patients are likely to be admitted in intensive care units (ICUs) and the evidence that their vitamin C levels usually reduce drastically (Carr et al., 2017; Hemilä & Chalker, 2019), there is no reason to doubt that vitamin C would not be effective against COVID-19. The potential role of vitamin C in shortening patients stay in ICUs by 8% was reported in a meta-analysis that included 12 trials with 1766 patients in ICU (Hemilä & Chalker, 2019). Likewise, another meta-regression analysis that included eight (8) trials found that vitamin C shortened the duration of mechanical ventilation in patients who required the longest ventilation (Hemilä & Chalker, 2020a, 2020b). Liu et al. (2020) therefore hypothesized that HIVC could be added to the treatment of ARDS and multiorgan dysfunction which are associated with COVID-19.

The role of zinc in enhancing immune function and reducing the risk of infections mainly as a result of its antiinflammatory property has also been reported (de Almeida Brasiel, 2020). A randomized, double-blind, placebo-controlled trial in nursing homes revealed that providing zinc supplements to older adults improved their immune response and provided protection against infection (Barnett et al., 2016). With regard to common colds, intake of zinc supplements was reported to shorten the duration of colds by approximately 33% (Rondanelli et al., 2018). In a meta-analysis that included a number of placebo-controlled zinc lozenge trials, it was revealed in five trials that common cold duration was reduced by 33% among participants who were administered with zinc doses of 80–92 mg/day. There was a further reduction in cold duration by 2% (i.e., 35%) in two trials in which participants received a higher zinc doses of 192–207 mg/day (Hemilä, 2017). Selenium (Se) is an essential trace mineral which is vital for particularly maintaining a well-balanced immune response. In an European cross-sectional study ($n = 1915$), COVID-19 patients showed a pronounced deficiency in total serum Se (mean ± SD, 50.8 ± 15.7 vs. 84.4 ± 23.4 μg/L) and SELENOP (3.0 ± 1.4 vs. 4.3 ± 1.0 mg/L) concentrations. A Se status below the 2.5th percentile of the reference population, i.e., [Se] < 45.7 μg/L and [SELENOP] < 2.56 mg/L, was observed in 43.4% and 39.2% of serum samples of COVID-19 patients, respectively. The Se status was significantly higher in samples from surviving COVID-19 patients as compared with nonsurvivors (Se; 53.3 ± 16.2 vs. 40.8 ± 8.1 μg/L, selenoprotein P (SELENOP); 3.3 ± 1.3 vs. 2.1 ± 0.9 mg/L (Moghaddam et al., 2020). Although the potential role of these micronutrients has been individually discussed, it is important to indicate their complementary roles in nutritional health, that is, they do not work in isolation, but rather mutually support and depend on each other.

Essential micronutrients and the omega-3 fatty acids eicosapentaenoic acid and docosahexaenoic acid are known to have the capacity to boost immunity against viral infections (Calder et al., 2020). Specifically, omega-3 PUFAs, mainly α-linolenic acid, docosahexaenoic acid, and eicosapentaenoic acid, inhibit the activation of immune cells while also actively enhancing specific immune functions like phagocytosis and neutrophil differentiation. This suggests that omega-3 PUFAs play a role in mediating immune function and thus may be vital as a supportive dietary therapy for prevention and treatment of flu-like viral infections, including COVID-19 (Akhtar et al., 2020).

Growing evidence suggests that functional foods which are products that contain different biologically active compounds when consumed, contributes to maintaining the optimal state of physical and mental health of the population. Functional foods contain biologically active compounds with the potential to improve health or to reduce the risk of disease (Butnariu & Sarac, 2019). These functional foods include tea components that may help optimize immunological responses such as improving defense functions and resistance to infections. Tea components such as Epigallocatechin-3-Gallate (EGCG) and garlic (*Allium sativum* L.) have been described as being gatekeepers of immune function (Wu, Lewis, Pae, & Meydani, 2019). Garlic contains diverse bioactive compounds, such as allicin, alliin, diallyl sulfide, diallyl disulfide, diallyl trisulfide, ajoene, and S-allyl-cysteine which have been shown to exhibit antiinflammatory, antibacterial, antifungal, immunomodulatory properties (Phan, Netzel, Chhim, Netzel, & Sultanbawa, 2019; Shang et al., 2019). Recently, the protective role of EGCG in diseases with uncontrolled immune activation such as the novel COVID-19 has been explored (Menegazzi et al., 2020). Menegazzi et al. (2020) argued and recommended that since EGCG can regenerate the natural immunological homeostasis in many autoimmune diseases it can be considered a potential safe natural supplement to counteract hyperinflammation development in COVID-19 patients.

Nutrition infection cycle

Nutrition has been reported to be closely associated with infection. Globally, nutritional deficiencies have been linked to a number of disease infections. Malnutrition is known to trigger immunodeficiency, predisposing the malnourished to several infectious diseases. Savino (2002) reported that thymus development is significantly affected in severely malnourished children leading to a compromised immune state and consequently a lasting reduction in peripheral lymphocyte counts (Savino, 2002). Both innate host defense mechanisms as well as acquired immunity (lymphocyte functions) are affected in patients with poor nutritional status (Schaible & Stefan, 2007). Consequently, this immunodeficiency results in the susceptibility to infections (Beisel, 1996) particularly those triggered commonly in persons with HIV/AIDS by opportunistic pathogens (Cegielski & McMurray, 2004; Field et al., 2001).

The multifaceted interaction of malnutrition and infections generates a prolong unfriendly environment of a vicious cycle which mutually favors the two entities. This vicious cycle of nutrition and infection is usually associated with a reduction in inflammatory response, a decrease in the ability to produce specific antibodies as well a decline in the activity of macrophages (Rodriguez-Morales, Bolivar-Mejía, Alarcón-Olave, & Calvo-Betancourt, 2016). Observations from epidemiological data have supported the contention that malnutrition and infection exacerbate each other. However, not all infections are influenced equally by nutrition (Chandra, 1983; Scrimshaw et al., 1968). There is sufficient evidence suggesting that certain infections like tuberculosis, diarrhea, and measles clinical outcomes are affected significantly by poor nutritional status whiles others like tetanus and viral encephalitis are minimally influenced (Chandra, 1996).

Two possible outcomes of the complex interaction between nutrition and infection are synergist and antagonistic effects. The former occurs when infection degenerates malnutrition or when poor nutrition status decreases immune response to infection. The latter occurs when the agent of multiplication is decreased by malnutrition (Rodriguez-Morales et al., 2016).

With regard to COVID-19, available data on the effect of nutrition on this infection is scarce. However, considering the key clinical features of COVID-19 which include cough, fever, sore throat, headache, fatigue, headache, and breathlessness suggest that it has similar features to a seasonal influenza infection (Guan et al., 2020). Hence, specific nutritional deficiencies in vitamins—A, C, D, and E—zinc, selenium, and omega-3 fatty acids may result in immune system dysfunction increasing one's susceptibility to COVID-19 infection. Vitamin D is involved in maintaining immunity and its deficiency has been reported to be associated with an increased risk of respiratory infection. This has led some researchers to hypothesize that vitamin D supplementation could hold promise as a preventive or therapeutic agent for COVID-19 (Martineau & Forouhi, 2020). Epidemiological studies assessing the relationship between vitamin D status and incidence and severity of COVID-19 are currently scarce in number (Martineau & Forouhi, 2020). In two ecological studies, an inverse association was reported between national estimates of vitamin D status and COVID-19 incidence and mortality in European countries (Ilie, Stefanescu, & Smith, 2020; Laird, Rhodes, & Kenny, 2020). Findings from a retrospective longitudinal study from Israel revealed an independent correlation between low vitamin D levels and subsequent incidence and severity of COVID-19 (Merzon et al., 2020).

Nutrition and infectivity

Beside genetic and environmental conditions which have been ascribed as an underlining factor leading to disease infections, recent findings have suggested that malnutrition is also another underestimated risk factor. In the quest to identify possible risk factors leading to autoimmune disease conditions, the vitamin D status of patients battling autoimmune gastritis was equated to those present in patients with *Helicobacter pylori*, lymphocytic gastritis, and in healthy controls. The analysis contended that low vitamin D was a possible risk factor for autoimmune diseases (Antico, Tozzoli, Giavarina, Tonutti, & Bizzaro, 2012). In probing the potency of multivitamin supplementation in mitigating disease infections in the aged population, Alexander et al. (2020) found that multivitamins effectively fight against infection in the aged population by reducing to a large extent, the length of infection (by a factor of 17.5). Contrarily the frequent usage of the supplement by the aged population in reducing incidence of infection was seen as insignificant and inconsistent in relation to its efficacy (El-Kadiki & Sutton, 2005).

Low calcifediol in the plasma has been linked with a possible high incidence of Inflammatory Bowel Disease (IBD) and related complications (Ananthakrishnan et al., 2013). This assertion follows after several databases were searched thoroughly for a possible association. After a meta-analysis of the existing literature, it was affirmed that there was over 60% incidence of vitamin D deficiency in IBD patients in comparison to healthy subjects (Del Pinto, Pietropaoli, Chandar, Ferri, & Cominelli, 2015). The role of vitamin A in fighting lower respiratory tract infections in infants below eight was evaluated. Reports from most studies suggested that retinol had no effect on prevalence of symptoms or occurrence of acute lower respiratory tract infections (LRTI). Chen et al.'s (2008) review of the effectiveness and safety of vitamin A for prevention of acute LRTI concluded that vitamin A has only a limiting effect in preventing LRTI; however, they do acknowledge its effect on populations with acute and chronic undernutrition and thus recommend against supplementation in all children to prevent acute LRTI (Chen et al., 2008). To validate claims suggesting a correlation between hypovitaminosis of calcifediol levels and severe acute lower respiratory infection, a total of 150 Indian children below age 5 were recruited. The study revealed that low vitamin D status in young infants coupled with a lack of exclusive breast feeding after the first trimester of birth triggered acute lower respiratory infection (ALRI) in children (Wayse, Yousafzai, Mogale, & Filteau, 2004).

A meta-analysis and meta-regression of ten (10) randomized trials revealed that zinc supplementation reduced the incidence of ALRI defined by specific clinical criteria [IRR 0.65, 95% confidence interval (CI) 0.52–0.82] (Roth, Richard, & Black, 2010). Similarly, Lassi, Moin, and Bhutta's (2016) systematic review reported that zinc supplementation reduced the incidence of pneumonia by 13% (fixed-effect risk ratio (RR) 0.87; 95% confidence interval (CI) 0.81 to 0.94, six studies, low-quality evidence) and prevalence of pneumonia by 41% (random-effects RR 0.59; 95% CI 0.35 to 0.99, one study, $n=609$, low-quality evidence). A study among Indian young children aged between 6 and 30 months found that the risk of ALRI was significantly higher among vitamin-D deficient (OR 1.26; 95% CI: 1.03 to 1.55) compared to vitamin-D-replete children in a six-month follow-up period (Chowdhury et al., 2017).

Nutrition and disease recovery

Timely provision of adequate nutrition in early phase of critical illness to minimize protein energy deficit has been suggested to improve clinical outcomes, particularly in lean and obese patients (Alberda et al., 2009). Heyland et al. (2015) postulate a possible greater impact of nutrition and exercise on physical recovery of survivors of critical illness but recommend the need for randomized trial testing in proving this relationship.

Earlier studies by Heighes, Doig, Sweetman, and Simpson (2010) highlighted evidence in favor of the timely supply of enteral nutrition in the terminally ill patients. The study reported a sharp decline in intestinal surgery-related deaths following the timely administration of enteral nutritional supports. Although existing data are limited and also inconsistent, data backing the crucial impacts of enteral nutrition and its outcome on severely sick patients cannot be overlooked Heighes et al. (2010).

Hyltander et al.'s (2005) study on timely enteral (EN) and parenteral (PN) feeding support and oral nutrition on recovery time during cancer treatment found the supply of supportive enteral and parenteral nutrition had no greater effect in contrast to oral nutrition when directed by a health care giver. The impact of the combination of PN and EN as against EN only was assessed in some terminally ill patients. Severely sick patients receiving EN alone saw a decline in length of hospitalization and infection. Subjects who received a combination of PN and EN saw no combined consequence following intake of one of the artificial nutritional supplement on death rate, duration in ICU, ventilation time, prealbumin and albumin (Shi, Wei, Huang, & Liao, 2018).

The potential role of healthy nutrition in enhancing recovery, reducing recurrence of terminal diseases, and thus increasing one's survival rate in conditions such as breast cancer (Reeves, Terranova, Eakin, & Demark-Wahnefried, 2014; Rock et al., 2015), endometrial cancer (Kitson et al., 2018; Koutoukidis,

Knobf, & Lanceley, 2015), and ovarian cancer (Beavis, Smith, & Fader, 2016; Thomson et al., 2014) has also been reported. With regard to the COVID-19 pandemic, it has been asserted that wider access to healthy foods should be a top priority and individuals should be mindful of healthy eating habits to reduce their susceptibility and also enhance recovery rate. In the case of severe COVID-19 patients who may have to be on admission in ICU for approximately 2 weeks or more, their dietary intakes become a key determinant for maintaining skeletal muscle and avoiding metabolic disturbances.

Additionally, severe COVID-19 patients suffer respiratory difficulties that result in another extra layer of complexity, preventing such patients from eating well.

Nutrition and respiratory illness

Several research works have reported some promising relationships among respiratory infection and nutritional status. Esposito, Baggi, Bianchini, Marchisio, and Principi (2013) summarized the vital role played by certain micronutrients in facilitating the body's production of antibiotics which goes a long way to protect the body against ARI. Low calcifediol levels in the plasma have been reported to be a potential risk factor contributing to an enhanced susceptibility to disease infection, particularly those associated with the respiratory system (Gibney et al., 2008; Laaksi et al., 2007; Roth et al., 2010). Gunville, Mourani, and Ginde (2013) reported that the modulatory effect of vitamin D on the body's function follows a cascade of events, where first an immune function is enhanced which in turn triggers antibody production which functions to resist and fight against infections.

Esposito and Lelii's (2015) review of studies also revealed that a concentration of between 20 ng/mL and 50 ng/mL of hydroxycholecalciferol (25[OH]D) is considered adequate to provide an immunomodulatory effect in childhood respiratory tract infections such as pediatric tuberculosis, acute otitis media, bronchiolitis, pharyngotonsillitis, and pneumonia. Zhang and coauthors reported the deficiency of fat-soluble vitamins such as vitamin D, A, and E as a possible risk factor for recurrent respiratory tract infections in children below 15 years of age considering the significantly low levels of micronutrients in recurrent RTI subjects (Zhang et al., 2016). Beside its role in encouraging weight gain in malnourished Chronic Obstructive Pulmonary Disease (COPD) patients, nutritional supports have been reported to also improve respiratory status and good health in a COPD population (Ferreira, Brooks, White, & Goldstein, 2012).

Nutrition and respiratory infectivity

Accumulated evidence over the past few decades from different sources suggests that micronutrients mediate host resistance infection. Several efforts have been directed at studying the possible effect of vitamin A intake on immune response to infections (Stephensen, Blount, Schoeb, & Park, 1993). Low vitamin A levels in experimental mouse models were observed to affect immune regulatory activities of the macrophages and neutrophils, as well as alter the barrier lining the epithelial tissues (Stephensen, 2001).

Chen et al. (2008) review of randomized control trials assessing the role of retinol in fighting LRTIs in children found no important influence of vitamin A on the incidence or occurrence of symptoms of LRTIs, following observations of eight different studies.

A case-control study to analyze the correlation between acute lower respiratory infection and vitamin D deficiency in neonates found low vitamin D status as a potential factor contributing to the risk of ALRI in newborns. They recommended adequate vitamin D supplementation during pregnancy especially in the winter (Karatekin, Kaya, Salihoğlu, Balci, & Nuhoğlu, 2009).

Similarly, a review on the efficacy of vitamin D supplements in fighting against the incidence of LRTIs and the modulating factors found to a large extent the effect of vitamin D intake in mitigating the risk of acute respiratory tract infections (Martineau et al., 2017). Subjects who received a routine supply of vitamin D supplements lacking extra bolus doses were shielded from ALRI during the analysis while those who received at least one bolus dose did not express protection against respiratory infections (varying odds fraction 0.86–1.10, 0.97; P for contact=0.05). However, varying degree of protection was observed among study subjects who received vitamin D in every day of the week. Participants with baseline calcifediol levels less than 25 nmol/L (varying odds fraction 0.17, 0.30–0.53) experienced stronger degree of protection than in those with baseline calcifediol levels greater than or equal to 25 nmol/L (varying odds fraction 0.60, 0.75–0.95; P for contact=0.006) (Martineau et al., 2017). Jolliffe, Griffiths, and Martineau (2013) reported vitamin D deficiency to be strongly associated with an enhanced vulnerability to respiratory-related infections although results of the RCT showed inconsistencies in variations in dosing regimens between participants. Conversely, after administering vitamin D supplements to children previously diagnosed with ARI, the results suggested that these nutritional interventions were not associated with the reduction of the incidence of ARIs. Notwithstanding, children previously diagnosed with asthma saw over 70% decrease in the event of asthma exacerbation after being exposed to vitamin D supplementation (Xiao et al., 2015).

Nutrition and immunity against respiratory illness

For more than a century now, greater consideration has been given to the role played by micronutrients on bodily functions. While their availability is known to improve immunity against infections, their deficiency has been reported to be correlated with an increase in the susceptibility to disease infection. The role of serum vitamin D levels' in disease activity was investigated in 39 participants suffering from asthma. Over 40% of asthmatic subjects recruited showed deficiency in serum vitamin D levels, while only 15% had adequate levels. The control participant did not express lower levels of the vitamin. The study suggested a negative association between vitamin D and interleukin-17 levels in young asthmatics and also described the availability of vitamin D in serum as a key factor in promoting the regulation of in vivo T cells between asthmatics (Maalmi et al., 2012). Probiotics and prebiotics administration have been found to trigger immunogenic response to influenza vaccines in the elderly as the rate of seroprotection in influenza H1N1, H3N2, and B subtypes improved dramatically in subjects who took prebiotics or probiotics (Lei et al., 2018). Lee and coauthors investigated the immunogenic influence of vitamin D against influenza. They observed no important effect of the vitamin on influenza infection, but conceded that it may have peculiar effects on immune response to different strains of the virus (Lee et al., 2018).

Fortes et al.'s (1998) randomized, controlled trial investigated the effect of vitamin A and zinc intake on immune function in aged population. Immune response to factors such as chronic diseases, depression, acute respiratory diseases, and smoking was assessed by performing immune test on counts of leucocytes, T-cell subsets, and lymphocytes. Zinc supplementation was found to increase the number of cytotoxic T-lymphocytes and $CD4^+DR^+$ T-cells while vitamin A intake decreased the number of $CD4^+$ T-cells and $CD3^+$ T-cells. The authors concluded that vitamin A supplementation had a deleterious effect in aged population.

A randomized control trial studying the effect of daily combination of vitamin E and multivitamin-mineral supplements on the severity and prevalence of respiratory tract infections among the elderly of over 60 years of age found the administration of both vitamin E and multivitamin-mineral to have a positive effect on the frequency and impact of acute respiratory infection among unhospitalized aged. However, an adverse effect of vitamin E was observed with disease severity (Graat, Schouten, & Kok, 2002). Meydani, Han, and Wu's (2005) review of the effect of the administration of vitamin E on immune response among aged revealed that vitamin E improved immune function as well as enhance the production of antibodies in response to the administration of vaccines. These improvements in immune function were linked to an enhanced resistance to influenza infection and a decreased risk factor for contracting upper respiratory infections in adult mice and human population. In a related study, a total of six hundred and seventeen (617) aged home residents were recruited in a clinical controlled trial which aimed at evaluating the impact of 1-year vitamin E administration on immune function, infection length, and incidence. The result showed to a large extent an improvement in immune response and the response to vaccines. Vitamin E administration was also found to be associated with a significant decrease in the occurrence of common cold and as well as a decline in the number of common cold cases among the adults (Meydani et al., 2004).

Over the past 2 decades, zinc supplements have been administered in an attempt to improve immunity against respiratory disease infections. Overbeck, Rink, and Haase (2008) review of existing literature summarizing the possible mechanism by which zinc affected various disease infections and response to vaccination reported that zinc administration affected immune function. The review, however, could not distinguish whether zinc solely modulated immune function and to what extent. Additionally, it was observed that zinc was ineffective in many vaccination trials as its effect on common cold and malaria is still not conclusive (Overbeck et al., 2008).

In an attempt to investigate the relationship between serum levels of trace elements and the susceptibility to asthma in adult population, a total of 270 adults comprising of 100 asthmatic patients and healthy individuals were enrolled. Serum levels of Zn, Mg, Cu, and Se were measured. The case-control study revealed higher levels of serum Cu and Se in healthy subjects than in asthmatic patients. On the contrary, serum zinc levels were found to be lower in controls than in asthmatics. It was concluded that the decrease in serum selenium and copper levels against increased zinc levels affected the function of antioxidant enzymes by decreasing to an extent the antioxidant capacity in asthmatic patients (Hussein, Yousif, & Saeed, 2008).

Nutrition and recovery from respiratory illness

Proactive management of infection has recently become a focal point in medical practice. Among the various approaches employed by health professionals which have been reported to be effective in mitigating complications arising from respiratory-related infections have always included the provision of specialized nutritional supports. Jackson, Lesho, and Peterson's (2000) meta-analysis of randomized control trials on zinc gluconate and common cold concluded a gap in evidence of its effectiveness. In order to synthesize evidence regarding the effectiveness of nutritional support in mitigating the incidence, morbidity, and mortality of childhood ALRI, a meta-analysis on RCT of nutritional interventions, antenatal and breastfeeding promotion, which measured one or more childhood ALRI outcome was conducted. The study revealed a drop in hospitalizations related to respiratory diseases. It was proposed that (1) zinc supplements are crucial in averting about a quarter of incidence of ALRI and ALRI-related mortality in zinc-deficient populations, (2) promoting exclusive breastfeeding lessens ALRI-related morbidity, (3) providing only iron supplements is ineffective in reducing ALRI incidence, and (4) ALRI incidence or mortality is unaffected by the supplementation of vitamin A outside the neonatal period (Roth, Caulfield, & Black, 2008).

The duration of illness in subjects who developed common acute respiratory infections was assessed after routine probiotics administration. Meta-analysis revealed that the incident of illness reduced significantly after respondents received probiotics. Similarly, the length of infection reduced significantly in participants who were administered than in subjects who took a placebo (King, Glanville, Sanders, Fitzgerald, & Varley, 2014). A review of the effect of probiotics on respiratory and gastrointestinal and nutritional outcomes in patients with Cystic Fibrosis (CF) concluded that, the routine administration of probiotics in a stable CF population is key in improving nutritional, gastrointestinal, and respiratory outcomes (Anderson, Miles, & Tierney, 2016).

Nutrition and COVID-19

Contemporary evidence on nutrition and COVID-19

The emergence of the novel corona virus disease has exposed lapses in nutrition and food security in many a population. Several schools of thought have recommended nutritional interventions as key in promoting patient recovery in the fight against the disease. It has also been suggested that an improved nutritional status reduces the risk of infection to a large extent (Beck, Handy, & Levander, 2004). Even though new vaccines are available, administration to everybody across the world will take sometime. The administration of nutrition supports therefore would be needed for better outcomes due to its availability and the established knowledge concerning its contribution to the fight against infection. There is enough evidence suggesting that an improved nutritional status promotes immunity to infections (Zabetakis, Lordan, & Norton, 2020). Maintaining a robust immune system at this material times is thus crucial to the fight against the pandemic. The possible effects of serving extra micronutrient supplementation to COVID-19 infected patients have been recently reviewed. Fortifying nutrition support with micronutrients or conditional amino acids has been suggested to improve outcome in COVID-19 infected individuals although evidences accentuating these facts are lacking (Rozga, Cheng, Moloney, & Handu, 2020). Vitamin D was confirmed as having antiviral properties responsible for protecting against respiratory-related infections such as COVID-19 (Hribar, Cobbold, & Church, 2020). Another study found that the continual administration of vitamin D triggers the antioxidant activity of glutathione enzymes (Lei et al., 2018) and facilitates the production of glutathione which is crucial in the treatment and prevention of COVID-19 (Mousavi, Bereswill, & Heimesaat, 2019; Colunga Biancatelli, Berrill, Catravas, & Marik, 2020; Wimalawansa, 2020). Interestingly, although several calls have been made with reference to the intake of probiotics with the hope of fighting COVID-19 infection, no clinical trial has backed these assertions till date. A possible correlation between pulmonary-related infections and microbiomes in the lung has been, however, underscored which relates bacterial metabolites to diets with a classical example being short chain fatty acids and lung microecological niche (Yang, Xing, Song, & Qian, 2020). Stachowska, Folwarski, Jamioł-Milc, Maciejewska, and Skonieczna-Żydecka (2020) proposed the administration of probiotics as a supportive intervention to coronavirus-infected patients who require antibiotic therapy but present symptoms of gastrointestinal infection.

Nutrition and immune development in COVID-19

It is well known that nutrition plays an important role in promoting immunity and protecting the body against diseases. Maggini et al. (2018) described the relationship between nutrition, immunity, and infection to be bidirectional in nature, and suggested that changing the components in any had a greater impact on the rests. Fruits and vegetables have been reported as important sources of phytonutrients and micronutrients which provides antiinflammatory and antioxidants agents vital in improving immune responses to disease infections (Calder et al., 2020; Zhang, Taylor, Bennett, Saad, & Rayman, 2020). In this period of the coronavirus outbreak, improving immune function against respiratory infections by administering nutrients with better prospects may be part of the needed solution in controlling the situation. Most recently, the role of vitamin D interventions as a booster of immune function in the resistance of respiratory infection was analyzed by conducting RCTs. The result confirmed the vitamin to boost immune function in deficient individuals against ARTIs (Martineau et al., 2017). Similarly, Zabetakis et al. (2020) recommended vitamin D as potent in reducing the incident of infections, including the novel coronavirus infection.

Nutrition and COVID-19 infectivity

In order to authenticate the numerous calls in the early parts of this year concerning the prospects of vitamin D supplementation on COVID-19 infectivity, publications on works featuring COVID-19 influenza and vitamin D were meticulously searched. Generally, epidemiological studies have reported that vitamin D deficiency is associated with viral respiratory tract infections (Ebadi & Montano-Loza, 2020). In most of the trials, vitamin D intake was linked to a decreased incidence of influenza while few reported otherwise. It was observed that coronavirus begun around the winter period, where serum calcifediol levels diminished considerably, on the other hand, cases of the infection were low during the summer period. Another observation was that a large portion of the aged population were victims of the infection, probably because most aged persons are more likely to be deficient in vitamin D as a result of being housebound or institutionalized and thus may not be exposed to sunlight in order for the skin to synthesize some invitro vitamin D. A meta-analysis incorporating data from 21,000 subjects across eight observational studies found that those with a serum vitamin D level <20 ng/mL (i.e., <50 nmoL/L) had a 64% increased risk of community-acquired pneumonia (Zhou, Luo, & Qin, 2019). Vitamin D agonist, calcitriol, exhibited defensive mechanisms against acute lung injury by modifying and controlling the expression of members of the renin-angiotensin system such as ACE2 in lung tissue (Xu et al., 2017). This supports and suggests that vitamin D deficiency can be a pathogenic factor in COVID-19 (Ebadi & Montano-Loza, 2020).

Likewise, persons who are deficient in vitamin D are predisposed easily to chronic diseases such as diabetes and cardiovascular diseases (Papandreou & Hamid, 2015). These observations were found to correspond with vitamin D deficiency and thus a recommendation in favor of vitamin D as a potent supplement in mitigating death rate and incidence of coronavirus and influenza infections (Grant et al., 2020; Han et al., 2016).

Selenium deficiency has been reported as crucial to viral infections (Guillin, Vindry, Ohlmann, & Chavatte, 2019). Fakhrolmobasheri, Nasr-Esfahany, Khanahmad, and Zeinalian (2020) reported that selenium may be relevant to the cause of COVID-19. The administration of this micronutrient is known to have positive impacts on immune function (Calder et al., 2020). It has been reported that subjects with low serum selenium levels are at risk of viral infections owing to higher pathogenic mutation rates which ultimately lead to a rapid evolution in pathogenic viral strains (Beck, 2006). Alexander et al.'s (2020) review on the need for possible micronutrient intervention to avert the risk of a chronic coronavirus infection with emphasis on vitamin D, zinc, and selenium found limited evidence for an association between the aforementioned micronutrients and coronavirus disease. It was however argued that since these micronutrients are known to be vital in promoting immune function, resisting viral infection, and reducing inflammations, their administration might offer protection against the novel coronavirus disease.

The protective role of zinc amid the COVID-19 pandemic has been discussed to a large extent. The micronutrient has been envisioned as a potential supportive intervention to overcome the current global crisis. This stems from the fact that zinc possesses immune modulatory characteristics coupled with an antiviral activity (Zhang et al., 2020). The combined effect of the cation form of the mineral (Zn^{2+}) with its ionophore pyrithione has been reported to alter SARS-coronavirus RNA polymerase activity and thereby decreasing its replication process (Te Velthuis et al., 2010).

It has been suggested that vitamin C administration may be effective in boosting the body's immune response to coronavirus infection (Khan, Parikh, Megala, & Predeteanu, 2020). Intravenous administration has been recommended for severe cases of COVID-19 infections, while the oral intake has been suggested to be effective in protecting against infection (Nilashi et al., 2020). Though various claims have been made in favor of vitamin C intake to battle COVID-19 infections, there is limiting evidence to buttress these speculations. Similarly, no current empirical data exist to validate claims that a higher intravenous dosage of vitamin C is effective in the management of COVID-19.

Nutrition and recoveries from COVID-19

A retrospective multicenter study of 212 cases by Alipio and Alipio (2020) to assess the possible clinical outcome of vitamin D supplementation on COVID-19 patient found serum calcifediol levels to significantly affect outcomes in the vast majority of cases with suboptimal vitamin D levels. Multinomial logistics regression analysis showed 8 times increase in the event of mild clinical outcome over a severe outcome as serum calcifediol levels increase ($P < 0.001$,

OR = 0.126), and an approximated 20 times increase in the event of mild clinical outcome over a critical clinical outcome. It was inferred that a drop in serum levels of calcifediol could exacerbate clinical outcomes, while a rise in levels enhances outcomes in COVID-19 infected subjects (Alipio & Alipio, 2020).

Vitamin C is highly acclaimed for its antioxidant properties in scavenging free radicals in the body and thereby protecting against oxidative damage. Its role also includes supporting the immune function of the body. Infection has the ability to decrease the levels of vitamin C and increase a person's requirement as the severity of the infection increases (Carr et al., 2017). In a review, Colunga Biancatelli, Berrill, and Marik (2020) suggest a combined prophylactic administration of vitamin C and quercetin in the prevention and early treatment of COVID-119. Currently, various studies are underway to determine the effectiveness of vitamin C on disease outcome among COVID-19 patients. However, in a recently published case series, it was noted that administration of 1 g of vitamin C every 8 h for 3 days significantly decreased inflammatory markers such as ferritin and D-dimer (Hiedra et al., 2020). Also, in a case report, a 74-year-old woman critically ill with COVID-19 recovered unusually early upon intravenous administration of high dose of vitamin C (Khan et al., 2020). The researchers postulated that vitamin C could be helpful in achieving rapid recovery, reducing length of time on a ventilator and stay at the ICU.

Selenium status was reported to be associated with a higher recovery rate from coronavirus infection early this year in China (Zhang et al., 2020). In a recent study, the association between serum selenium levels and the risk of COVID-19 related mortality was assessed. An X-ray fluorescence and selenoprotein analysis was performed on the serum samples obtained from a total of 33 coronavirus-infected subjects. Deficient levels of serum selenium levels were observed in the samples. Additionally, when serum levels were compared between COVID-19 survivors and nonsurvivors, the former showed higher Se levels than the latter. Serum levels in survivors were restored to normal levels while nonsurvivors saw a sharp decline in Se levels (Moghaddam et al., 2020). In a similar study, the relationship between regional selenium status and COVID-19 outcomes was investigated. The study employed Stata prtest to compare COVID-19 related recovery and death rates and assessed the association between recovery rates and regional Se serum levels using linear regression models. Interregional differences in cure rate were observed: regions with low selenium consumption rates had lower cure rates compared to other provinces. Higher death rates were, however, recorded in regions with low consumption. Thus it was concluded that selenium administration was crucial in COVID-19 recovery rate (Zhang et al., 2020).

Nutrition for optimal mental health during COVID-19

The current COVID-19 pandemic brings specific challenges and problems associated with the mental health status of both affected and healthy persons and even frontline health professionals who care for COVID-19 patients. The pandemic has been reported to have taken a heavy toll on the dietary intakes and nutritional status of people, mainly a result of not only being affected but the psychological trauma that accompanies being affected with COVID-19. Poor diet can be detrimental to mental health and as such dietary interventions hold promise for reducing symptoms of depression across the population. Therefore this section considers the critical role that certain foods and nutrients play in the prevention, management, and recovery from the common mental health-related problems associated with COVID-19.

COVID-19 patients may be confronted by emotional disorders, anxiety, distress, eating disorders, and depression which can take its toll on their sleeping patterns (insomnia), nutritional status, and rate of recovery. A study that evaluated the symptoms of patients with eating disorders during the pandemic found that 37.5% reported symptoms of worsening eating disorder and 56.2% reported additional anxiety symptoms (Fernández-Aranda et al., 2020),

Rogers and colleagues' systematic review revealed that COVID-19 patients on admission in health facilities experienced psychological problems. They included confusion (36 [27.9%; 95% CI 20.5–36.0] of 129 patients), depressed mood (42 [32.6%; 24.7–40.9] of 129), anxiety (46 [35.7%; 27.6–44.2] of 129), impaired memory (44 [34.1%; 26.2–42.5] of 129), and insomnia (54 [41.9%; 22.5–50.5] of 129). Even after recovery (postillness stage) there were still such experiences of depressed mood (35 [10.5%; 95% CI 7.5–14.1] of 332 patients), insomnia (34 [12.1%; 8.6–16.3] of 280), anxiety (21 [12.3%;7.7–17.7] of 171), irritability (28 [12.8%; 8.7–17.6] of 218), memory impairment (44 [18.9%; 14.1–24.2] of 233), and fatigue feeling (61 [19.3%; 15.1–23.9] of 316) (Rogers et al., 2020).

It is also possible that affected persons who are cared for in the ICU are very likely to develop certain psychological trauma. These include feelings of anger, sadness and helplessness, severe irritation, problems with sleeping, and extreme stress. Findings from previous studies indicate that COVID-19 patients reported gloomy feelings, lack of interest in happening in their immediate environment, and losses in their appetite. A systematic review on COVID-19 and mental health consequences reported a high level of posttraumatic stress symptoms (PTSS) (96.2%) and significantly higher level of depressive symptoms ($p=0.016$) among COVID-19 patients (Vindegaard & Benros, 2020).

A broad body of studies associate social isolation and loneliness to both poor mental health outcomes, especially because of the challenge of overcoming the difficulties associated with adapting to the new lifestyle of the quarantine. In addition, research on the psychological impact of quarantine outbreaks of diseases suggests that such isolations and confinements can result in negative mental health outcomes. Specifically, there is also a cause for alarm considering the possibility of suicidal ideation during this time, given that isolation is a risk factor for suicide.

Research that has been conducted to elucidate the relationship between diet and mental health is scarce (Choda et al., 2020). However, some studies have reported that increased consumption of fruits, vegetables, fish, poultry, dairy products, unprocessed meat, and whole grains is associated with a reduced susceptibility to depression (Lai et al., 2014; Lang, Beglinger, Schweinfurth, Walter, & Borgwardt, 2015; Schefft, Kilarski, Bschor, & Koehler, 2017). Several nutrients such as calcium, magnesium, zinc, folate, vitamins D and B12, and n-3 polyunsaturated fatty acids (PUFA) have been suggested to be effective in the management of depression (Lang et al., 2015; Schefft et al., 2017). For example, in a recent prospective cohort study that was conducted among 4701 participants who were followed for 5 years, it was revealed that regular intake of rich food sources of calcium such as dairy products resulted in better mental health outcomes among Japanese adults (Choda et al., 2020). Another systematic review revealed twelve (12) antidepressant nutrients that are associated with the prevention and treatment of depressive disorders (LaChance & Ramsey, 2018). The twelve (12) nutrients are folate, iron, long-chain omega-3 fatty acids (EPA and DHA), magnesium, potassium, selenium, thiamine, vitamin A, vitamin B6, vitamin B12, vitamin C, and zinc. These nutrients are present in foods sources such as oysters and mussels, various seafoods, and organ meats for animal foods. They also include plant food sources such as leafy greens, lettuces, peppers, and cruciferous vegetables (cabbage, cauliflower, broccoli, brussels sprouts) (LaChance & Ramsey, 2018). With regard to meat consumption, in a systematic review, eleven (11) out of eighteen (18) studies demonstrated that meat abstention was associated with poorer psychological health. The most rigorous studies demonstrated that the prevalence or risk of depression and/or anxiety were significantly greater in participants who avoided meat consumption (Dobersek et al., 2020).

A systematic review and dose-response meta-analysis of prospective studies found that high-quality diet, regardless of type (i.e., healthy/prudent or Mediterranean) which contained vegetables and fish sources, was associated with a lower risk of depressive symptoms over time (odds ratios ranged 0.64–0.78 in a linear dose-response fashion [$P<0.01$]) (Molendijk, Molero, Sánchez-Pedreño, Van der Does, & Martínez-González, 2018). A meta-analysis involving sixteen (16) eligible randomized controlled trials reported that dietary interventions significantly reduced depressive symptoms ($g=0.275$, 95% CI=0.10 to 0.45, $P=0.002$). Similar effects were observed among high-quality trials ($g=0.321$, 95% CI=0.12 to 0.53, $P=0.002$) and when compared with both inactive ($g=0.308$, 95% CI=0.02 to 0.60, $P=0.038$) and active controls ($g=0.174$, 95% CI=0.01 to 0.34, $P=0.035$) (Firth et al., 2019).

Nutrition in management of COVID-19

Malnutrition is known to extend the length of infection as well as increase the overall number of times spent in a health center during an ailment. As vaccines trials are still underway, and much attention is being given to nutritional interventions as possible remedies in the fight against COVID-19, rehabilitation departments must step up their game in the diagnosis, treatment, and prevention of malnutrition in hospitalized coronavirus-infected patients, so as to improve prognosis and patient recovery (Barazzoni et al., 2020; Volkert et al., 2019). Any attempt to underestimate the intervening role of nutrition in the fight against coronavirus infection must be downplayed since the recovery and chances of survival as well as the rehabilitation of patient is also dependent on nutritional support (Brugliera et al., 2020).

San Raffaele Scientific Institute, early this year, hosted some 50 COVID-19 infected patients at its Rehabilitation Centre. Participants, after testing positive for functional independence measure and nasopharyngeal swab test, were recruited for admission with the aim of assessing the managerial effect of nutrition on COVID-19 patient. A multidisciplinary team took care of patient's nutritional status and swallowing function during the rehabilitation period. The cohort expressed an approximated average Functional Independence Measure (FIM) value of 77.0 with some degree of dysphagia in more than 90% of COVID-19 infected patients. A dysphagia rate of about 50% was reported in a previous communication after orotracheal intubation. While less than 30% of patients exhibited a minimal incidence of malnutrition, 45% of the recruited patients expressed an elevated risk indicating that the recovery of COVID-19 patients was also dependent on nutritional supplementations coupled with effective swallowing training techniques (Brugliera et al., 2020).

A systematic review performed between February and April 2020 revealed that micronutrient deficiencies, especially vitamins A, B complex, C, and D, zinc, iron, and selenium, are common among COVID-19 patients and could plausibly increase their risk of death. A recommendation was made to consider the judicious use of need-based micronutrient supplementation, alongside existing micronutrient fortification program, in the management of this global pandemic (Akhtar et al., 2020). For COVID-19 patients in rehabilitation centers, it has been recommended that another supportive therapy that must be considered is the use of probiotics, particularly in case of intestinal issues among some COVID-19 patients. In addition, adequate hydration must be maintained particularly in patients confronted by frequent episodes of diarrhea and vomiting in order to prevent electrolyte imbalances (Brugliera et al., 2020).

Conclusion

The role of nutrition in the human defense system cannot be overemphasized as nutrition, diet, and nutritional status is an important determinant of the body's immunity. Malnutrition is known to trigger immunodeficiency, predisposing the malnourished to several infectious diseases.

Existing evidence has established relationship between disease infectivity, mortality, and micronutrient deficiencies. Numerous micronutrients, including vitamins A, D, C, E, zinc, iron, copper, and selenium, are critically essential as they mutually support each other in the immune protection and response process. The role of vitamin C in the prevention and management of respiratory infections cannot be overemphasized. Zinc's role in enhancing immune function and reducing the risk of infections mainly as a result of its antiinflammatory property has also been established. Selenium (Se) is an essential trace mineral which is vital for particularly maintaining a well-balanced immune response. Although the potential role of these micronutrients has been individually discussed, it is important to note their complementary roles in nutritional health as they do not work in isolation. Growing evidence suggests that functional foods which include tea components may help optimize immunological responses such as improving defense functions and resistance to infections. The effect of probiotics and prebiotics on health is also known.

The COVID-19 pandemic is a stressful time and it can be especially challenging when managing concerns around eating. With the occurrence of such pandemics and its associated psychological problems, dietary interventions may be immensely helpful and effective as part of the prevention, management, and treatment strategies. This review has highlighted the need to consume adequate amounts of particular nutrients and foods, especially calcium, dairy products, vegetables, vitamin D, carotene, and n-3 PUFA which have been found to lead to better mental health.

Timely provision of adequate nutrition in early phase of critical illness to minimize protein energy deficit has been suggested to improve clinical outcomes, particularly in lean and obese patients. With regard to the COVID-19, a wider access to healthy foods should be a top priority and individuals should be mindful of healthy eating habits to reduce their susceptibility and also enhance recovery rate.

References

Akhtar, S., Das, J. K., Ismail, T., Wahid, M., Saeed, W., & Bhutta, Z. A. (2020). Nutritional perspectives for the prevention and mitigation of COVID-19. *Nutrition Reviews*, *323*.

Alberda, C., Gramlich, L., Jones, N., Jeejeebhoy, K., Day, A. G., Dhaliwal, R., et al. (2009). The relationship between nutritional intake and clinical outcomes in critically ill patients: Results of an international multicenter observational study. *Intensive Care Medicine*, *35*(10), 1728–1737.

Alexander, J., Tinkov, A., Strand, T. A., Alehagen, U., Skalny, A., & Aaseth, J. (2020). Early nutritional interventions with zinc, selenium and vitamin D for raising anti-viral resistance against progressive COVID-19. *Nutrients*, *12*(8), 2358.

Alipio, M. M., & Alipio, M. M. (2020). *Vitamin D supplementation could possibly improve clinical outcomes of patients infected with Coronavirus-2019 (COVID-2019) (082)* (pp. 1–9).

Ananthakrishnan, A. N., Cagan, A., Gainer, V. S., Cai, T., Cheng, S. C., Savova, G., et al. (2013). Normalization of plasma 25-hydroxy vitamin D is associated with reduced risk of surgery in Crohn's disease. *Inflammatory Bowel Diseases*, *19*(9), 1921–1927.

Anderson, J. L., Miles, C., & Tierney, A. C. (2016). Effect of probiotics on respiratory, gastrointestinal and nutritional outcomes in patients with cystic fibrosis: A systematic review. *Journal of Cystic Fibrosis*. https://doi.org/10.1016/j.jcf.2016.09.004.

Antico, A., Tozzoli, R., Giavarina, D., Tonutti, E., & Bizzaro, N. (2012). Hypovitaminosis D as predisposing factor for atrophic type A gastritis: A case-control study and review of the literature on the interaction of vitamin D with the immune. *System*, *25*, 355–364. https://doi.org/10.1007/s12016-011-8255-1.

Barazzoni, R., Bischoff, S. C., Breda, J., Wickramasinghe, K., Krznaric, Z., Nitzan, D., et al. (2020). ESPEN expert statements and practical guidance for nutritional management of individuals with SARS-CoV-2 infection. *Clinical Nutrition, 39.*

Barnett, J. B., Dao, M. C., Hamer, D. H., Kandel, R., Brandeis, G., Wu, D., et al. (2016). Effect of zinc supplementation on serum zinc concentration and T cell proliferation in nursing home elderly: A randomized, double-blind, placebo-controlled trial. *The American Journal of Clinical Nutrition, 103*(3), 942–951.

Beavis, A. L., Smith, A. J. B., & Fader, A. N. (2016). Lifestyle changes and the risk of developing endometrial and ovarian cancers: Opportunities for prevention and management. *International Journal of Women's Health, 8*, 151.

Beck, M. A. (2006). Selenium and viral infections. In *Selenium* (pp. 287–298). Boston, MA: Springer.

Beck, M. A., Handy, J., & Levander, O. A. (2004). Host nutritional status: The neglected virulence factor. *Trends in Microbiology, 12*(9), 417–423.

Beisel, W. R. (1996). Nutrition and immune function: Overview. *The Journal of Nutrition, 126*(Suppl_10), 2611S–2615S.

Bhaskaram, P. (2001). Immunobiology of mild micronutrient deficiencies. *British Journal of Nutrition, 85*(S2), S75–S80.

Bottari, B., Castellone, V., & Neviani, E. (2020). Probiotics and COVID-19. *International Journal of Food Sciences and Nutrition*, 1–7.

Brugliera, L., Castellazzi, P., Cimino, P., Arcuri, P., Negro, A., Houdayer, E., et al. (2020). *Nutritional management of COVID-19 patients in a rehabilitation unit* (pp. 860–863).

Butnariu, M., & Sarac, I. (2019). Functional food. *International Journal of Nutrition, 3*(3), 7.

Calder, P. C., Carr, A. C., Gombart, A. F., & Eggersdorfer, M. (2020). Optimal nutritional status for a well-functioning immune system is an important factor to protect against viral infections. *Nutrients, 12*(4), 1181.

Campbell, K. (2020). *How some probiotic scientists are working to address COVID-19.* https://isappscience.org/tag/COVID-19/. (Accessed 4 May 2020).

Carr, A. C., Rosengrave, P. C., Bayer, S., Chambers, S., Mehrtens, J., & Shaw, G. M. (2017). Hypovitaminosis C and vitamin C deficiency in critically ill patients despite recommended enteral and parenteral intakes. *Critical Care, 21*(1), 1–10.

Cegielski, J. P., & McMurray, D. N. (2004). The relationship between malnutrition and tuberculosis: Evidence from studies in humans and experimental animals. *The International Journal of Tuberculosis and Lung Disease, 8*(3), 286–298.

Chandra, R. K. (1983). Nutrition, immunity, and infection: Present knowledge and future directions. *Lancet, 1.*

Chandra, R. K. (1996). Nutrition, immunity and infection: From basic knowledge of dietary manipulation of immune responses to practical application of ameliorating suffering and improving survival. *Proceedings of the National Academy of Sciences, 93*(25), 14304–14307.

Chen, H., Zhuo, Q., Yuan, W., Wang, J., Wu, T., Chen, H., et al. (2008). *Vitamin A for preventing acute lower respiratory tract infections in children up to seven years of age* (Review). https://doi.org/10.1002/14651858.CD006090.pub2.www.cochranelibrary.com.

Choda, N., Wakai, K., Naito, M., Imaeda, N., Goto, C., Maruyama, K., et al. (2020). Associations between diet and mental health using the 12-item general health questionnaire: Cross-sectional and prospective analyses from the Japan multi-institutional collaborative cohort study. *Nutrition Journal, 19*(1), 2.

Chowdhury, R., Taneja, S., Bhandari, N., Sinha, B., Upadhyay, R. P., Bhan, M. K., et al. (2017). Vitamin-D deficiency predicts infections in young north Indian children: A secondary data analysis. *PLoS One, 12*(3), e0170509.

Colunga Biancatelli, R. M. L., Berrill, M., Catravas, J. D., & Marik, P. E. (2020). Quercetin and vitamin C: An experimental, synergistic therapy for the prevention and treatment of SARS-CoV-2 related disease (COVID-19). *Frontiers in Immunology*, *11*, 1451.

Colunga Biancatelli, R. M. L., Berrill, M., & Marik, P. E. (2020). The antiviral properties of vitamin C. *Expert Review of Anti-Infective Therapy*, *18*.

de Almeida Brasiel, P. G. (2020). The key role of zinc in elderly immunity: A possible approach in the COVID-19 crisis. *Clinical Nutrition ESPEN*, *38*, 65–66.

Del Pinto, R., Pietropaoli, D., Chandar, A. K., Ferri, C., & Cominelli, F. (2015). Association between inflammatory bowel disease and vitamin D deficiency: A systematic review and meta-analysis. *Inflammatory Bowel Diseases*, *21*(11), 2708–2717.

Dobersek, U., Wy, G., Adkins, J., Altmeyer, S., Krout, K., Lavie, C. J., et al. (2020). Meat and mental health: A systematic review of meat abstention and depression, anxiety, and related phenomena. *Critical Reviews in Food Science and Nutrition*, 1–14.

Ebadi, M., & Montano-Loza, A. J. (2020). Perspective: Improving vitamin D status in the management of COVID-19. *European Journal of Clinical Nutrition*, 1–4.

El-Kadiki, A., & Sutton, A. J. (2005). Role of multivitamins and mineral supplements in preventing infections in elderly people: Systematic review and meta-analysis of randomised controlled trials. *BMJ*, *330*(7496), 871.

Enaud, R., Prevel, R., Ciarlo, E., Beaufils, F., Wieërs, G., Guery, B., et al. (2020). The gut-lung axis in health and respiratory diseases: A place for inter-organ and inter-kingdom crosstalks. *Frontiers in Cellular and Infection Microbiology*, *10*, 9.

Esposito, S., Baggi, E., Bianchini, S., Marchisio, P., & Principi, N. (2013). Role of vitamin D in children with respiratory tract infection. *International Journal of Immunopathology and Pharmacology*, *26*.

Esposito, S., & Lelii, M. (2015). Vitamin D and respiratory tract infections in childhood. *BMC Infectious Diseases*, *15*(1), 487.

Fakhrolmobasheri, M., Nasr-Esfahany, Z., Khanahmad, H., & Zeinalian, M. (2020). Selenium supplementation can relieve the clinical complications of COVID-19 and other similar viral infections. *International Journal for Vitamin and Nutrition Research*, *1*(1), 1–3.

Fernández-Aranda, F., Casas, M., Claes, L., Bryan, D. C., Favaro, A., Granero, R., et al. (2020). COVID-19 and implications for eating disorders. *European Eating Disorders Review*, *28*(3), 239.

Ferreira, I. M., Brooks, D., White, J., & Goldstein, R. (2012). Nutritional supplementation for stable chronic obstructive pulmonary disease. *The Cochrane Database of Systematic Reviews*, *12*.

Field, A. E., Coakley, E. H., Must, A., Spadano, J. L., Laird, N., Dietz, W. H., et al. (2001). Impact of overweight on the risk of developing common chronic diseases during a 10-year period. *Archives of Internal Medicine*, *161*(13), 1581–1586.

Firth, J., Marx, W., Dash, S., Carney, R., Teasdale, S. B., Solmi, M., et al. (2019). The effects of dietary improvement on symptoms of depression and anxiety: A meta-analysis of randomized controlled trials. *Psychosomatic Medicine*, *81*(3), 265.

Fortes, C., Forastiere, F., Agabiti, N., Fano, V., Pacifici, R., Virgili, F., et al. (1998). The effect of zinc and vitamin A supplementation on immune response in an older population. *Journal of the American Geriatrics Society*, *46*(1), 19–26.

Gibney, K. B., MacGregor, L., Leder, K., Torresi, J., Marshall, C., Ebeling, P. R., et al. (2008). Vitamin D deficiency is associated with tuberculosis and latent tuberculosis infection in immigrants from sub-Saharan Africa. *Clinical Infectious Diseases*, *46*(3), 443–446.

Global Nutrition Report. (2020). https://globalnutritionreport.org/reports/2020-global-nutrition-report/. (Accessed 14 July 2020).

Gombart, A. F., Pierre, A., & Maggini, S. (2020). A review of micronutrients and the immune system-working in harmony to reduce the risk of infection. *Nutrients*, *12*(1), 236.

Graat, J. M., Schouten, E. G., & Kok, F. J. (2002). Effect of daily vitamin E and multivitamin-mineral supplementation on acute respiratory tract infections in elderly persons: A randomized controlled trial. *JAMA*, *288*(6), 715–721.

Grant, W. B., Lahore, H., Mcdonnell, S. L., Baggerly, C. A., French, C. B., Aliano, J. L., et al. (2020). Evidence that vitamin D supplementation could reduce risk of influenza and COVID-19 infections and deaths. *Nutrients*, 1–19.

Grueber, C. E., Gray, L. J., Morris, K. M., Stephen, J., & Senior, A. M. (2018). Intergenerational effects of nutrition on immunity: A systematic review and meta-analysis. *Biological Reviews of the Cambridge Philosophical Society*, *93*, 1108–1124. https://doi.org/10.1111/brv.12387.

Guan, W. J., Ni, Z. Y., Hu, Y., Liang, W. H., Ou, C. Q., He, J. X., et al. (2020). Clinical characteristics of coronavirus disease 2019 in China. *New England Journal of Medicine*, *382*(18), 1708–1720.

Guillin, O. M., Vindry, C., Ohlmann, T., & Chavatte, L. (2019). Selenium, selenoproteins and viral infection. *Nutrients*, *11*(9), 2101.

Gunville, C. F., Mourani, P. M., & Ginde, A. A. (2013). The role of vitamin D in prevention and treatment of infection. *Inflammation & Allergy-Drug Targets*, *12*(4), 239–245. Formerly Current Drug Targets-Inflammation & Allergy.

Han, J. E., Jones, J. L., Tangpricha, V., Brown, M. A., Hao, L., Hebbar, G., et al. (2016). High dose vitamin D administration in ventilated intensive care unit patients: A pilot double blind randomized controlled trial. *Journal of Clinical & Translational Endocrinology*, *4*, 59–65.

Heighes, P. T., Doig, G. S., Sweetman, E. A., & Simpson, F. (2010). An overview of evidence from systematic reviews evaluating early enteral nutrition in critically ill patients: More convincing evidence is needed. *Anaesthesia and Intensive Care*, *38*, 167–174.

Hemilä, H. (2017). Zinc lozenges and the common cold: A meta-analysis comparing zinc acetate and zinc gluconate, and the role of zinc dosage. *JRSM Open*, *8*(5), 2054270417694291.

Hemilä, H., & Chalker, E. (2019). Vitamin C can shorten the length of stay in the ICU: A meta-analysis. *Nutrients*, *11*(4), 708.

Hemilä, H., & Chalker, E. (2020a). Vitamin C as a possible therapy for COVID-19. *Infection & Chemotherapy*, *52*.

Hemilä, H., & Chalker, E. (2020b). Vitamin C may reduce the duration of mechanical ventilation in critically ill patients: A meta-regression analysis. *Journal of Intensive Care*, *8*(1), 15.

Heyland, D. K., Stapleton, R. D., Mourtzakis, M., Hough, C. L., Morris, P., Deutz, N. E., et al. (2015). Combining nutrition and exercise to optimize survival and recovery from critical illness: Conceptual and methodological issues. *Clinical Nutrition*. https://doi.org/10.1016/j.clnu.2015.07.003.

Hiedra, R., Lo, K. B., Elbashabsheh, M., Gul, F., Wright, R. M., Albano, J., et al. (2020). The use of IV vitamin C for patients with COVID-19: A case series. *Expert Review of Anti-Infective Therapy*, 1–3.

Hribar, C. A., Cobbold, P. H., & Church, F. C. (2020). Potential role of vitamin D in the elderly to resist COVID-19 and to slow progression of Parkinson's disease. *Brain Sciences*, 6–13. https://globalnutritionreport.org/reports/2020-global-nutrition-report/.

Hussein, M. M., Yousif, A. A., & Saeed, A. M. (2008). Serum levels of selenium, zinc, copper and magnesium in asthmatic patients: A case control study. *Sudan Journal of Medical Sciences*, *3*(1), 45–48.

Hyltander, A., Bosaeus, I., Svedlund, J. A. N., Liedman, B., Hugosson, I., Wallengren, O. L. A., et al. (2005). Supportive nutrition on recovery of metabolism, nutritional state, health-related quality of life, and exercise capacity after major surgery: A randomized study. *Clinical Gastroenterology and Hepatology*, *3565*(05), 466–474.

Ilie, P. C., Stefanescu, S., & Smith, L. (2020). The role of vitamin D in the prevention of coronavirus disease 2019 infection and mortality. *Aging Clinical and Experimental Research*, *32*, 1195–1198.

Jackson, J. L., Lesho, E., & Peterson, C. (2000). Zinc and the common cold: A meta-analysis revisited. *The Journal of Nutrition*, *130*(5), 1512S–1515S.

Jayawardena, R., Sooriyaarachchi, P., Chourdakis, M., Jeewandara, C., & Ranasinghe, P. (2020). Enhancing immunity in viral infections, with special emphasis on COVID-19: A review. *Diabetes and Metabolic Syndrome: Clinical Research & Reviews*, *14*.

Jolliffe, D. A., Griffiths, C. J., & Martineau, A. R. (2013). Vitamin D in the prevention of acute respiratory infection: Systematic review of clinical studies. *The Journal of Steroid Biochemistry and Molecular Biology*, *136*, 321–329.

Karatekin, G., Kaya, A., Salihoğlu, Ö., Balci, H., & Nuhoğlu, A. (2009). Association of subclinical vitamin D deficiency in newborns with acute lower respiratory infection and their mothers. *European Journal of Clinical Nutrition*, *63*(4), 473–477.

Khan, H. M. W., Parikh, N., Megala, S. M., & Predeteanu, G. S. (2020). Unusual early recovery of a critical COVID-19 patient after administration of intravenous Vitamin C. *The American Journal of Case Reports*, *21*, e925521-1.

King, S., Glanville, J., Sanders, M. E., Fitzgerald, A., & Varley, D. (2014). Effectiveness of probiotics on the duration of illness in healthy children and adults who develop common acute respiratory infectious conditions: A systematic review and meta-analysis. *British Journal of Nutrition*, 41–54. https://doi.org/10.1017/S0007114514000075.

Kitson, S., Ryan, N., MacKintosh, M. L., Edmondson, R., Duffy, J. M., & Crosbie, E. J. (2018). Interventions for weight reduction in obesity to improve survival in women with endometrial cancer. *Cochrane Database of Systematic Reviews*, (2).

Koutoukidis, D. A., Knobf, M. T., & Lanceley, A. (2015). Obesity, diet, physical activity, and health-related quality of life in endometrial cancer survivors. *Nutrition Reviews*, *73*(6), 399–408.

Laaksi, I., Ruohola, J. P., Tuohimaa, P., Auvinen, A., Haataja, R., Pihlajamäki, H., et al. (2007). An association of serum vitamin D concentrations <40 nmol/L with acute respiratory tract infection in young Finnish men. *The American Journal of Clinical Nutrition*, *86*(3), 714–717.

LaChance, L. R., & Ramsey, D. (2018). Antidepressant foods: An evidence-based nutrient profiling system for depression. *World Journal of Psychiatry*, *8*(3), 97.

Lai, J. S., Hiles, S., Bisquera, A., Hure, A. J., McEvoy, M., & Attia, J. (2014). A systematic review and meta-analysis of dietary patterns and depression in community-dwelling adults. *The American Journal of Clinical Nutrition*, *99*(1), 181–197.

Laird, E., Rhodes, J., & Kenny, R. A. (2020). Vitamin D and inflammation: Potential implications for severity of COVID-19. *Irish Medical Journal*, *113*, 81.

Lang, U. E., Beglinger, C., Schweinfurth, N., Walter, M., & Borgwardt, S. (2015). Nutritional aspects of depression. *Cellular Physiology and Biochemistry*, *37*(3), 1029–1043.

Lassi, Z. S., Moin, A., & Bhutta, Z. A. (2016). Zinc supplementation for the prevention of pneumonia in children aged 2 months to 59 months. *Cochrane Database of Systematic Reviews*, (12).

Lee, M., Lin, C., Lei, W., Chang, H., Lee, H., Yeung, C., et al. (2018). Does vitamin D deficiency affect the immunogenic responses to influenza vaccination? A systematic review and meta-analysis. *Nutrients*, *25*, 1–12. https://doi.org/10.3390/nu10040409.

Lei, W., Shih, P., & Liu, S. (2018). Effect of probiotics and prebiotics on immune response to influenza vaccination in adults: A systematic review and meta-analysis of randomized controlled trials. *Nutrients*. https://doi.org/10.3390/nu9111175.

Liu, F., Zhu, Y., Zhang, J., Li, Y., & Peng, Z. (2020). Intravenous high-dose vitamin C for the treatment of severe COVID-19: Study protocol for a multicentre randomised controlled trial. *BMJ Open*, *10*(7), e039519.

Maalmi, H., Tangour, E., & Hamzaoui, K. (2012). The impact of vitamin D deficiency on immune T cells in asthmatic children: A case-control study. *Journal of Asthma and Allergy*, *5*, 11–19.

Maggini, S., Pierre, A., & Calder, P. C. (2018). Immune function and micronutrient requirements change over the life course. *Nutrients*, *10*(10), 1531.

Mak, J. W., Chan, F. K., & Ng, S. C. (2020). Probiotics and COVID-19: One size does not fit all. *The Lancet Gastroenterology & Hepatology*, *5*.

Martineau, A. R., & Forouhi, N. G. (2020). Vitamin D for COVID-19: A case to answer? *The Lancet Diabetes & Endocrinology*, *8*(9), 735–736.

Martineau, A. R., Jolliffe, D. A., Hooper, R. L., Greenberg, L., Aloia, J. F., Bergman, P., et al. (2017). Vitamin D supplementation to prevent acute respiratory tract infections: Systematic review and meta-analysis of individual participant data. *British Medical Journal*. https://doi.org/10.1136/bmj.i6583.

Menegazzi, M., Campagnari, R., Bertoldi, M., Crupi, R., Di Paola, R., & Cuzzocrea, S. (2020). Protective effect of Epigallocatechin-3-Gallate (EGCG) in diseases with uncontrolled immune activation: Could such a scenario be helpful to counteract COVID-19? *International Journal of Molecular Sciences*, *21*(14), 5171.

Merzon, E., Tworowski, D., Gorohovski, A., Vinker, S., Golan Cohen, A., Green, I., et al. (2020). Low plasma 25 (OH) vitamin D level is associated with increased risk of COVID-19 infection: An Israeli population-based study. *The FEBS Journal*, *287*(17), 3693–3702.

Meydani, S. N., Han, S. N., & Wu, D. (2005). Vitamin E and immune response in the aged: Molecular mechanisms and clinical implications. *Immunological Reviews*, *205*(1), 269–284.

Meydani, S. N., Leka, L. S., Fine, B. C., Dallal, G. E., Keusch, G. T., Singh, M. F., et al. (2004). Vitamin E and respiratory tract infections in elderly nursing home residents: A randomized controlled trial. *JAMA*, *292*(7), 828–836.

Moghaddam, A., Heller, R. A., Sun, Q., Seelig, J., Cherkezov, A., Seibert, L., et al. (2020). Selenium deficiency is associated with mortality risk from COVID-19. *Nutrients*, *12*(7), 2098.

Molendijk, M., Molero, P., Sánchez-Pedreño, F. O., Van der Does, W., & Martínez-González, M. A. (2018). Diet quality and depression risk: A systematic review and dose-response meta-analysis of prospective studies. *Journal of Affective Disorders*, *226*, 346–354.

Moreira, A., Kekkonen, R. A., Delgado, L., Fonseca, J., Korpela, R., & Haahtela, T. (2007). Nutritional modulation of exercise-induced immunodepression in athletes: A systematic review and meta-analysis. *European Journal of Clinical Nutrition*, 443–460. https://doi.org/10.1038/sj.ejcn.1602549.

Mousavi, S., Bereswill, S., & Heimesaat, M. M. (2019). Immunomodulatory and antimicrobial effects of vitamin C. *European Journal of Microbiology and Immunology*, *9*(3), 73–79.

Naja, F., & Hamadeh, R. (2020). Nutrition amid the COVID-19 pandemic: A multi-level framework for action. *European Journal of Clinical Nutrition*, 1–5.

Nilashi, M., Samad, S., Shahmoadi, L., Ahmadi, H., Akbari, E., & Rashid, T. A. (2020). The COVID-19 infection and the immune system: The role of complementary and alternative medicines. *Biomedical Research*, *31*(3). 0970-938X.

Overbeck, S., Rink, L., & Haase, H. (2008). Modulating the immune response by oral zinc supplementation: A single approach for multiple diseases. *Archivum Immunologiae et Therapiae Experimentalis*, *56*(1), 15–30.

Papandreou, D., & Hamid, Z. T. N. (2015). The role of vitamin D in diabetes and cardiovascular disease: An updated review of the literature. *Disease Markers*, *2015*.

Phan, A. D. T., Netzel, G., Chhim, P., Netzel, M. E., & Sultanbawa, Y. (2019). Phytochemical characteristics and antimicrobial activity of Australian grown garlic (*Allium Sativum* L.) cultivars. *Foods*, *8*(9), 358.

Reeves, M. M., Terranova, C. O., Eakin, E. G., & Demark-Wahnefried, W. (2014). Weight loss intervention trials in women with breast cancer: A systematic review. *Obesity Reviews*, *15*(9), 749–768.

Rock, C. L., Flatt, S. W., Byers, T. E., Colditz, G. A., Demark-Wahnefried, W., Ganz, P. A., et al. (2015). Results of the exercise and nutrition to enhance recovery and good health for you (ENERGY) trial: A behavioral weight loss intervention in overweight or obese breast cancer survivors. *Journal of Clinical Oncology*, *33*(28), 3169.

Rodriguez-Morales, A. J., Bolivar-Mejía, A., Alarcón-Olave, C., & Calvo-Betancourt, L. S. (2016). Nutrition and infection. In *Encyclopedia of food and health* (1st ed.). Elsevier Ltd. https://doi.org/10.1016/B978-0-12-384947-2.00491-8. Issue September 2017.

Rogers, J. P., Chesney, E., Oliver, D., Pollak, T. A., McGuire, P., Fusar-Poli, P., et al. (2020). Psychiatric and neuropsychiatric presentations associated with severe coronavirus infections: A systematic review and meta-analysis with comparison to the COVID-19 pandemic. *The Lancet Psychiatry*, *7*.

Rondanelli, M., Miccono, A., Lamburghini, S., Avanzato, I., Riva, A., Allegrini, P., et al. (2018). Self-care for common colds: The pivotal role of vitamin D, vitamin C, zinc, and echinacea in three main immune interactive clusters (physical barriers, innate and adaptive immunity) involved during an episode of common colds—Practical advice on dosages and on the time to take these nutrients/botanicals in order to prevent or treat common colds. *Evidence-based Complementary and Alternative Medicine*, *2018*.

Roth, D. E., Caulfield, L. E., & Black, R. E. (2008). Acute lower respiratory infections in childhood: Opportunities for reducing the global burden through nutritional interventions. *Bulletin of the World Health Organization*. https://doi.org/10.2471/BLT.07.049114.

Roth, D. E., Richard, S. A., & Black, R. E. (2010). Zinc supplementation for the prevention of acute lower respiratory infection in children in developing countries: Meta-analysis and meta-regression of randomized trials. *International Journal of Epidemiology*, *39*(3), 795–808.

Rozga, M., Cheng, F. W., Moloney, L., & Handu, D. (2020). Effects of micronutrients or conditional amino acids on COVID-19-related outcomes: An evidence analysis center scoping review. *Journal of the Academy of Nutrition and Dietetics*. https://doi.org/10.1016/j.jand.2020.05.015.

Savino, W. (2002). The thymus gland is a target in malnutrition. *European Journal of Clinical Nutrition*, *56*(3), S46–S49.

Schaible, U. E., & Stefan, H. E. (2007). Malnutrition and infection: Complex mechanisms and global impacts. *PLoS Medicine*, *4*(5), e115.

Schefft, C., Kilarski, L. L., Bschor, T., & Koehler, S. (2017). Efficacy of adding nutritional supplements in unipolar depression: A systematic review and meta-analysis. *European Neuropsychopharmacology*, *27*(11), 1090–1109.

Scrimshaw, N. S., Taylor, C. E., Gordon, J. E., & World Health Organization. (1968). *Interactions of nutrition and infection*. World Health Organization.

Shang, A., Cao, S. Y., Xu, X. Y., Gan, R. Y., Tang, G. Y., Corke, H., et al. (2019). Bioactive compounds and biological functions of garlic (*Allium sativum* L.). *Foods*, *8*(7), 246.

Shi, J., Wei, L., Huang, R., & Liao, L. (2018). Effect of combined parenteral and enteral nutrition versus enteral nutrition alone for critically ill patients. *Medicine*, *97*.

Sicotte, M., Langlois, É. V., Aho, J., Ziegler, D., & Zunzunegui, M. V. (2014). Association between nutritional status and the immune response in HIV + patients under HAART: Protocol for a systematic review. *Systematic Reviews*, 1–8.

Stachowska, E., Folwarski, M., Jamioł-Milc, D., Maciejewska, D., & Skonieczna-Żydecka, K. (2020). Nutritional support in coronavirus 2019 disease. *Medicina*, *56*(6), 289.

Stephensen, C. B. (2001). Vitamin A, infection, and immune function. *Annual Review of Nutrition, 21*(1), 167–192.

Stephensen, C. B., Blount, S. R., Schoeb, T. R., & Park, J. Y. (1993). Vitamin A deficiency impairs some aspects of the host response to influenza A virus infection in BALB/c mice. *The Journal of Nutrition, 123*(5), 823–833.

Te Velthuis, A. J., van den Worm, S. H., Sims, A. C., Baric, R. S., Snijder, E. J., & van Hemert, M. J. (2010). Zn2 + inhibits coronavirus and arterivirus RNA polymerase activity in vitro and zinc ionophores block the replication of these viruses in cell culture. *PLoS Pathogens, 6*(11), e1001176.

Thomson, C. A., Crane, T. E., Wertheim, B. C., Neuhouser, M. L., Li, W., Snetselaar, L. G., et al. (2014). Diet quality and survival after ovarian cancer: Results from the women's health initiative. *Journal of the National Cancer Institute, 106*(11).

Vindegaard, N., & Benros, M. E. (2020). COVID-19 pandemic and mental health consequences: Systematic review of the current evidence. *Brain, Behavior, and Immunity, 89*.

Volkert, D., Beck, A. M., Cederholm, T., Cruz-Jentoft, A., Goisser, S., Hooper, L., et al. (2019). ESPEN guideline on clinical nutrition and hydration in geriatrics. *Clinical Nutrition, 38*(1), 10–47.

Wayse, V., Yousafzai, A., Mogale, K., & Filteau, S. (2004). Association of subclinical vitamin D deficiency with severe acute lower respiratory infection in Indian children under 5 y. *European Journal of Clinical Nutrition*, 563–567. https://doi.org/10.1038/sj.ejcn.1601845.

Wimalawansa, S. J. (2020). Global epidemic of coronavirus—COVID-19: What can we do to minimize risks. *European Journal of Biomedical, 7*(3), 432–438.

Wu, D., Lewis, E. D., Pae, M., & Meydani, S. N. (2019). Nutritional modulation of immune function: Analysis of evidence, mechanisms, and clinical relevance. *Frontiers in Immunology, 9*, 3160.

Xiao, L., Xing, C., Yang, Z., Xu, S., Wang, M., Du, H., et al. (2015). Vitamin D supplementation for the prevention of childhood acute respiratory infections: A systematic review of randomised controlled trials. *The British Journal of Nutrition, 25*, 1026–1034. https://doi.org/10.1017/S000711451500207X.

Xu, J., Yang, J., Chen, J., Luo, Q., Zhang, Q., & Zhang, H. (2017). Vitamin D alleviates lipopolysaccharide-induced acute lung injury via regulation of the renin-angiotensin system. *Molecular Medicine Reports, 16*(5), 7432–7438.

Yang, D., Xing, Y., Song, X., & Qian, Y. (2020). The impact of lung microbiota dysbiosis on inflammation. *Immunology, 159*(2), 156–166.

Zabetakis, I., Lordan, R., & Norton, C. (2020). COVID-19: The inflammation link and the role of nutrition in potential mitigation. *Nutrients, 2*, 1–28. Figure 1.

Zhang, J., Taylor, E. W., Bennett, K., Saad, R., & Rayman, M. P. (2020). Association between regional selenium status and reported outcome of COVID-19 cases in China. *The American Journal of Clinical Nutrition, 111*(6), 1297–1299.

Zhang, X., Ding, F., Li, H., Zhao, W., Jing, H., Yan, Y., et al. (2016). Low serum levels of vitamins A, D, and E are associated with recurrent respiratory tract infections in children living in northern china: A case control study. *PLoS One*, 1–9. https://doi.org/10.1371/journal.pone.0167689.

Zhou, Y. F., Luo, B. A., & Qin, L. L. (2019). The association between vitamin D deficiency and community-acquired pneumonia: A meta-analysis of observational studies. *Medicine, 98*(38).

Zurita, M. F., Cárdenas, P. A., Sandoval, M. E., Peña, C., Fornasini, M., Flores, N., et al. (2020). Analysis of gut microbiome, nutrition and immune status in autism spectrum disorder: A case-control study in Ecuador. *Gut Microbes, 11*(3), 453–464. https://doi.org/10.1080/19490976.2019.1662260.

Chapter 13

Physical activity as a counteracting measure to mitigate the harmful effects of COVID-19 lockdowns: Special focus on healthy children, adolescents, adults, elderly, athletes, and people with Down syndrome

Monoem Haddad[a], Zied Abbes[a,*], Amine Ghram[b,c,*], Germina Cosma[d], and Karim Chamari[e]

[a]*Department of Physical Education, College of Education, Qatar University, Doha, Qatar,* [b]*Department of Exercise Physiology, Faculty of Physical Education and Sport Sciences, University of Tehran, Tehran, Iran,* [c]*Department of Cardiac Rehabilitation, Tehran Heart Center, Tehran University of Medical Sciences, Tehran, Iran,* [d]*Department of Theory and Methodology of Motor Activities, University of Craiova, Craiova, Romania,* [e]*Aspetar, Qatar Orthopaedic and Sports Medicine Hospital, Doha, Qatar*

Introduction

The World Health Organization (WHO) defines health as "a state of complete physical, mental, and social well-being and not merely the absence of disease or infirmity" (World Health Organization, 2020). Physical inactivity has been identified as the fourth leading risk factor for global mortality (6% of deaths globally). This follows high blood pressure (13%), tobacco use (9%), and high blood glucose (6%). Overweight and obesity are responsible for 5% of global mortality (World Health Organization, 2009). There is a growing awareness and concern surrounding potential public health threats posed by a lack of physical activity as well as the benefits of sustained engagement in physical activity (Waddington, 2000).

* These two authors contributed equally.

Mental Health Effects of COVID-19. https://doi.org/10.1016/B978-0-12-824289-6.00010-6

Scientific evidence shows major beneficial effects of physical activity on health. Physical activity reduces the risk of most chronic diseases (Advisory Committee, 2008; World Health Organization, 2010), including cardiovascular disease, overweight and obesity, type 2 diabetes, and several cancers. Furthermore, physical activity improves musculoskeletal health and psychological well-being (Warburton, Nicol, & Bredin, 2006).

Routine physical activity is also associated with improved psychological well-being (for example, through reduced stress, anxiety, and depression) (Warburton, Gledhill, & Quinney, 2001). Psychological well-being is particularly important for the prevention and management of cardiovascular disease, but it also has key implications for the prevention and management of other chronic diseases such as diabetes, osteoporosis, hypertension, obesity, cancer, and depression.

Recent analyses by the WHO and US Centers for Disease Control and Prevention have underscored a growing recognition that the economic impact of physical inactivity is worldwide. Moreover, a joint report by the World Heart Federation and WHO suggested that 60%–85% of the world's population, including developing countries, is not physically active enough to gain health benefits (Mackay & Mensah, 2004). A study by Cadilhac et al. (2011) on an Australian population reported that a feasible reduction in the prevalence of physical inactivity can lead to total potential opportunity cost savings of AUD 258 million, with 37% of the savings arising in the health sector. The largest savings would benefit individuals, followed by the health sector, business, and government.

National and international public health policies that manage physical inactivity are rapidly developing. The WHO's Global Strategy on Diet, Physical Activity, and Health (World Health Organization, 2004) sends a clear message about the importance of policies promoting physical activity. Additionally, numerous policy documents such as the European Union's Physical Activity Guidelines (EU Working Group, 2008) and the Healthy People 2020 Objectives of the United States Department of Health and Human Services (US Department of Health and Human Services, 2020) convey strong support for physical activity promotion initiatives.

On January 31, 2020, the World Health Organization (WHO) declared the outbreak of a novel coronavirus responsible for an infection called COVID-19 as a global public health emergency (Yousfi, Bragazzi, Briki, Zmijewski, & Chamari, 2020). Changes have been felt on all levels: social, economic, cultural, sports, and so on. Those changes arose due to the appearance of SARS-CoV-2, a new coronavirus, first identified on December, 12, 2019 (Zhu et al., 2020), in an outbreak of pneumonia in Wuhan, Hubei province, the largest city (> 11 million) in central China, which is an important transportation hub, industry, and trade center, that has the largest railway station, airport, and port in central China (Wilson & Chen, 2019). SARS-CoV-2 has spread rapidly worldwide. As of August 7, 2020, an estimated 19,272,197 people had contracted this virus and 717,918 people died (Worldometers, 2020) as a consequence.

To minimize the risk of contamination, various protective measures have been introduced by authorities, including closing schools and universities, and bans on travel, cultural and sporting events, and social gatherings (Parnell, Widdop, Bond, & Wilson, 2020). These actions will negatively affect people's physical activity behaviors, with more time spent at home, self-isolating and sitting watching screens. The COVID-19 pandemic has had an effect on the physical health, well-being, sleeping patterns, and quality of life of different populations: children, adults, elderly, athletes, and those with Down syndrome. Therefore implementing an adapted physical training program at home during this pandemic can decrease the negative physiological and psychological impact of sedentary behaviors.

Preventing COVID-19 spread

Since there are no currently approved treatments for COVID-19, prevention is crucial. Following the global spread of the COVID-19 pandemic, health care authorities have adopted nonpharmacological measures, implementing self-isolation, social distancing, quarantine, and even lockdown of entire communities and territories as well as travel restrictions (Wilder-Smith & Freedman, 2020). In addition, physical and social distancing measures, lockdown of businesses, schools, and universities, and precautionary actions such as staying at home, avoiding going out and gathering, wearing masks, and avoiding contacting anyone with symptoms of cold or influenza are required to better prevent and control the spread of COVID-19 (Li, Hu, & Liu, 2020). At the community level, people should avoid crowded areas and postpone nonessential travel to places with ongoing transmission. They should practice cough hygiene by coughing in their sleeve/tissue rather than hands and wash their hands every 15–20 min (Singhal, 2020).

The absence of specific preventive or therapeutic medical interventions for COVID-19 infection, along with its rapid transmission rate and apparently substantial undocumented contamination and transmission numbers, has led to scientifically sound recommendations that individuals must stay home to avoid social interactions and restrain the disease spread, thereby reducing pressure on health systems worldwide. Despite being effective for infection control, this strategy has potential behavioral and clinical repercussions (Peçanha, Goessler, Roschel, & Gualano, 2020). These public health preventive measures have disrupted many regular aspects of life, including sports and physical activity (UN, 2020).

Consequences of COVID-19 on health

COVID-19's high transmission rate affects high-risk clinical populations and alters physical and mental health. The current pandemic poses serious public health problems (Zarocostas, 2020), deepens psychological problems such as stress, anxiety, depression symptoms (Khan et al., 2020), insomnia, panic behavior, fear, and hopelessness (Khan et al., 2020), and impairs sexual activity (Jacob et al., 2020). Moreover, during an infectious disease outbreak, particularly in the presence of inaccurate or exaggerated information from the media, health anxiety can become excessive. At an individual level, this can manifest as maladaptive behaviors (repeated medical consultations, avoiding health care even if genuinely ill, or hoarding items) (Asmundson & Taylor, 2020).

The wide scope and spread of COVID-19 could lead to a true mental health crisis, especially in countries with high caseloads (Dong & Bouey, 2020) that would require both large-scale psychosocial crisis interventions and the incorporation of mental health care in future disaster management plans. Further, preventive measures such as gloves, masks, and headcovers during the widespread lockdown may increase stress in the general population and advising infected individuals to stay isolated inside their homes rather than hospitals may also increase the stress burden on family members due to the fear of infection. Several stressor factors including duration of quarantine, fear of infection, frustration and boredom, and inadequate supplies and information may increase the negative health consequences during the COVID-19 pandemic (Brooks et al., 2020).

Sedentary behavior, bed rest, and physical inactivity during COVID-19 lockdown

Due to the spread of COVID-19, people's lifestyles have changed. People are obliged to stay home which increases the sedentary behavior (i.e., "any waking behavior characterized by an energy expenditure ≤ 1.5 MET (the energy cost) while in a sitting or reclining posture") (Mansoubi et al., 2015) and the physical inactivity levels. Fitbit Inc. (a US-based company that develops wearable devices tracking an individual's physical activity levels) recently shared physical activity data from 30 million users that demonstrated a substantial reduction (ranging from 7% to 38%) in average step counts in almost all countries during the week ending March 22, 2020, compared to the same period in 2019 (Fitbit News, 2020).

Bed rest, limb immobilization, and cessation of exercise during the COVID-19 pandemic could result in deleterious effects of inactivity in restricted living environments. Sedentary behavior, bed rest, and physical inactivity contribute to low levels of energy expenditure and are a health risk factor. Sedentary behavior including screen time and sitting time is associated with the deterioration of physical and mental health (Zhai, Zhang, & Zhang, 2015), sleep-related breathing disorders (Kline, Krafty, Mulukutla, & Hall, 2017), and increased risk of insomnia and sleep disturbance (Yang, Shin, Li, & An, 2017). Bed rest has a negative impact on health including losing muscle size, strength, and power (Ferrando, Lane, Stuart, Davis-Street, & Wolfe, 1996; Trappe et al., 2008); impaired postural control (Mulder et al., 2014; Reschke et al., 2009; Viguier, Dupui, & Montoya, 2009); and increased incidence of falls (Mulder et al., 2014) and muscle atrophy (Bowden Davies et al., 2019).

Thus it is necessary to avoid sedentary behavior, bed rest, and physical inactivity by implementing physical activity in an individual's lifestyle. Physical activity and exercise, as effective countermeasures, could help attenuate the harmful effects caused by living isolated/confined, protect individuals from deconditioning, and attenuate inactivity-induced muscle atrophy.

Why are physical activity and sports important for health?

To confront the COVID-19 lockdown, individuals should be aware of safety, feasibility, and efficacy of physical activity and sport to achieve better health outcomes and improve their daily life activities. Physical activity plays a fundamental role in protecting against disease and provides biological and psychological benefits. Physical activity has proven to be beneficial for improving clinical conditions that are most frequently associated with severe COVID-19 (Dwyer, Pasini, De Dominicis, & Righi, 2020).

The American College of Sports Medicine (ASCM) released information on how to remain active during COVID-19 (ASCM, 2020). The college highlighted the positive impact of regular physical exercise on improving the immunological system in humans, highlighting that physically active people have a lower risk of developing chronic degenerative diseases, which is pertinent, as those who are affected are at a higher risk if infected by SARS-CoV-2 (De Oliveira Neto, De Oliveira Tavares, Schuch, & Lima, 2020; Pedersen & Saltin, 2015). Exercise and physical activity lower blood pressure; improve lipoprotein profiles, C-reactive protein, and other CHD biomarkers; enhance insulin sensitivity; and play an important role in weight management (US Department of Health and Human Services, 2020). Of particular relevance to older adults, exercise preserves bone mass and reduces the risk of falling (Nelson et al., 2007).

Considering the positive effects of physical activity on the general and cardiovascular health state, it is advisable that people continue to exercise at home. Treadmills, stationary bikes, and rowing machines are good tools. Using fitness balls, elastic bands, and weights is also advisable. Even going up and down stairs can help. Whenever possible, local authorities should consider allowing some outdoor activities with sufficient interpersonal distance (more than 1.5 m).

It is recommend to use online technology to prescribe and monitor exercise, such as mobile telephone messages, apps, email, video calls, or other Internet-based strategies (De Oliveira Neto et al., 2020). This chapter focuses in detail on the importance of physical activity and exercise for reducing the harmful effects of living in restricted environments due to the pandemic for different types of populations.

Physical activity and sports in healthy adults

The ACSM recommends a comprehensive exercise program including cardiorespiratory, resistance, flexibility, and neuromotor exercise with sufficient volume and quality as outlined in this document for apparently healthy adults of all ages. Reducing total time spent in sedentary pursuits and interspersing short bouts of physical activity and standing between periods of sedentary activity should be goals for all adults irrespective of their exercise habits. Exercise performed in this manner improves physical and mental health and/or fitness in most populations (Garber et al., 2011).

We recommend that adults exercise with at least a light physical activity intensity instead of spending time watching television. Following such recommendation can reduce the risk of type 2 diabetes and cardiovascular disease (Healy et al., 2007). People should be engaged in 7 h per week of moderate to vigorous physical activity and only 1 h of daily television viewing time to lower the risk of cardiovascular mortality (Matthews et al., 2012).

According to the 2007 American Heart Association and ACSM recommendations (Haskell et al., 2007), all healthy adults need moderate intensity aerobic physical activity for a minimum of 30 min 5 days each week or vigorous intensity aerobic activity for a minimum of 20 min 3 days each week to promote and maintain their health. According to the World Health Organization (WHO, 2010), adults should practice a minimum of 150 min of moderate intensity or 75 min of vigorous intensity aerobic activity or their equivalent combination per week, in addition muscle-strengthening activities at least 2 days a week.

Physical activity and sports in elderly

The health benefits of physical activity, specifically for older adults, have been comprehensively studied. For older adults, physical activity can be beneficial for physical (Paterson, Jones, & Rice, 2007), mental (Bishop, Lu, & Yankner, 2010), and social (Sirven & Debrand, 2008) health. Being isolated/confined and increased sitting time may decrease strength, alter flexibility, and affect the functional performance of tasks that hinder a healthy lifestyle. Therefore exercise is the basis for improving individuals' functional skills.

Home-based physical exercise is essential for confronting the COVID-19 pandemic to maintain and improve health-related physical fitness components in older people (Ghram et al., 2020), which can be used safely by other populations during this period of uncertainty (Jiménez-Pavón, Carbonell-Baeza, & Lavie, 2020). Regular exercise is also beneficial for the immune system (Yousfi et al., 2020). Moderate intensity exercise at home (for example, walking) can help prevent aspiration pneumonia and falls in older adults (Matsumoto, Takatori, Nishida, & Matsushita, 2015; Takatori et al., 2016), increase antibody titer in response to influenza vaccination in older adults (Kohut et al., 2004), reduce the mortality of mice infected by influenza virus (Lowder, Padgett, & Woods, 2005), increase hemagglutination inhibition (antibody titer) in older adults with and without vaccine history (Vieira et al., 2008), and improve influenza seroprotection, overall illness severity, and sleep disturbance in older adults (Woods et al., 2009). These data indicate the importance of highlighting the impact of exercise training on immunity in the elderly population.

Neuromotor exercise training incorporates motor skills such as balance, coordination, gait, agility, and proprioceptive training (Garber et al., 2011) and also is beneficial for older persons, especially to improve balance, agility, and muscle strength and reduce the risk of falls (Liu-Ambrose et al., 2004, 2008; Logghe et al., 2010; Nelson et al., 2007; Wu, 2002). A new physical training program based on mind-body practices and a focus on the breath and mind to achieve deep states of relaxation has been recently defined as meditative movement (Larkey, Jahnke, Etnier, & Gonzalez, 2009) and includes tai chi, qigong, yoga, other less familiar forms. These practices involve varying combinations of neuromotor, resistance, and flexibility exercises (Garber et al., 2011) and have beneficial effects on both physical and psychological health in older people (Chen et al., 2020). These exercises are more suitable than other types of exercise for older adults (Ghram et al., 2020). They are executed via slow controlled movements and result in a minimal risk of injuries (Chen et al., 2020). Tai chi, the most widely studied neuromotor activity, can be effective at improving balance, agility, motor control, proprioception, and quality of life, reducing stress, anxiety, depression, and mood disturbance and increasing self-esteem (Chin, Van Uffelen, Riphagen, & Van Mechelen, 2008; Jahnke, Larkey, Rogers, Etnier, & Lin, 2010; Li, Xu, & Hong, 2008; Verhagen, Immink, Van Der Meulen, & Bierma-Zeinstra, 2004; Wang et al., 2010).

Many medical centers recommend how to use mind-body exercises such as Harvard Medical School and National Health Service. Qigong plays a role in the prevention, treatment, and rehabilitation of respiratory infections, such as COVID-19 (Feng, Tuchman, Denninger, Fricchione, & Yeung, 2020) and can help to enhance the antibody responses to influenza vaccination in older adults (Yang et al., 2007). Moderate intensity Pilates exercise can increase the salivary flow rate and S-IgA secretion (Hwang, Park, & Lim, 2016) and improve both cognitive and functional abilities as well as balance in older women (García-Garro et al., 2020). Flexibility plays a fundamental role in the elderly's functional capacity (Stathokostas, Mcdonald, Little, & Paterson, 2013) and can be improved by yoga (Im, Bang, & Seo, 2019), Yang-style tai chi (Zou, Wang, Tian, Wang, & Shu, 2017), Pilates (Curi, Haas, Alves-Vilaça, & Fernandes, 2018), and resistance exercises (Carneiro et al., 2015) in elderly women.

Using available options in any house is recommended: resistance training through bodyweight exercises such as squats holding a chair, sitting, and getting up from the chair or going up and down a step, transporting items with light and moderate weights, aerobic exercises such as walking inside the house, dancing or balance exercise such as walking on a line on the floor, walking on the toes or heels, walking heel to toe, and stepping over obstacles (Jiménez-Pavón et al., 2020). Therefore it is imperative to advise older people to engage in regular physical activity to boost their immune system and decrease the rate of falls and injuries. In addition, we recommend performing mind-body interventions (for example, tai chi, yoga, and Pilates) that are more suitable than other types of exercise for older adults and executed by slow controlled movements that result in a minimal risk of injuries (Chen et al., 2020).

Poor health as a limitation to participation is a unique determinant for this age group and needs to be considered. As such, to enable older adults to derive the health benefits sports can provide, age appropriate playing opportunities are required, especially in more exertive sports, to accommodate older adults who may have age-related reduced physical capabilities (Jenkin et al., 2017).

Physical activity and sports in children and adolescents

Physical activity decreases sedentary time as well as sedentary behavior and is effective at reducing body mass index in children who are overweight or obese. Thus it is important to encourage children not only to decrease their sedentary time, but also change their diet and increase their physical activity levels. In addition, children's family can encourage them to lose weight in response to physical interventions, thereby leading to behavior changes, which highlights the parent's influential role in supporting and managing children's behaviors.

The present pandemic has necessitated family isolation, but children must move their bodies. Exercise in children is beneficial for their mental and physical health and helps them cope with COVID-19. According to the World Health Organization (WHO, 2010), children and adolescents should do at least 1 h of physical activity every day, which should include moderate and vigorous intensity aerobic activities and muscle- and bone-strengthening activities. Young people who exercise have lower levels of depression, stress, and psychological distress and higher levels of positive self-image, life satisfaction, and psychological well-being (Rodriguez-Ayllon et al., 2019). Evidence shows the greater positive effects of exercise on academic performance (De Greeff, Bosker, Oosterlaan, Visscher, & Hartman, 2018) and cognitive development (Carson et al., 2016) in physically active children compared to their physical inactive peers. Just 40 min per day of vigorous aerobic exercise could improve symptoms of sleep-related breathing disorders in overweight 7–11-year-old children (Davis, Tkacz, Gregoski, Boyle, & Lovrekovic, 2006).

Autism spectrum disorder (ASD) is a heterogeneous neurodevelopmental disorder with qualitative impairments in social and communication skills, repetitive behaviors, and a range of motor sensory difficulties (Bello-Mojeed, Ani, Lagunju, & Omigbodun, 2016). Low levels of motor skills in individuals with ASD can decrease their participation in physical activities and sports (Cairney, Hay, Faught, Corna, & Flouris, 2006) and increase the rate of sedentary-related diseases (Pan, 2011). Investigations have demonstrated the beneficial effects of engaging in physical exercise and sports training across a wide variety of skills in children with autism spectrum disorders (Movahedi, Bahrami, Marandi, & Abedi, 2013; Pitetti, Rendoff, Grover, & Beets, 2007). Karate training can improve communication skills (Bahrami, Movahedi, Marandi, & Sorensen, 2016) and aquatic programs can promote motor skills and physical fitness (Pan, 2011) in children with ASD.

Physical activity and sports in athletes

The preventive measures recommended by health authorities and governments to decelerate the propagation of COVID-19 resulted in the suspension of sports training and competitions (Herrero-Gonzalez et al., 2020). The organizational consequences of quarantine/isolation are absence of organized training and competition, lack of communication among athletes and coaches, inability to move freely, lack of adequate sunlight exposure, and inappropriate training conditions (Jukic, 2020). Professional athletes have been unable to train as usual during home confinement, and it is thought that they will have to return to sports competitions in most countries once the risk of infection has been adequately reduced (Herrero-Gonzalez et al., 2020). As the pandemic runs its course, uncertainties persist regarding exercise safety, resumption of sporting activity, and managing infected athletes (Yeo, 2020).

Based on the current scientific knowledge, we strongly recommend encouraging athletes to reset their mindset to understand quarantine as an opportunity for development, organizing appropriate guidance, educating and encourage athletes to apply appropriate preventive behavior and hygiene measures to promote immunity and ensure good living isolation conditions. Athletes' living space should be equipped with cardio and resistance training equipment (such as a portable bicycle or rowing ergometer). Some forms of body mass resistance circuit-based training can promote aerobic adaptation. Sports skills training should be organized based on the athlete's needs. Personalized conditioning training should be carried out with an emphasis on neuromuscular performance.

To reduce the harmful effects of home isolation in athletes, they should be encouraged to perform physical activities (for example, walking, running, or other individual sports in which an adequate interpersonal distance can be maintained) (Lippi, Henry, & Sanchis-Gomar, 2020). Video- or app-guided equipment-free aerobics or strength training can also be performed at home and should be encouraged (Lippi et al., 2020). Physical activity as an immunotherapy can enhance immunity rather than suppress immune competency among athletes (Campbell & Turner, 2018; Kakanis et al., 2010). Moderate intensity aerobic exercise (push-ups, pull-ups, and crunches followed by a 2-min run, biceps curls, dips, and shoulder presses to target smaller muscles) in outdoor environments with special attention to maintaining a safe distance from others and surfaces may be a proper alternative.

In addition, coaches and fitness trainers should encourage athletes during quarantine or self-isolation to follow adequate training regimens including endurance (for example, aerobics and calisthenics) and resistance exercises (for example, strengthening the core and limbs with body weights) (Yousfi et al., 2020). Indeed, they should highlight the necessity to ascertain the extent of immune decline in athletes due to extreme exercise training (overtraining/excessive training). Moreover, athletes are encouraged to practice distraction techniques such as meditation and quiet rest that are effective at reducing anxiety (Katula, Blissmer, & Mcauley, 1999).

Before returning to outdoor physical activities, medical examinations are advised for athletes to be eligible to participate in competitions after the ban on sports activities is lifted. Athletes with positive COVID-19 tests should refrain from exercise for at least 7 days. Following resolution of symptoms for 7 days, progressive return to training over an additional 7 days is advised (Yeo, 2020). In addition to preseason physical and medical examinations defined by the UEFA's medical regulations, two consecutive negative RT-qPCR COVID-19 pharyngeal swabs over a 5-day interval should be conducted as well as examining the immune response of athletes for antibodies (IgM and IgG) against the virus or viral antigens are necessary (Primorac, Matišić, Molnar, Bahtijarević, & Polašek, 2020).

On March 20, 2020, the Royal Spanish Football Federation created a task force composed of sports physicians, sports scientists, and strength and conditioning coaches to establish guidelines to resume football activities after the COVID-19 pandemic (Herrero-Gonzalez et al., 2020). The framework encompasses three levels of guidelines: (1) clinical measures to assess players' health status after the lockdown and procedures to reduce the probability of COVID-19 infection during training and competition, (2) training recommendations to develop strategies for injury prevention and physiological readaptation, and (3) proposals for the competition calendar and allowance of changes of in-game regulations (Herrero-Gonzalez et al., 2020).

Physical activity in individuals with Down syndrome

Why do those with Down syndrome have a major risk of being infected with SARS COV 2?

Down syndrome, a congenital syndrome also known as trisomy 21, is a genetic disorder caused by an additional partial or full copy of 21 chromosomes (Rafii, Kleschevnikov, Sawa, & Mobley, 2019). Almost 95% of individuals with Down syndrome have complete trisomy 21, 3%–4% are manifested due to translocations, and the remaining 1%–2% of cases are caused by mosaicism in which an individual has a mixture of cell types with and without extra chromosomes (Nussbaum, Mcinnes, & Willard, 2016). This syndrome is associated with a wide range of cognitive and physiological deficiencies that include short stature, obesity, macroglossia, hypotonia, and delays in motor and neurological development (Dumortier & Bricout, 2020). In addition to intellectual disabilities, those with Down syndrome have other weaknesses such as slower processing speeds, poor inhibitory control, shorter attention spans, less working memory capacity, motor skills dysfunctions (Adams & Oliver, 2010; Chen & Ringenbach, 2019; Daunhauer et al., 2014; Sugimoto, Bowen, Meehan, & Stracciolini, 2016), autoimmune thyroid (Iughetti et al., 2014), celiac disease (Marild et al., 2013), and/or type 1 diabetes (Bergholdt, Eising, Nerup, & Pociot, 2006).

Although the survival for those with Down syndrome has been improved in recent decades with the betterment of social and health care systems (Day, Strauss,

Shavelle, & Reynolds, 2005; Glasson et al., 2002), the mortality rate of those with Down syndrome remains higher than the general population (Hill et al., 2003).

These characteristics cause those with Down syndrome who have other associated conditions to be at major risk in case of SARS-CoV-2 infection.

Espinosa (2020) warned that people with Down syndrome should be considered at a high risk of developing more serious symptoms and high hospitalization rates, secondary bacterial infections, intensive care, and mortality from SARS-CoV-2 infections compared to the general population.

How physical exercise can improve those with Down syndrome

Social isolation and staying at home encourages sedentary behavior and reduces levels of physical activity, but also increases the risk of some diseases (Ekelund, Tarp, Steene-Johannessen, & Al, 2019).

As discussed before, it is advisable to avoid high sedentary behavior during isolation and view internal activities as an opportunity to stay healthy (Carvalho, Moreira, De Oliveira, Landim, & Neto, 2020). Nevertheless, the results of studies regarding physical activity conducted in the general population cannot be translated to those with intellectual disabilities because the predictive value of physical condition for survival can be different for those with intellectual disabilities (Oppewal & Higenkamp, 2019).

Gradually adjusting those with Down syndrome to the systematic practice of physical exercise and movement in their free time assumes modeling, awareness, and active participation. Thus physical activity acquires a formative character, which together with other educational factors (family and youth organizations) make their actions convergent. In this context, some studies suggest that those with Down syndrome are less physically active than those without Down syndrome (Matute-Liorente, Gonzalez-Aguero, Gomez-Cabello, Vicente-Rodriguez, & Casajus, 2013). Pitetti, Baynard, and Agiovlasitis (2013) suggest that effective physical activity promotion for those with Down syndrome should be multifactorial (i.e., adapted to their physiological, cognitive, and psychosocial profiles).

Physical activities are meant to inspire and challenge people to experience the joy of movement to develop positive attitudes as individuals or part of a group to improve their quality of life through an active lifestyle, which is mandatory for those with Down syndrome need. In the context of the pandemic and the protective measures established by authorities, it is assumed that those with Down syndrome who are sedentary have suffered considerably. It might be caused by the needs to belong to a community and to the limitation of some activities in special centers. Indeed, during the isolation period, all specific centers were closed and physical activities were carried out only with the support of families based on, at the most, online instructions provided by specialists.

Those with Down syndrome have difficulty maintaining balance, which is necessary for posture control, especially in a standing or walking position

(Malak, Kostiukow, Wasielewska, Mojs, & Samborski, 2015). To improve the components of their coordination capacity, those with Down syndrome need physical exercise to stimulate it. Alsakhawi and Elshafey (2019) demonstrated that core stability exercises and treadmill training significantly improved balance in children with Down syndrome.

Many studies reported that the level of physical condition of those with Down syndrome is even lower than that of those with intellectual disabilities (Block, 1991; Burns & Gunn, 1993) and thus requires permanent intervention on the motor capacity of those with Down syndrome. It was also proven that a lack of exercise in the lifestyle of those with Down syndrome can increase their risk of health problems such as obesity, diabetes, or Alzheimer's disease (Zigman & Lott, 2007). Many studies indicated that moderate to vigorous physical activity may be effective at maintaining cognitive components, including attention, memory, and executive function in adults with Alzheimer's disease (DeFina et al., 2013; Erickson, Weinstein, & Lopez, 2012).

Through their content, the forms of organization and practice of physical exercises necessarily require some mental processes and features. For example, to understand the purpose, structure, and sequence of elements of a physical exercise, it is necessary to be aware of the movement and pay attention of those who perform them.

In a 2017 study, the positive influence that dance-specific methods have on the motor and functional capacity of adults with Down syndrome was shown (Cosma, Dragomir, Nanu, Brabiescu, & Cosma, 2017). Dance lessons also resulted in positive effects on physical, cognitive, and psychological benefits for those with Down syndrome (Reinders, Bryden, & Fletcher, 2015), for breast cancer patients and Parkinson's (Lelievre, Tuchowski, & Rolland, 2015), but benefits have also been identified on self-esteem, body satisfaction, and depression on those with Down syndrome (Santana, Adorno, & Teixeira-Machado, 2018).

Conclusion

Notwithstanding variations in individual tolerance to living in confined environments, there is marked consistency of public health measures on psychological and physiological health effects. In addition, physical exercise can be considered a viable tool for the management, treatment, and health maintenance of those living in confined environments and/or experiencing limited movement because of the COVID-19 pandemic. In this unique situation, physical activity can be delivered through a multitude of technological tools, such as physical activity trackers and applications for smart watches and phones, that can help improve the delivery of supervised physical activity interventions. This chapter summarized the potential beneficial effects of physical activity in healthy children, adolescents, adults, elderly, but also on specific populations, as athletes and those with Down syndrome.

References

Adams, D., & Oliver, C. (2010). The relationships between acquired impairments of executive function and behaviour change in adults with Down syndrome. *Journal of Intellectual Disability Research, 54*, 393–405.

Alsakhawi, R., & Elshafey, M. (2019). Effect of core stability exercises and treadmill training on balance in children with down syndrome: Randomized controlled trial. *Advances in Therapy, 36*, 2364–2373.

ACSM. (2020). *Staying active during the coronavirus pandemic*. Available: https://www.exerciseismedicine.org/assets/page_documents/EIM_Rx%20for%20Health_%20Staying%20Active%20During%20Coronavirus%20Pandemic.pdf (Accessed 29 May 2020).

Asmundson, G. J. G., & Taylor, S. (2020). Coronaphobia: Fear and the 2019-nCoV outbreak. *Journal of Anxiety Disorders, 70*.

Bahrami, F., Movahedi, A., Marandi, S. M., & Sorensen, C. (2016). The effect of karate techniques training on communication deficit of children with autism spectrum disorders. *Journal of Autism and Developmental Disorders, 46*, 978–986.

Bello-Mojeed, M., Ani, C., Lagunju, I., & Omigbodun, O. (2016). Feasibility of parent-mediated behavioural intervention for behavioural problems in children with Autism Spectrum Disorder in Nigeria: A pilot study. *Child and Adolescent Psychiatry and Mental Health, 10*, 28.

Bergholdt, R., Eising, S., Nerup, J., & Pociot, F. (2006). Increased prevalence of Down's syndrome individuals with type 1 diabetes in Denmark: A nationwide population-based study. *Diabetologia, 49*, 1179–1182.

Bishop, N., Lu, T., & Yankner, B. A. (2010). Neural mechanisms of ageing and cognitive decline. *Nature, 464*, 529–535.

Block, M. E. (1991). Motor development in children with Down syndrome: A review of the literature. *Adapted Physical Activity, 8*, 179–209.

Bowden Davies, K. A., Pickles, S., Sprung, V. S., Kemp, G. J., Alam, U., Moore, D. R., et al. (2019). Reduced physical activity in young and older adults: Metabolic and musculoskeletal implications. *Therapeutic Advances in Endocrinology and Metabolism, 10*. 2042018819888824.

Brooks, S. K., Webster, R. K., Smith, L. E., Woodland, L., Wessely, S., Greenberg, N., et al. (2020). The psychological impact of quarantine and how to reduce it: Rapid review of the evidence. *The Lancet, 395*, 912–920.

Burns, Y., & Gunn, P. (1993). *Down syndrome: Moving through life*. London: Chapman and Hall.

Cadilhac, D. A., Cumming, T. B., Sheppard, L., et al. (2011). The economic benefits of reducing physical inactivity: An Australian example. *International Journal of Behavioral Nutrition and Physical Activity, 8*, 99. https://doi.org/10.1186/1479-5868-8-99.

Cairney, J., Hay, J., Faught, B. E., Corna, L. M., & Flouris, A. D. (2006). Developmental coordination disorder, age and play: A test of the divergence in activity-deficit with age hypothesis. *Adapted Physical Activity Quarterly, 23*, 261.

Campbell, J. P., & Turner, J. E. (2018). Debunking the myth of exercise-induced immune suppression: Redefining the impact of exercise on immunological health across the lifespan. *Frontiers in Immunology, 9*, 648.

Carneiro, N. H., Ribeiro, A. S., Nascimento, M. A., Gobbo, L. A., Schoenfeld, B. J., Júnior, A. A., et al. (2015). Effects of different resistance training frequencies on flexibility in older women. *Clinical Interventions in Aging, 10*, 531.

Carson, V., Hunter, S., Kuzik, N., Wiebe, S. A., Spence, J. C., Friedman, A., et al. (2016). Systematic review of physical activity and cognitive development in early childhood. *Journal of Science and Medicine in Sport, 19*, 573–578.

Carvalho, P. M. M., Moreira, M. M., De Oliveira, M. N. A., Landim, J. M. M., & Neto, M. L. R. (2020). The psychiatric impact of the novel coronavirus outbreak. *Psychiatry Research, 286*, 112902.

Chen, F. T., Etnier, J. L., Chan, K. H., Chiu, P. K., Hung, T. M., & Chang, Y. K. (2020). Effects of exercise training interventions on executive function in older adults: A systematic review and meta-analysis. *Sports Medicine, 50*(8), 1451–1467.

Chen, C., & Ringenbach, S. (2019). The effect of acute exercise on the performance of verbal fluency in adolescents and young adults with Down syndrome: A pilot study. *Journal of Intellectual Disability Research, 63*, 614–623.

Chin, A. P. M. J., Van Uffelen, J. G., Riphagen, I., & Van Mechelen, W. (2008). The functional effects of physical exercise training in frail older people: A systematic review. *Sports Medicine, 38*, 781–793.

Cosma, G., Dragomir, M., Nanu, M., Brabiescu, C. L., & Cosma, A. (2017). The influence of the dance for people with down syndrome. *Social Sciences and Law: Vol. 10. Bulletin of the Transilvania University of Brasov* (pp. 83–88).

Curi, V. S., Haas, A. N., Alves-Vilaça, J., & Fernandes, H. M. (2018). Effects of 16-weeks of Pilates on functional autonomy and life satisfaction among elderly women. *Journal of Bodywork and Movement Therapies, 22*, 424–429.

Daunhauer, L. A., Fidler, D. J., Hahn, L., Will, E., Lee, N. R., & Susan, H. (2014). Profiles of everyday executive functioning in young children with Down syndrome. *American Journal on Intellectual and Developmental Disabilities, 119*, 303–318.

Davis, C. L., Tkacz, J., Gregoski, M., Boyle, C. A., & Lovrekovic, G. (2006). Aerobic exercise and snoring in overweight children: A randomized controlled trial. *Obesity, 14*, 1985–1991.

Day, S. M., Strauss, D. J., Shavelle, R. M., & Reynolds, R. J. (2005). Mortality and causes of death in persons with Down syndrome in California. *Developmental Medicine & Child Neurology, 47*, 171–176.

De Greeff, J. W., Bosker, R. J., Oosterlaan, J., Visscher, C., & Hartman, E. (2018). Effects of physical activity on executive functions, attention and academic performance in preadolescent children: A meta-analysis. *Journal of Science and Medicine in Sport, 21*, 501–507.

De Oliveira Neto, L., De Oliveira Tavares, V. D., Schuch, F. B., & Lima, K. C. (2020). Coronavirus pandemic (SARS-COV-2): Pre-exercise screening questionnaire (PESQ) for telepresential exercise. *Frontiers in Public Health, 8*, 146.

DeFina, L. F., Willis, B. I., Radford, N. B., Gao, A., Leonard, D., Haskell, M., et al. (2013). The association between midlife cardiorespiratory fitness levels and later-life dementia cohort study. *Annals of Internal Medicine, 158*, 162–168.

Dong, L., & Bouey, J. (2020). Public mental health crisis during COVID-19 pandemic, China. *Emerging Infectious Diseases, 27*, 1016–1018.

Dumortier, L., & Bricout, V.-A. (2020). Obstructive sleep apnea syndrome in adults with down syndrome: Causes and consequences. Is it a "chicken and egg" question? *Neuroscience and Biobehavioral Reviews, 108*, 124–138.

Dwyer, M. J., Pasini, M., De Dominicis, S., & Righi, E. (2020). Physical activity: Benefits and challenges during the COVID-19 pandemic. *Scandinavian Journal of Medicine & Science in Sports, 30*, 1291–1294.

Ekelund, U., Tarp, J., Steene-Johannessen, J., & Al, E. (2019). Dose-response associations between accelerometry measured physical activity and sedentary time and all cause mortality: Systematic review and harmonised meta-analysis. *BMJ, 2019*, 366.

Erickson, K., Weinstein, A. M., & Lopez, O. L. (2012). Physical activity, brain plasticity, and Alzheimer's disease. *Archives of Medical Research, 43*, 615–621.

Espinosa, J. (2020). Down syndrome and COVID-19: A perfect storm? *Cell Reports Medicine*, *1*, 1–8.

EU Working Group. (2008). Recommended policy actions in support of health-enhancing physical activity. In *"Sport & health" EU physical activity guidelines*.

Feng, F., Tuchman, S., Denninger, J. W., Fricchione, G. L., & Yeung, A. (2020). Qigong for the prevention, treatment, and rehabilitation of COVID-19 infection in older adults. *The American Journal of Geriatric Psychiatry: Official Journal of the American Association for Geriatric Psychiatry*. https://doi.org/10.1016/j.jagp.2020.1005.1012.

Ferrando, A. A., Lane, H. W., Stuart, C. A., Davis-Street, J., & Wolfe, R. R. (1996). Prolonged bed rest decreases skeletal muscle and whole body protein synthesis. *American Journal of Physiology-Endocrinology and Metabolism*, *270*, E627–E633.

Fitbit News. (2020). *The impact of coronavirus on global activity*. Available: https://blog.fitbit.com/covid-19-global-activity/ (Accessed 29 May 2020).

Garber, C. E., Blissmer, B., Deschenes, M. R., Franklin, B. A., Lamonte, M. J., Lee, I.-M., et al. (2011). Quantity and quality of exercise for developing and maintaining cardiorespiratory, musculoskeletal, and neuromotor fitness in apparently healthy adults: Guidance for prescribing exercise. *Medicine & Science in Sports & Exercise*, *43*, 1334–1359.

García-Garro, P. A., Hita-Contreras, F., Martínez-Amat, A., Achalandabaso-Ochoa, A., Jiménez-García, J. D., Cruz-Díaz, D., et al. (2020). Effectiveness of a Pilates training program on cognitive and functional abilities in postmenopausal women. *International Journal of Environmental Research and Public Health*, *17*, 3580.

Ghram, A., Briki, W., Mansoor, H., Al-Mohannadi, A. S., Lavie, C. J., & Chamari, K. (2020). Home-based exercise can be beneficial for counteracting sedentary behavior and physical inactivity during the COVID-19 pandemic in older adults. *Postgraduate Medicine*. https://doi.org/10.1080/00325481.2020.

Glasson, E. J., Sullivan, S. G., Hussain, R., Petterson, B., Montgomery, P. D., & Bittles, A. H. (2002). The changing survival profile of people with Down's syndrome: Implications for genetic counselling. *Clinical Genetics*, *62*, 390–393.

Haskell, W. L., Lee, I. M., Pate, R. R., Powell, K. E., Blair, S. N., Franklin, B. A., et al. (2007). Physical activity and public health: Updated recommendation for adults from the American College of Sports Medicine and the American Heart Association. *Medicine and Science in Sports and Exercise*, *39*, 1423–1434.

Healy, G. N., Dunstan, D. W., Salmon, J., Cerin, E., Shaw, J. E., Zimmet, P. Z., et al. (2007). Objectively measured light-intensity physical activity is independently associated with 2-h plasma glucose. *Diabetes Care*, *30*, 1384–1389.

Herrero-Gonzalez, H., Martín-Acero, R., Del Coso, J., Lalín-Novoa, C., Pol, R., Martín-Escudero, P., et al. (2020). Position statement of the Royal Spanish Football Federation for the resumption of football activities after the COVID-19 pandemic (June 2020). *British Journal of Sports Medicine*. https://doi.org/10.1136/bjsports-2020-102640.

Hill, D. A., Gridley, G., Cnattingius, S., Mellemkjaer, L., Linet, M., Adami, H. O., … Fraumeni, J. F., Jr. (2003). Mortality and cancer incidence among individuals with Down syndrome. *Archives of Internal Medicine*, *163*(6), 705–711.

Hwang, Y., Park, J., & Lim, K. (2016). Effects of Pilates exercise on salivary secretory immunoglobulin A levels in older women. *Journal of Aging and Physical Activity*, *24*, 399–406.

Im, J. Y., Bang, H. S., & Seo, D. Y. (2019). The effects of 12 weeks of a combined exercise program on physical function and hormonal status in elderly Korean women. *International Journal of Environmental Research and Public Health*, *16*, 4196.

Iughetti, L., Predieri, B., Bruzzi, P., Predieri, F., Vellani, G., Madeo, S. F., et al. (2014). Ten-year longitudinal study of thyroid function in children with Down syndrome. *Hormone Research in Paediatrics*, *82*, 113–121.

Jacob, L., Smith, L., Butler, L., Barnett, Y., Grabovac, I., Mcdermott, D., et al. (2020). COVID-19 social distancing and sexual activity in a sample of the British Public. *The Journal of Sexual Medicine*. https://doi.org/10.1016/j.jsxm.2020.1005.1001.

Jahnke, R., Larkey, L., Rogers, C., Etnier, J., & Lin, F. (2010). A comprehensive review of health benefits of qigong and tai chi. *American Journal of Health Promotion*, *24*, e1–e25.

Jenkin, C. R., Eime, R. M., Westerbeek, H., et al. (2017). Sport and ageing: A systematic review of the determinants and trends of participation in sport for older adults. *BMC Public Health*, *17*, 976.

Jiménez-Pavón, D., Carbonell-Baeza, A., & Lavie, C. J. (2020). Physical exercise as therapy to fight against the mental and physical consequences of COVID-19 quarantine: Special focus in older people. *Progress in Cardiovascular Diseases*, *63*(3), 386–388. https://doi.org/10.1016/j.pcad.2020.03.009.

Jukic, I. E. A. (2020). Strategies and solutions for team sports athletes in isolation due to COVID-19. *Sports (Basel, Switzerland)*, *8*(4), 56. https://doi.org/10.3390/sports8040056.

Kakanis, M. W., Peake, J., Brenu, E. W., Simmonds, M., Gray, B., Hooper, S. L., et al. (2010). The open window of susceptibility to infection after acute exercise in healthy young male elite athletes. *Exercise Immunology Review*, *16*, 119–137.

Katula, J. A., Blissmer, B. J., & Mcauley, E. (1999). Exercise intensity and self-efficacy effects on anxiety reduction in healthy, older adults. *Journal of Behavioral Medicine*, *22*, 233–247.

Khan, S., Siddique, R., Li, H., Ali, A., Shereen, M. A., Bashir, N., et al. (2020). Impact of coronavirus outbreak on psychological health. *Journal of Global Health*, *10*, 010331.

Kline, C. E., Krafty, R. T., Mulukutla, S., & Hall, M. H. (2017). Associations of sedentary time and moderate-vigorous physical activity with sleep-disordered breathing and polysomnographic sleep in community-dwelling adults. *Sleep and Breathing*, *21*, 427–434.

Kohut, M. L., Arntson, B. A., Lee, W., Rozeboom, K., Yoon, K.-J., Cunnick, J. E., et al. (2004). Moderate exercise improves antibody response to influenza immunization in older adults. *Vaccine*, *22*, 2298–2306.

Larkey, L., Jahnke, R., Etnier, J., & Gonzalez, J. (2009). Meditative movement as a category of exercise: Implications for research. *Journal of Physical Activity & Health*, *6*, 230–238.

Lelievre, A., Tuchowski, F., & Rolland, Y. (2015). La danse, une therapie pour la personne agee. *Revue de la litterature, Les cahiers de l'anne egerontologique*, *7*, 177–187.

Li, H., Hu, M., & Liu, S. (2020). The need to improve the laws and regulations relevant to the outbreak of COVID-19: What might be learned from China? *Journal of Global Health*, *10*(1), 010328. https://doi.org/10.7189/jogh.10.010328.

Li, J. X., Xu, D. Q., & Hong, Y. (2008). Effects of 16-week Tai Chi intervention on postural stability and proprioception of knee and ankle in older people. *Age and Ageing*, *37*, 575–578.

Lippi, G., Henry, B. M., & Sanchis-Gomar, F. (2020). Physical inactivity and cardiovascular disease at the time of coronavirus disease 2019 (COVID-19). *European Journal of Preventive Cardiology*. https://doi.org/10.1177/2047487320916823.

Liu-Ambrose, T., Donaldson, M. G., Ahamed, Y., Graf, P., Cook, W. L., Close, J., et al. (2008). Otago home-based strength and balance retraining improves executive functioning in older fallers: A randomized controlled trial. *Journal of the American Geriatrics Society*, *56*, 1821–1830.

Liu-Ambrose, T., Khan, K. M., Eng, J. J., Janssen, P. A., Lord, S. R., & Mckay, H. A. (2004). Resistance and agility training reduce fall risk in women aged 75 to 85 with low bone mass: A 6-month randomized, controlled trial. *Journal of the American Geriatrics Society*, *52*, 657–665.

Logghe, I. H., Verhagen, A. P., Rademaker, A. C., Bierma-Zeinstra, S. M., Van Rossum, E., Faber, M. J., et al. (2010). The effects of Tai Chi on fall prevention, fear of falling and balance in older people: A meta-analysis. *Preventive Medicine*, *51*, 222–227.

Lowder, T., Padgett, D. A., & Woods, J. A. (2005). Moderate exercise protects mice from death due to influenza virus. *Brain, Behavior, and Immunity*, *19*, 377–380.

Mackay, J., & Mensah, G. (2004). *Atlas of heart disease and stroke*. Geneva: World Health Organization.

Malak, R., Kostiukow, A., Wasielewska, A., Mojs, E., & Samborski, W. (2015). Delays in motor development in children with Down syndrome. *Medical Science Monitor*, *21*, 1904–1910.

Mansoubi, M., Pearson, N., Clemes, S. A., et al. (2015). Energy expenditure during common sitting and standing tasks: Examining the 1.5 MET definition of sedentary behaviour. *BMC Public Health*, *516*, 15. https://doi.org/10.1186/s12889-015-1851-x.

Marild, K., Stephansson, O., Grahnquist, L., Cnattingius, S., Soderman, G., & Ludvigsson, J. F. (2013). Down syndrome is associated with elevated risk of celiac disease: A national case-control study. *The Journal of Pediatrics*, *163*, 237–242.

Matsumoto, D., Takatori, K., Nishida, M., & Matsushita, S. (2015). Effects of home-based exercise with expiratory muscle training on the prevention of falls and aspiration pneumonia in community-dwelling older adults. *Physiotherapy*, *101*, e963–e964.

Matthews, C. E., George, S. M., Moore, S. C., Bowles, H. R., Blair, A., Park, Y., et al. (2012). Amount of time spent in sedentary behaviors and cause-specific mortality in US adults. *The American Journal of Clinical Nutrition*, *95*, 437–445.

Matute-Liorente, A., Gonzalez-Aguero, A., Gomez-Cabello, A., Vicente-Rodriguez, G., & Casajus, J. (2013). Physical activity and cardiorespiratory fitness in adolescents with Down syndrome. *Nutrición Hospitalaria*, *28*, 1151–1155.

Movahedi, A., Bahrami, F., Marandi, S. M., & Abedi, A. (2013). Improvement in social dysfunction of children with autism spectrum disorder following long term Kata techniques training. *Research in Autism Spectrum Disorders*, *7*, 1054–1061.

Mulder, E., Linnarsson, D., Paloski, W., Rittweger, J., Wuyts, F., Zange, J., et al. (2014). Effects of five days of bed rest with and without exercise countermeasure on postural stability and gait. *Journal of Musculoskeletal and Neuronal Interactions*, *14*, 359–366.

Nelson, M. E., Rejeski, W. J., Blair, S. N., Duncan, P. W., Judge, J. O., King, A. C., et al. (2007). Physical activity and public health in older adults: Recommendation from the American College of Sports Medicine and the American Heart Association. *Medicine and Science in Sports and Exercise*, *39*, 1435–1445.

Nussbaum, R., Mcinnes, R., & Willard, H. F. (2016). *Thompson & Thompson genetics in medicine*. Philadelphia, PA: Elsevier.

Oppewal, A., & Higenkamp, T. I. M. (2019). Physical fitness is predictive for 5-year survival in older adults with intellectual disabilities. *Journal of Applied Research in Intellectual Disabilities*, *32*, 958–966.

Pan, C.-Y. (2011). The efficacy of an aquatic program on physical fitness and aquatic skills in children with and without autism spectrum disorders. *Research in Autism Spectrum Disorders*, *5*, 657–665.

Parnell, D., Widdop, P., Bond, A., & Wilson, R. (2020). *COVID-19, networks and sport. Managing sport and Leisure*. Taylor & Francis Online.

Paterson, D. H., Jones, G. R., & Rice, C. L. (2007). Ageing and physical activity: Evidence to develop exercise recommendations for older adults. This article is part of a supplement entitled "Advancing physical activity measurement and guidelines in Canada: A scientific review and evidence-based foundation for the future of Canadian physical activity guidelines" *Applied Physiology, Nutrition, and Metabolism and the Canadian Journal of Public Health*, S69–S108. 18213941.

Peçanha, T., Goessler, K. F., Roschel, H., & Gualano, B. (2020). Social isolation during the COVID-19 pandemic can increase physical inactivity and the global burden of cardiovascular disease. *American Journal of Physiology. Heart and Circulatory Physiology*, *318*, H1441–H1446.

Pedersen, B. K., & Saltin, B. (2015). Exercise as medicine—Evidence for prescribing exercise as therapy in 26 different chronic diseases. *Scandinavian Journal of Medicine & Science in Sports*, *25*(Suppl. 3), 1–72.

Physical Activity Guidelines Advisory Committee. (2008). *Physical activity guidelines*. Washington, DC: US Department of Health and Human Services.

Pitetti, K., Baynard, T., & Agiovlasitis, S. (2013). Children and adolescents with Down syndrome, physical fitness and physical activity. *Journal of Sport and Health Science*, *2*, 47–57.

Pitetti, K. H., Rendoff, A. D., Grover, T., & Beets, M. W. (2007). The efficacy of a 9-month treadmill walking program on the exercise capacity and weight reduction for adolescents with severe autism. *Journal of Autism and Developmental Disorders*, *37*, 997–1006.

Primorac, D., Matišić, V., Molnar, V., Bahtijarević, Z., & Polašek, O. (2020). Pre-season football preparation in the era of COVID-19: Croatian Football Association Model. *Journal of Global Health*, *10*, 010352.

Rafii, M., Kleschevnikov, A., Sawa, M., & Mobley, W. (2019). *Down syndrome*.

Reinders, N., Bryden, P. J., & Fletcher, P. C. (2015). Dancing with Down syndrome: A phenomenological case study. *Research in Dance Education*, *16*, 291–307.

Reschke, M. F., Bloomberg, J. J., Paloski, W. H., Mulavara, A. P., Feiveson, A. H., & Harm, D. L. (2009). Postural reflexes, balance control, and functional mobility with long-duration head-down bed rest. *Aviation, Space, and Environmental Medicine*, *80*, A45–A54.

Rodriguez-Ayllon, M., Cadenas-Sánchez, C., Estévez-López, F., Muñoz, N. E., Mora-Gonzalez, J., Migueles, J. H., et al. (2019). Role of physical activity and sedentary behavior in the mental health of preschoolers, children and adolescents: A systematic review and meta-analysis. *Sports Medicine*, *49*, 1383–1410.

Santana, T. L. S., Adorno, E. T., & Teixeira-Machado, L. (2018). Dance and quality of life promotion in down syndrome: A view on depressive ad self-esteem aspects. *International Journal of Research*, *6*, 37–46.

Singhal, T. (2020). A review of coronavirus disease-2019 (COVID-19). *Indian Journal of Pediatrics*, *87*, 281–286.

Sirven, N., & Debrand, T. (2008). Social participation and healthy ageing: An international comparison using SHARE data. *Social Science & Medicine*, *67*, 2017–2026.

Stathokostas, L., Mcdonald, M. W., Little, R., & Paterson, D. H. (2013). Flexibility of older adults aged 55–86 years and the influence of physical activity. *Journal of Aging Research*, *2013*, 8. https://doi.org/10.1155/2013/743843.

Sugimoto, D., Bowen, S. L., Meehan, W. P., & Stracciolini, A. (2016). Effects on neuromuscular training on children and young adults with Down syndrome: Systematic review and meta-analysis. *Research in Developmental Disabilities*, *55*, 197–206.

Takatori, K., Matsumoto, D., Nishida, M., Matsushita, S., Noda, T., & Imamura, T. (2016). Benefits of a novel concept of home-based exercise with the aim of preventing aspiration pneumonia and falls in frail older women: A pragmatic controlled trial. *BMJ Open Sport & Exercise Medicine*, *2*(1), e000127. https://doi.org/10.1136/bmjsem-2016-000127.

Trappe, S., Creer, A., Minchev, K., Slivka, D., Louis, E., Luden, N., et al. (2008). Human soleus single muscle fiber function with exercise or nutrition countermeasures during 60 days of bed rest. *American Journal of Physiology-Regulatory, Integrative and Comparative Physiology*, *294*, R939–R947.

UN. (2020). *The impact of COVID-19 on sport, physical activity and well-being and its effects on social development*. Available: https://www.un.org/development/desa/dspd/2020/05/covid-19-sport/ (Accessed 4 June 2020).

US Department of Health and Human Services. (2020). *Healthy people*. Available: http://www.healtypeople.gov/2020/topicsobjectives2020 (Accessed 29 May 2020).

Verhagen, A. P., Immink, M., Van Der Meulen, A., & Bierma-Zeinstra, S. M. (2004). The efficacy of Tai Chi Chuan in older adults: A systematic review. *Family Practice*, *21*, 107–113.

Vieira, V., Keylock, K. T., Lowder, T., Zelkovich, W., Dumich, S., Colantuano, K., et al. (2008). 83. Effects of exercise training on the immune response to influenza vaccination in older adults: A randomized controlled trial. *Brain Behavior and Immunity*, *4*, 26.

Viguier, M., Dupui, P., & Montoya, R. (2009). Posture analysis on young women before and after 60 days of – 6° head down bed rest (Wise 2005). *Gait & Posture*, *29*, 188–193.

Waddington, I. (2000). *Sport, health and drugs: A critical sociological perspective*. Oxford: Taylor & Francis.

Wang, C., Bannuru, R., Ramel, J., Kupelnick, B., Scott, T., & Schmid, C. H. (2010). Tai Chi on psychological well-being: Systematic review and meta-analysis. *BMC Complementary and Alternative Medicine*, *10*, 23.

Warburton, D. E., Gledhill, N., & Quinney, A. (2001). Musculoskeletal fitness and health. *Canadian Journal of Applied Physiology*.

Warburton, D. E., Nicol, C. W., & Bredin, S. S. (2006). Health benefits of physical activity: The evidence. *CMAJ*, *174*(6), 801–809. https://doi.org/10.1503/cmaj.051351.

WHO. (2010). *Global recommendations on physical activity for health*. Available: http://whqlibdoc.who.int/publications/2010/9789241599979_eng.pdf (Accessed 22 May 2020).

Wilder-Smith, A., & Freedman, D. O. (2020). Isolation, quarantine, social distancing and community containment: Pivotal role for old-style public health measures in the novel coronavirus (2019-nCoV) outbreak. *Journal of Travel Medicine*, *27*.

Wilson, M., & Chen, L. (2019). Travelers give wings to novel coronavirus (2019nCoV). *Journal of Translational Medicine*, 1–3. 2020 published online.

Woods, J. A., Keylock, K. T., Lowder, T., Vieira, V. J., Zelkovich, W., Dumich, S., et al. (2009). Cardiovascular exercise training extends influenza vaccine seroprotection in sedentary older adults: The immune function intervention trial. *Journal of the American Geriatrics Society*, *57*, 2183–2191.

World Health Organization. (2004). *Global strategy on diet, physical activity and health*. WHO.

World Health Organization. (2009). *Global health risks: Mortality and burden of disease attributable to selected major risks*. (Geneva).

World Health Organization. (2010). *Global recommendations on physical activity for health*. https://www.who.int/publications/i/item/9789241599979 (Accessed 29 May 2020).

World Health Organization. (2020). *Water, sanitation, hygiene, and waste management for the COVID-19 virus*. Available: https://apps.who.int/iris/bitstream/handle/10665/331499/WHO-2019-nCoV-IPC_WASH-2020.2-eng.pdf?sequence=1&isAllowed=y (Accessed 29 May 2020).

Worldometers. (2020). https://www.worldometers.info/coronavirus/ (Accessed 29 May 2020).

Wu, G. (2002). Evaluation of the effectiveness of Tai Chi for improving balance and preventing falls in the older population—A review. *Journal of the American Geriatrics Society*, *50*, 746–754.

Yang, Y., Shin, J. C., Li, D., & An, R. (2017). Sedentary behavior and sleep problems: A systematic review and meta-analysis. *International Journal of Behavioral Medicine*, *24*, 481–492.

Yang, Y., Verkuilen, J., Rosengren, K. S., Mariani, R. A., Reed, M., Grubisich, S. A., et al. (2007). Effects of a Taiji and Qigong intervention on the antibody response to influenza vaccine in older adults. *The American Journal of Chinese Medicine*, *35*, 597–607.

Yeo, T. J. (2020). Sport and exercise during and beyond the COVID-19 pandemic. *European Journal of Preventive Cardiology*, *27*(12), 1239–1241. https://doi.org/10.1177/2047487320933260.

Yousfi, N., Bragazzi, N. L., Briki, W., Zmijewski, P., & Chamari, K. (2020). The COVID-19 pandemic: How to maintain a healthy immune system during the lockdown—A multidisciplinary approach with special focus on athletes. *Biology of Sport*, *37*(3), 211–216.

Zarocostas, J. (2020). How to fight an infodemic. *Lancet*, *395*, 676.

Zhai, L., Zhang, Y., & Zhang, D. (2015). Sedentary behaviour and the risk of depression: A meta-analysis. *British Journal of Sports Medicine*, *49*, 705–709.

Zhu, N., Zhang, D., Wang, W., Li, X., Yang, B., Song, J., et al. (2020). China Novel Coronavirus Investigating and Research Team. A novel coronavirus from patients with pneumonia in China, 2019. *The New England Journal of Medicine*, *382*, 727–733.

Zigman, W., & Lott, I. (2007). Alzheimer's disease in Down syndrome: Neurobiology and risk. *Mental Retardation and Development Disabilities Research Reviews*, *13*, 237–246.

Zou, L., Wang, C., Tian, Z., Wang, H., & Shu, Y. (2017). Effect of Yang-style Tai Chi on gait parameters and musculoskeletal flexibility in healthy Chinese older women. *Sports*, *5*, 52.

Chapter 14

Parenting through the COVID-19 pandemic

Natalie M.V. Morrison[a,b] and Ben. W. Morrison[c]
[a]School of Medicine, Western Sydney University, Penrith, NSW, Australia, [b]Translational Health Research Institute, Western Sydney University, Penrith, NSW, Australia, [c]Department of Psychology, Macquarie University, Macquarie Park, NSW, Australia

Introduction

The COVID-19 pandemic has presented individuals the world over with a host of confronting realities and challenges without precedent. Parents are arguably in one of the most taxing positions as they face many responsibilities leveled at them as individual adults, but by way of being a parent their circle of concern is inevitably broadened as they renegotiate how and what "parenting" is in the pandemic climate. Parents are finding that multitasking is taking on a whole new meaning as they negotiate a collision of roles—many of which they feel particularly unskilled in undertaking (e.g., a home-schooling teacher, or a guidance or pastoral counselor), in a growingly isolated world full of social distancing, lockdowns, curfews, and quarantining requirements. The nature of many of these new roles, and the inevitable importance of these (e.g., their child's academic progression and mental wellbeing), and the sheer number of time competition between these make for a highly stressful environment. The pre-COVID-19 capacity to undertake the parenting role meant that many of these tasks were shared between many other adults in the family (i.e., extended or blended grandparents and stepparents, etc.) and the immediate social systems (e.g., teachers, religious leaders, social and sporting groups). With access to these support systems becoming limited during the pandemic, and with many other coping strategies rendered unworkable (e.g., "time out" with friends or engaging in other social activities), parents find themselves at high risk of parental burnout. Such burnout poses a risk to their own physical and mental health, both immediate and long term, and may compromise their capacity to adequately parent, resulting in risks for their children in the form of neglect or abuse (Griffith, 2020; Humphreys, Myint, & Zeanah, 2020). Fortunately for most parents the challenges presented by the COVID-19 pandemic, while still stressful, are experienced in a more balanced way allowing for psychological growth within the family.

Mental Health Effects of COVID-19. https://doi.org/10.1016/B978-0-12-824289-6.00008-8

This chapter will explore the unique positioning of parents within the family unit and how such a structure might impose both a greater scope of concern but also a source of strength. The chapter will consider the imitable stressors experienced by parents and the dynamic coping strategies available to parents to navigate this period. Finally, a reflection on the varying familial outcomes, including parental burnout, family violence, and posttraumatic growth will be undertaken in an attempt to highlight why, and how, families may experience such diversity in positive and negative outcomes during the COVID-19 pandemic.

The changing landscape of parenting

Independent to the COVID-19 pandemic, the role of a parent in 2020 is varied and dynamic in nature. Such a need for adaptability comes on the back of the growing number of structures representing family units and how the members of such structures work together. The 1980's picture of the "typical" nuclear family including members with well-defined gendered roles is no longer the norm (Bengtson, 2001), with a growing number of structures now representing the "modern typical" family, which involves a sharing of working, caring, and household duties between all family members. It is worth taking a brief lesson in history here to appreciate why the modern family is in a position of strength to deal with the COVID-19 pandemic.

While the timeline for family structure prevalence is varied worldwide, the broad transitions between these structures over time share some global parallels. For instance, the reliance on extended family structures reminiscent of Eastern cultures was a hallmark of the World War and Depression periods throughout most of the Western world. Here many members of one family (grandparents, parents, children, cousins, aunts, and uncles) were brought together under the single roof—in part to reduce expenditure on assets that could now be shared among more family members, but also because the increased family numbers could contribute to a larger family endeavor (e.g., farming and assisted child rearing arrangements)—earning the brand the "corporate family." Throughout the 1960s to 1990s the larger extended families became more eroded in line with social shifts encouraging independence from family, international travel, gender equality, and equal rights all individually advantageous movements however with respect to family structure certainly a time for a transition toward the smaller nuclear family arrangement (Hertz & Marshall, 2001; Ruggles, 1994). According to United States census data, prior to 1900 approximately 90% of children grew up in extended/corporate family structures; however, less than 20% were in such a structure by 2010 (Pew Research Centre, 2015).

This shift, "looking backwards to move forwards" if you will, does incorporate a more contemporary addition to the concept of the extended family. With divorce rates now over 50% in many Western countries the family constitution now readily includes multiple parents and stepparents; the 2020's version of the extended family expands further to include "blended" families—the *blended and extended family* (see Portrie & Hill, 2016). Herein lies a nexus. While extended families of the past benefited from the financial and social supports of having many families under the one roof but with clear *designations and division* for individual roles (e.g., who are the grandparents, who are the parents, who are the children) the more contemporary extended family must navigate and determine the *sharing* of such roles. Tricky—yes. However, the rapidly changing family structure may have inadvertently armed families, and parents, with adaptability, psychological flexibility, and sophisticated interrelational skills that will enable them to successfully navigate the unprecedented, and quickly shifting, COVID-19 pandemic landscape far more effectively than more simplistic family structures of the near past. The more malleable composition of the family might well be a savior as all these areas of consideration and compromise required to build this new functioning blended and extended family encourage the development of psychological flexibility and adaptability, which are being reported as features key to family and individual resilience during the pandemic (Szabo, Richling, Embry, Biglan, & Wilson, 2020).

Concomitant with the evolving family landscape is a shift in parenting roles, where sometimes families are needing to incorporate four or more parents and stepparents into the decision-making hierarchy and process. While such a situation could easily be a source of disharmony (i.e., "too many cooks in the kitchen") when well managed this system has heightened resilience, taking strength actually from the more extended or corporate family units reminiscent of the early 1900s, as it offers more options for financial, social, and emotional support (Ruggles, 1994). Key to this system offering these profound benefits is an appreciation of what constitutes principles of "good parenting."

Being "a parent" is, at its most minimalist profile, about an adult sharing a relationship with a child (Grose, 2010)—this relationship may stem from a biological (i.e., being the genetic contributor of the child) and/or social (i.e., providing care for the child) origin. Being a "good parent" requires the provision of a host of additional long-term practical, emotional, and social opportunities for the child within an environment of safety and security (Fave, 2004). Good parenting is known to have a basis in consistency and routine (Boston University, 2017) which is essential for children to experience a level of perceived control in their lives. This sense of control is an essential building block for developing a sense of independence as they grow (Dijkstra & Homan, 2016; Grose, 2010). In a sense good parenting is about fostering an environment where parents essentially make themselves redundant. Within a growing landscape of independence, children become less reliant on their parents as their sole source of engagement in the world as they are encouraged to socialize in school-type environments and in other social settings (e.g., sporting and religious groups) (Feldman, 2016) and even in the more contemporary online environment (Vaala & Bleakley, 2015). In the background good parents play a role in modeling many of the interactive behaviors for their children—modeling that alters and adapts as their children grow older and gradually master a growing tool kit of skills (Schrodt, Witt, & Messersmith, 2008). Good parenting also involves a recognition that each child in a family is different and so parenting practices must not be preestablished and instead share a plasticity so as to create a best fit for each child to develop in directions and in ways consistent with their needs (Newland & Crnic, 2017). The best parents are those that can help children build growth mindsets (Mueller, Rowe, & Zuckerman, 2017)—making themselves adaptable and effort focused rather than being exclusively achievement driven. In this way, best practice sees a reliance on positive reinforcement and when required considered and consistent discipline that is mindful of the developmental expectations of their child (Gardner, Shaw, Dishion, Burton, & Supplee, 2007). Together all these skills allow parents to provide opportunities for the children to experience a diversity of activities to capture their children's interest and in a way that difficulties are reappraised as challenges, which in turn underpin the development of resilience in their children.

The *provision of opportunity* is a key ingredient of parenting that should not be undervalued. Again, at the risk of sounding repetitive, it has never been considered that a good parent could, or should, personally provide all the opportunities a child needs to grow into a healthy and functioning adult. Rather, a good parent merely needs to provide connections and experiences with other people, and it is from these connections that many of the necessary opportunities arise. These other connections were inherent in the older extended and corporate family structures of the early 1900s but over the last 30 years have now been more commonly provided by other community structures within which a family functions, for instance, educational systems, religious settings, and sporting associations to name a few. In this way a parent provides direction and support to their child in engaging in these nonfamilial settings. These various systems are key to a child's development but a child's engagement with these systems is very much reliant on the guidance that they receive from their parents.

The COVID-19 landscape has created a world wherein parenting is fundamentally changed. However, the effects of the pandemic are experienced quite differently across different families (Marques, Moraes, Hasselmann, Deslandes, & Reichenheim, 2020; Szabo et al., 2020) and as such, a good place to start is in appreciating why it is that families are impacted differentially from individuals before attempting to understand what makes each family unique from every other family.

Relational models of the parent-child dynamic

As already established, parents are not the exclusive providers of all the experiences necessary for child development. Throughout time varying family structures have created a situation where the growth and development of a child is promoted ultimately by parents but executed via the many levels of relationships the child and parents have within the world in which they live. Bronfenbrenner's (1981) Ecological Systems Theory highlights how a child develops supported by the various connections made available in their world—most influentially are the child's parents, their school, their religious connections, and their peers. Beyond this, a host of school, community, medical, social, political, and economic systems and philosophies play key supporting roles in facilitating this development (see Fig. 1 for a pictorial representation).

The importance of the parent-child relationship in terms of development specifically is made clear in Bowen's (1966) Family System's Model. The family systems approach has, for a long time, been utilized in psychological trauma treatment by reenvisaging the experience of trauma to any single member as a stressor on the family as a whole. Herein a family is considered as a "cohesive emotional unit" rather than as individual members—in this way any disruption to an individual's circumstances will have a ripple effect through the entire unit as relational ties and ensuing family member behaviors, wax and wane in response to the disturbance. Depicted in the literature is the notion that

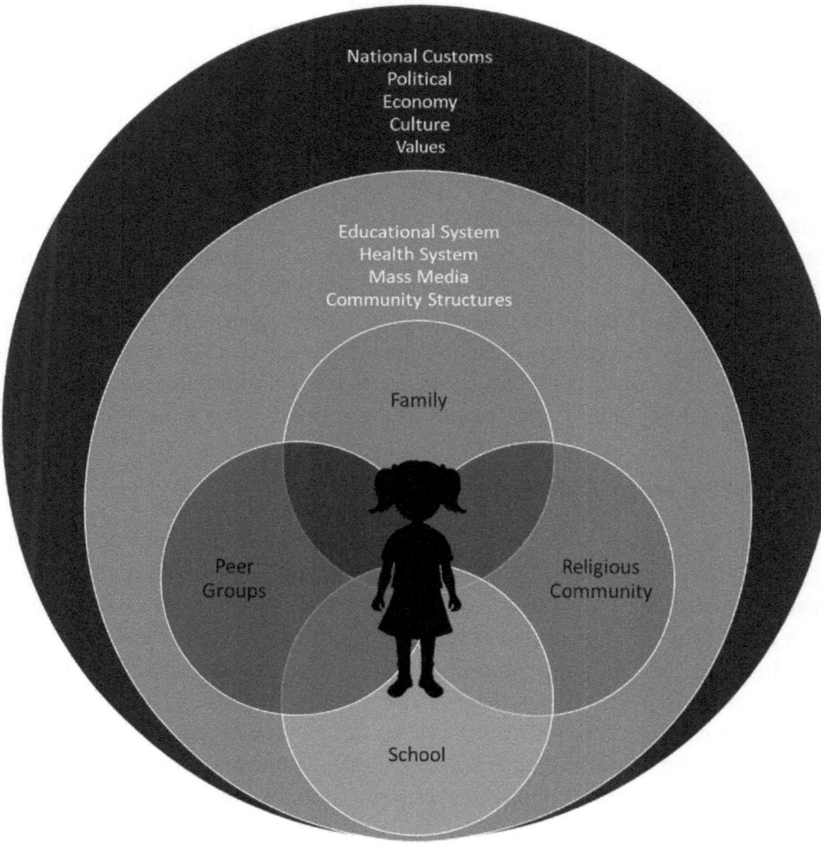

FIG. 1 Pictorial representation of Bronfenbrenner's Ecological Model of Child Development illustrating the various interrelating systems that support and underlie child development.

a particularly distressing event may be "contagious" meaning that even those who did not personally experience the event may report thoughts and emotions similar to those who did directly witness it, highlighting the capacity for such disturbance to spread through a family system (Kilroy, Egan, Maliszewska, & Sarma, 2014). Despite this, fundamental to the Family Systems Model is that, as a unit, the family is seen to be more resilient as a single entity than any individual member is alone, as the remaining members of the unit can provide a cushioning to the disturbance or distress experienced by any single member.

The COVID-19 period presents an interesting demand on this model as the compensatory nature of the framework is undermined when all members are independently under pressure from a range of sources. This means that the critical absorption feature is ameliorated when all members are essentially individually compromised. While Patterson (2002) reported that a shared family trauma can actually result in enhanced perceptions of cohesion and bonding between family members and effectively strengthen the bonds within the family system, the COVID-19 pandemic cannot be routinely viewed as a "traumatic event." Rather the COVID-19 pandemic, by way of its indefinite timeframe, consists of many varying events that are differentially experienced by all members of the family, and as such the ripples experienced throughout the family system are not uniform making for a tumultuous and challenging period for the family unit (Rolland, 2020). To date no clear articulation of the impacts of such family-level trauma has been made (Horesh & Brown, 2018) despite there existing many real-world examples of such system-level trauma, for instance that seen during war (Qouta, Punamäki, & El Sarraj, 2008), poverty (Strohschein & Gauthier, 2017), and natural disasters (Kelley et al., 2010; Stanke, Murray, Amlôt, Nurse, & Williams, 2012). However, a good place to start is in establishing an understanding of the many challenges faced by families during this time and by then considering how these each might individually impact on parents who are ultimately the "managers" of their family units, before making a larger collective appraisal.

COVID-19 parental stressors

The global COVID-19 pandemic is a stressor with its origins outside the family system itself, but given the novelty and uncertainty surrounding the virus it creates a multitude of stressful situations that families navigate on a daily basis. Even families who have not been directly exposed to the virus itself are likely to be impacted by the many indirect effects of the pandemic (Van Baval et al., 2020). Recent reports indicate that 91% of parents, in addition to the concerns of the virus itself, have experienced a series of changes during this period, with 44% saying their lives have changed to a significant level during the pandemic (see Griffith, 2020), resulting in changes to their mood and stress levels (Horesh & Brown, 2018). For many parents though, it is the simultaneous juggling of many atypical stressors that results in exponentially growing feelings of distress (Fontanesi et al., 2020; Ghosh, Dubey, Chatterjee, & Dubey, 2020).

These direct and indirect circumstances give rise to parental stress, which may have serious adverse implications to a parent's mental health (Patrick et al., 2020), their physical health (Grose, 2010), their use of alcohol and other substances (Pelham & Lang, 1999), and their parenting practices (Beckerman, van Berkel, Mesman, & Alink, 2016). In turn, such impacts on parents are felt by their children (Griffith, 2020; Humphreys et al., 2020) with the COVID-19 period marked by increased emotional and behavioral sequelae among children whose parents are distressed (Spinelli, Lionetti, Pastore, & Fasolo, 2020). Of course, the distress felt by children, both as a result of the parenting they are receiving and the virus itself (see Haig-Ferguson, Cooper, Cartwright, Loades, & Daniels, 2020) further agitates their emotional state and regulation. In turn the ensuing behaviors are then felt by their parents and consequently increases in parental stress are seen (Mikolajczak, Gross, Stinglhamber, Lindahl Norberg, & Roskam, 2020). This seemingly vicious cycle is well explained in the Family Systems Model (Carr, 2016).

As previously recognized parents are themselves individuals in their own right, and as such, many of the changes and stressors resulting from COVID-19 already identified in this book apply to parents also. However, by way of the presence of dependent children and the associated responsibilities of the care of these children, the scope of a parent's concern is widened, and many unique changes and stressors brought to bear. It is these which are of primary interest here.

Health anxiety

Parents' concerns around the infectious nature of COVID-19 are not unwarranted. Despite early research suggesting children to be fairly immune to the COVID-19 virus (Lee, Hu, Chen, Huang, & Hsueh, 2020; Ludvigsson, 2020), more recent data demonstrates that children can indeed become significantly ill with COVID-19 and that for a small number COVID-19 may be lethal—particularly for those with other preexisting health conditions (Eastin & Eastin, 2020). Additionally, research is suggesting that other respiratory-related illnesses among children have risen during the COVID-19 pandemic leading to well informed academics, researchers, and clinicians suggesting a direct link between the two (Ahmed et al., 2020). Despite these findings, the risk profile of children still does appear lower than for other populations; however, parents may find themselves uncomforted by population-wide statistics (Liu, Bao, Huang, Shi, & Lu, 2020). It is also important to recognize that children themselves share significant concerns about the virus (Huang & Zhao, 2020) and that these are associated with increases in diagnosed mental illness in this younger population. The health and wellbeing of a child is a fundamental concern of parents with childhood sickness known to be a leading cause of distress in families (Miles, Carter, Spicher, & Hassanein, 1984). Parents with an unwell child, particularly one experiencing a potentially life threatening disease, are more likely to themselves present with a related, or even unrelated, physical illness, sleep problems, anxiety and/or depression (Lindstrom, Aman, & Norberg, 2010; Mikolajczak, Brianda, Avalosse, & Roskam, 2018), and discord in the marital relationship (Pai et al., 2007). As such the fear and worry caused by the presence of COVID-19 has a hugely destabilizing impact on parents' wellbeing.

The COVID-19 pandemic also gives rise to a host of preemptive anxieties—concerns about cleanliness and virus exposure. Here, even with currently healthy children parents worry about the hygiene practices of their children, who are notoriously poorer at managing the social distancing, handwashing, and general hygiene practices so critical to stemming the spread of a virus like COVID-19 (Willmott et al., 2016). Moreover, with the aforementioned lower risk profile for children many countries are maintaining and reimplementing in-person school attendance as a priority meaning that parents are no longer able to exert control over many aspects of their child's interactions with others. It is often noted that a reduced sense of control over their children's lives can amplify the stress experienced by parents (Duxbury, Higgins, & Lee, 1994) and conversely that increases in perceived control can reduce parental distress (Brown, Doom, Lechuga-Peña, Watamura, & Koppels, 2020; Humphreys et al., 2020).

The anxiety around virus transmission is also especially sensitive for those parents who also form part of the frontline defense against the virus. The thousands of frontline workers, particularly those in health care, find themselves in a situation where they are personally at a higher risk of contracting the virus due to their working environment but are then faced with returning to their children each night with concerns about whether they might someday infect their family (Humphreys et al., 2020). The stress felt by health care workers during this time is shown to be far greater for those with families than for those without families (Xiang et al., 2020).

Role collision and navigation

The worker

For those parents not in essential roles many are finding themselves working from home on a more permanent basis. Herein, the structure of the workday is significantly altered as meetings move online, technology difficulties arise, reduced workplace support is available, and many of the day-to-day interactions of the work environment are lost. Working from home represents a significant disruption to structure, which is a primary cause of stress (Griffith, 2020). While more generally the workplace, where the average adult will spend up to one-third of their life in (World Health Organisation, 1994), has been evidenced as a source of psychological distress—particularly during periods of significant change and uncertainty (Rolland, 2020)—it might also be a place where mental health can be bolstered—particularly for parents. Several authors highlight how parents, during times of stress, may engage in "escape" behaviors to afford them times away from parenting duties (Lindstrom et al., 2010; Mikolajczak, Gross,

& Roskam, 2019) and in this way the workplace might well afford them an oasis in the midst of the pandemic stress but which is made unavailable due to quarantine, lockdown, and social distancing periods. An essential balance between the stressful and protective features of the workplace may be lost.

While the change in structure to the working day is not unique to parents, the specifics of that change do present additional challenges for parents as they find themselves needing to achieve a balance between their own work and the provision of care (including home-schooling) to their children. Parents have shouldered a particularly delicate burden throughout the pandemic with many still continuing their expected weekly hours of work in the home environment while now also managing their children's care or education in the context of unprecedented school and day care closures that have extended over many months (American Psychological Association, 2020). More than a third of parents in the US have reported that they are struggling to balance work and childcare responsibilities (Patrick et al., 2020; Pew Research Centre, 2020).

Despite the challenge's parents face with the balancing of work and children, the flexibility provided by work-from-home arrangements may also be a saving grace. Many parents who do not have the capacity to undertake their work from home, being classified as 'essential workers,' report struggles sourcing childcare for their younger children and supervision for older children who might also require home-schooling support.

The teacher

Since the beginning of the pandemic parents across the world have been faced with the realities of educating their own children from within the home environment. For some this represents more extended periods and their communities come under enforced lockdowns; however, for others, these periods may only be days in length following isolated COVID-19 cases appearing in the local school environment requiring school closure, cleaning and contact tracing efforts in advance of a swift reopening. To this end, the extent of education delivery by parents is quite varied. However, in a similar vein to the preemptive concerns around health, many parents have found themselves preparing for the inevitabilities of educating their children to at least some degree.

The capacity of parents to provide such education is likely to be perceived as somewhat of an insult to the many educators around the world who have spent years training to be teachers. Parents, with no explicit training in teaching, have suddenly needed to take on what could be considered one of the most critical roles in their child's life. These parents report concerns with not knowing the materials or being confident in how to teach them (Parczewska, 2020). Many parents operate under an assumption that their children require 7 h of schooling a day (Morrow, 2019) while teachers estimate that the 7-h school day is broken up into much smaller subperiods of didactic learning and much larger periods of discovery and peer-to-peer learning (Poole-Boykin, 2020). In this way parents are often unaware of the developmental capabilities of their children in terms of attention and concentration. This mismatch between parental expectation of "study hours" and their child's usual school routine has been identified as a source of parent-child stress (Poole-Boykin, 2020). For parents with younger aged school children the assistance required in learning is greater and the manner in which a child absorbs the information is also at a developmental point far removed from the way in which their parents now learn—meaning a common ground and understanding is often times absent.

For children undertaking home learning the support materials provided by schools is highly variable—with some schools offering live classroom sessions complemented by home learning packs with timetabled activities, other schools provide learning materials to be navigated by children (and their parents) while others still provide general links to resources that children and parents may access at their own leisure. Such variability is highly problematic as it means that age cohorts across jurisdictions may not be achieving the same academic milestones across the academic year, posing systemic problems for education systems as more school-as-usual practices resume. For parents this is an obvious area of concern but not all parents find themselves in the same position to assist their children (American Psychological Association, 2020). Long before the COVID-19 pandemic it was well established that low socioeconomic status (SES) families typically include parents who (i) themselves have received lower quality educations undermining their capacity to "bridge the gap" and/or (ii) are financially unable to take time off work to assist in such schooling. The parental stress emerging from such a situation is well documented and the poorer education and social outcomes for their children is unfortunately also clear (Doyle, 2020).

In addition to concerns about their own capacity to deliver home learning materials, parents are now privy to the performance of their children in a far more direct way than before. While some report great satisfaction in being able to watch their children learning (Morris, 2020), others are reporting a heightened sense of worry as they observe their child struggling with the materials (Morrow, 2019; Parczewska, 2020). Such a struggle might well be a typical and transient stage of learning while for others it might be indicative of more substantive difficulties. The problem faced by parents is that without pedagogy training they are unable to decipher to which group their child belongs.

The guidance counselor

The practicalities surrounding home-schooling are not isolated to academic features either. The social environment provided at school is an essential ingredient in childhood and adolescent development. For young children their peers provide an opportunity to learn the skills of turn taking, working in teams and emotional regulation, for primary aged children their peers provide them with challenges to try new activities, to develop empathy, and to learn theory of mind, while for adolescents their peers become a source of comfort outside the home and indeed represent a network through which new adult-like relationship can be built (Meadows, 2018). Teacher also plays a role in social development by representing a family-external authority figure and emotional guide for children and adolescents. Even within a school environment caring roles are divided between multiple staff—teachers, counselors, principals—because the boundaries for one role might need to be different for another role (e.g., a teacher might require strict behavioral rules in a classroom setting to establish equality between students while a counselor might have more relaxed boundaries with specific students based on their personal circumstances). Certainly, this time of upheaval means that children are more likely to engage in emotional, oppositional, or boundary testing behaviors, which are likely to engender harsher parenting styles even when parents are unstressed themselves. In the presence of such a multitude of additional stressors, such parenting styles are likely to contribute to parent-child relationships that are inconsistent, unstable, and mistrustful (Ackerman, Kogos, Youngstrom, Schoff, & Izard, 1999).

The pandemic has leveled many significant changes at the feet of children and adolescents who are themselves still learning the sophisticated coping strategies of their parents that would enable them to more adequately cope (Coyne et al., 2020; Kliewer et al., 2006). As such, parents find they are required to bridge this gap and play the role of a counselor in helping their children navigate the changes and associated emotional issues. Brown et al. (2020) reported that 21% to 47% of parents reported that their children had experienced significant changes because of COVID-19. The changes in routine are particularly problematic for young children who derive a sense of control in their lives from such routine. In its absence children often find themselves unsettled, irritable, and anxious (Humphreys et al., 2020). Older children too are finding long-held expectations being crushed by the pandemic as established "rites of passage" are being delayed or canceled like special birthdays (e.g., Sweet 16), religious rituals (e.g., bar mitzvahs or communions), or educational milestones (e.g., graduations). For these children, such changes have a destabilizing effect on mood (Humphreys et al., 2020; Wang, Zhang, Zhao, Zhang, & Jiang, 2020) and potentially confer a heightened risk for suicidal ideation (Buitron et al., 2016; Loades et al., 2020).

To date only one published study was available on suicide rates of children and adolescents during the pandemic which promisingly suggested no ensuing increase in suicidal behaviors was evident among a Japanese cohort (Isumi, Doi, Yamaoka, Takahashi, & Fujiwara, 2020). With such significant impacts on their children, parents are feeling the pressure as they attempt to personally deliver support across all of these domains reporting that "if it's not me, who will do it," "someone has to and I am the only one" indicating that unreasonable or not, they feel that they are ultimately responsible for protecting and soothing their child through this period of pain and loss (Morris, 2020; Spinelli et al., 2020). It is worth noting that such "loss" is not exclusively experienced by their child either—parents themselves speak of the importance of such events in the lives of their child as being major events in their own lives (American Psychological Association, 2020).

Financial burden

The pandemic has resulted in record rates of unemployment with more than half of Americans reporting being financially impacted by the pandemic, including losing their job, being laid off, or experiencing reduced income (Pew Research Centre, 2020). For many parents, the COVID-19 period has resulted in significant hardships being placed on their families. Unemployment, worldwide, is at an all-time high—with 70% of American reporting financial hardship compared to only 46% 12 months previously (American Psychological Association, 2020). For parents such financial hardship is more distressing as generally the cost of living is higher as they support dependents not capable of deriving their own income and the cost of relocating homes to reduce expenditure is more difficult than for singles and childless couples (e.g., the sheer volume of belongings, school enrolments issues, etc.) (American Psychological Association, 2020). For family's poverty and homelessness the often inevitable outcome of job losses is of significant concern given the ensuing heightened risk for family violence (Humphreys et al., 2020). We will discuss this more later.

Sleep deprivation

While sleep might appear to represent a category quite unlike those discussed to this point it is clearly identified as an issue of increased concern during the pandemic (Hurley, 2020). While presentation numbers specific to parents are not available it is well appreciated that parents already represent an at-risk population with respect to lost sleep (Wang et al., 2020). Parents share a similar underlying risk profile for sleep disorders (e.g., insomnia) as their childless peers; however, disordered sleeping among parents is compounded by the disruptions they experience as a result of their children's sleep problems also. With many of the quarantine and isolation measures in place during the pandemic, the energy (both physical and cognitive) typically expelled by children in the school environment exists in surplus making the typical sleep routine ineffective (Wang et al., 2020). Moreover, the additional screen time children are exposed to is an additional aspect that might reduce sleep quality and quantity for children placing greater strain on parents (Wang et al., 2020). Pre-COVID-19 the average hours of sleep per night for a parent were less than for their childless peers (Meltzer & Montgomery-Downs, 2011) so it is highly likely that this figure is now even worse. As sleep is considered essential for cognitive activities (Fortier-Brochu, Beaulieu-Bonneau, Ivers, & Morin, 2012) and is associated with immune function (Taylor, Lichstein, & Durrence, 2003), it is clear that parents are at risk in both of these areas. Many studies have demonstrated that reduced sleep is associated with poorer parenting practices; parents become less tolerant and more irritable, are less capable of dealing with stressful situations, make less considered choices and often times engage in harsher disciplining behaviors (Chary, McQuillan, Bates, & Deater-Deckard, 2018; Cooklin, Giallo, & Rose, 2012; McCann, Bull, & Winzenberg, 2015).

Family separation

Previously we discussed the potential benefits that blended and extended family structures could yield during this pandemic. However, when periods of lockdown have been initiated throughout the world, these very families find themselves now spread across multiple households with members unable to engage in typical fashion. For some families this requires only minor adjustments and compromises to facilitate ongoing virtual interaction between all family members, but for other families such geographic separation requires far more substantive changes. For instance, in households with a single parent who is an essential worker the capacity to maintain any level of custody of their child during this time might be impossible, requiring extensive periods of separation between the child and this parent. For other families coparenting in across multiple households might no longer be possible requiring significant changes to the household routines. Changes in living circumstances, particularly where a parent's separation may not be cordial, are considered among the most stressful events one can experience (Coleman & Glenn, 2010). To date, we do know that children who have been separated from their parents due to quarantine requirements during this pandemic (i.e., when their parent is hospitalized with COVID-19) demonstrate significantly poor psychosocial outcomes (Ghosh et al., 2020).

Separation between blended and extended families and indeed even to remote areas of cultural significance are particularly problematic for many indigenous communities. For instance, in Australia this "connection to land" is fundamental to the daily lives of its First Peoples ('Yotti' Kingsley, Townsend, Phillips, & Aldous, 2009) and the quarantining measures put in place by federal and state governments have meant that many indigenous Australians have been unable to maintain such connections. For indigenous families the capacity to connect with their children is crucial but under many of the quarantining regulations such contact has been prevented. Historically such separation has been associated with poor mental health outcomes (The National Inquiry Into the Separation of Aboriginal and Torres Strait Islander Children From Their Families, 1997) and such poor mental health outcomes are related with increased substance use and instances of incarceration (Heffernan, Andersen, Dev, & Kinner, 2012). As such, while data relating specifically to the COVID-19 period is not yet known, there is good reason to be particularly concerned about this population.

Parental burnout

The combination of stressors that are faced by parents as they attempt to multitask and manage colliding roles (Fontanesi et al., 2020) throughout this pandemic leaves them at particular risk of psychological exhaustion and "parental burnout" (Mikolajczak et al., 2019). This intense period of exhaustion is crucially related to one's role as a parent, sidelining the stressors that might be contributed by other sources (e.g., work) and heartbreakingly renders one doubtful of their capacity to be a good parent during this period of chronic stress (Mikolajczak et al., 2019). It is not representative of the typical stress that is associated with parenting (e.g., the daily hassles of getting ready for school on time or completing homework before TV in the evenings) but rather is the result of additional ongoing exposure to atypical stressors impacting the family unit (Mikolajczak et al., 2019).

For some this period of overwhelming fear or burden results in significant anxiety and worry accompanied by a host of physiological sensations (e.g., ranging from more transient periods of a racing heart or sweating through to more chronic headaches and stomach complaints) and a sense of being "unable to act" or of "treading water" (Murray, 2003). Others may seek time away from their family (withdrawal) due to a lack of energy or as an avoidance mechanism (Mikolajczak et al., 2019). For a smaller, but nonetheless significant, number of parents this burnout results in intense feelings of anger marked by an insensitivity to the needs of those of indeed a harshness in their interactions with their children and significant others (Coyne et al., 2020; Humphreys et al., 2020). These fight (anger), flight (withdrawal), and freeze (anxiety) behaviors may lead parents to be absent, neglectful, or even violent in their interactions with their children. Interestingly the presence of parental burnout confers a risk value 4 times, 10 times, and 25 times more for each absence, neglect, and abuse compared to other types of burnout experienced by nonparenting related stressors (e.g., work burnout) (Mikolajczak et al., 2018). Cross-sectional findings suggest that parental burnout is associated with depressive symptoms, addictive behaviors, sleep disorders, and couple conflicts (Mikolajczak et al., 2020). This meaning that many of the above-mentioned stressors faced by parents have an interacting and somewhat spiraling influence on one another.

Pre-COVID-19 studies of stress within families demonstrate that parenting during periods of high stress is marked with insensitivity in interrelation behaviors, a lack of responsiveness to others needs, the withdrawal from others and routines in the home, high reactivity and irritability to low stakes situations, reduced warmth in relationships, and an increase in negativity, harshness, and punitiveness in parenting behaviors (Marques et al., 2020; Usher, Bhullar, Durkin, Gyamfi, & Jackson, 2020). As a result the parent-child relationship can significantly suffer (Prime, Wade, & Browne, 2020) with longer period of detachment and more extreme levels of harshness indicative of longer term parent-child conflict, which may continue long past the conclusion of the stressful event itself (Humphreys et al., 2020).

Those parents most at risk of burnout are those with high expectations of themselves as a parent and perfectionistic qualities (Kawamoto, Furutani, & Alimardani, 2018), those who have preexisting emotional and stress regulation issues or poor parenting practices (Mikolajczak et al., 2018), those who lack support from a coparent or other networks involved with the care of their child (Griffith, 2020). Clearly a number of these risk profiles are consistent with the environment created during the pandemic; parents trying to undertake many diverse roles for their children to a quality generally expected following the completion of a university level course (e.g., teaching) during a time where their typical social support networks are unavailable to them and their children. Moreover this time is a period where all members of the family are spending increasing periods of time together, often under lockdown conditions, preventing them from escaping the family hot pot.

Family violence

Research into family violence during this pandemic is in its infancy—with numbers only beginning to be available as private and government agencies begin to document the results of the chronic stress imposed by the ongoing virus control measures (Usher et al., 2020). New Zealand reported that family violence has escalated during the pandemic in a similar way to that evidenced following other large-scale crises in the country (Johnston, 2020). In nearby Australia as lockdown measures were put in place, overall crime across the country dropped as much as 40% while domestic violence incidents increased by 5% (Kagi, 2020). As well known, reported domestic violence numbers is a gross underestimate of the actual social problem of domestic abuse and neglect. Perhaps more telling is that during this same period in Australia Google searches relating to domestic violence support rose by 75% (Poate, 2020). Globally the numbers paint a similarly discouraging picture; the United States, the United Kingdom, China, and Brazil (Campbell, 2020;Usher et al., 2020 ; van Gelder et al., 2020) showing that the pandemic period is associated with increasing levels of family violence independent of country, religion, political, and social structures.

Fortunately for most parents the navigation through this pandemic will not dissolve into such a period of distress for themselves and their children so as to lead to any form of domestic violence or neglect within the home (Prime et al., 2020). However, in the presence of so many psychological and economic stressors being placed on parents during this time, the incidence of parental burnout is unfortunately more prevalent than typical (Griffith, 2020; Humphreys et al., 2020). In Australia, the lockdown period was shown to be associated with an increased rise in alcohol sales (Colbert, Wilkinson, Thornton, & Richmond, 2020) highlighting the problems of engagement with negative coping strategies (e.g., alcohol and other substances). Such a combination—stressors in the company of negative coping strategies—is a "perfect storm" for family violence (Usher et al., 2020; van Gelder et al., 2020). Moreover, the isolating features of the pandemic add an additional layer of risk to the family violence picture.

A substantial body of research now exists about the impact of continued close contact between family members during periods of stress showing heightened prevalence of aggressive and violent behaviors (Brown et al., 2020; Marques et al., 2020; van Gelder et al., 2020). Add to this that access to assistance services is limited and the opportunity to access more helpful coping strategies (e.g., grandparents, parental time outs) is a rarity (Brown et al., 2020). As such, risk is higher during this period and the mechanisms required to offset this risk are few. Unfortunately the pandemic also relegates useless one of the key combatants in preventing child abuse and neglect—the schools and teachers who provide a safety for children and who act as a primary identifier of such abuse and neglect (Brown et al., 2020). With school closures this critical mechanism means many children are spending additional time in the neglectful or abusive environment with no people available to maintain a watchful eye over them.

On the back of such figures relating to familial violence during the COVID-19 pandemic now being made available and ensuing research providing an understanding of the underlying causes, a call is now being placed for governments and nongovernment agencies to build purpose-built services—services that can operate within the constraints of the isolative pandemic period (Coyne et al., 2020; Humphreys et al., 2020; Patrick et al., 2020).

Parental coping through COVID-19

Note all research emanating from the COVID-19 period with respect to parents and children suggests an inevitable decline into illness, emotional distress, and/or violence as a result of the many challenges presented directly or indirectly by the pandemic. Certainly, as discussed by (Horesh & Brown, 2018) the appraisals made by an individual about an experience can influence whether adaptive, or maladaptive, behaviors follow. These outcomes are well explained by the Transactional Stress Model (Lazarus, 1984). The Transaction Stress Model describes a process of cognitive appraisal whereby the experience of *stress* arises from two critical phases—the first being whether the specifics of the event are deemed of concern or danger to the individual while the second is concerned with whether the individual feels capable to managing the concern of danger.

In terms of appreciating the impact of COVID-19 on parents, and families, the critical undertaking that must first occur is to define and describe the various specifics of the event (i.e., what potential stressors are present). Many of these stressors have been overviewed before. Some families, while exposed to the same events as others just will not find themselves as concerned about the potential outcomes in the same way as others (Coyne et al., 2020; Prime et al., 2020; Szabo et al., 2020). For instance, while some might be concerned about the impact school closures might have on their children's education, other families might well see this as an opportunity to focus learning in other domains (e.g., cooking, gardening, and other exploratory activities). Obviously, the different ways the same experience might be interpreted at this initial appraisal stage will determine whether it is deemed as a stressor or not.

The second appraisal stage is where those families who have determined the experience to be a stressor evaluate the different resources available to them to decide whether or not they can meet the demands of the stressor. As such, a family who might have a parent who has had training as a teacher might feel they hold adequate resources to combat the stressor while another family who has two parents who are both essential workers and cannot easily provide the attention to their children to assist in their home-schooling at this time. The latter family is more likely to experience heightened stress during this period compared to the former. As such, it is important to examine the coping strategies for families in an effort to examine how it is they can manage the demands of the stressors they are faced with.

Coping strategies can work in two ways firstly, by allowing a parent to directly address the stressor at hand often with practical solutions or secondly, by reducing levels of stress more generally by "destressing," freeing up emotional and cognitive resources to now direct toward developing solutions for the stressors (Biggs, Brough, & Drummond, 2017).

The very nature of the pandemic has resulted in many parents experiencing significant physical boundaries to accessing their pre-COVID-19 social support networks. *Social supports* are essential for parents as they seek out other adults sometimes to assist directly with concerns they have about their children or methods of parenting while at other times the assistance is more indirect as parents engage with peers as a way to disengage from highly stressful family situations (Paster, Brandwein, & Walsh, 2009). As a result of social distancing and isolation measures, the many platforms for facilitating such engagement are lost—coffee in the afternoon, a catch up over lunch or dinner, time at the gym—and as mentioned previously, even within the workplace. Even capacity to engage with their most primary peer support—their coparent—can be compromised as times for "adulting" (going out for dinner, to the movies, having a quiet time in the home while children are visiting with friends or at extracurricular activities) are eroded. The pandemic has seen a rise of virtual gatherings between friends (Howard, 2020), which have been noted to provide a reasonable alternative to face to face in some settings during this time (Barsom, Feenstra, Bemelman, Bonjer, & Schijven, 2020), although the pre-COVID-19 literature suggests the social quality of such interactions is substantially different (Webster, 2020). It remains to be seen whether over time, and with continued practice, such virtual interactions might become more natural and therefore permit enhanced social quality more akin to face-to-face interactions.

Where peer interactions can provide a platform for destressing, parents also engage in many other activities designed to reduce their baseline levels of stress. Attending the gym; going for a walk or run; going to a beautician, hairdresser, or barber; attending sporting events; playing in sporting teams; and even reading a book are all legitimate stress coping strategies. Many of their leisure and self-care activities either cannot be undertaken due to isolation and social distancing government requirements or can no longer be undertaken as independently with so many individuals in the one space (Coyne et al., 2020).

Parents also have been forced into reduced, if any, contact with family members outside of their home location (e.g., grandparents). It is often these extended family members who provide additional childcare support to allow parents the time to work, to engage in their own social outings, and even to enable periods of relaxation (Griffith, 2020). In the absence of this support it is unsurprising that parents feel enormous pressure to provide all of the care for their children without being afforded any opportunity to recharge their own energy levels or to destress in the midst of such burden.

Of course, parents, as adults, do have a large repertoire of coping behaviors available to them—ones they have crafted and mastered over time that are particularly individual to them (reference). Parents who can practice flexible thinking (Coyne et al., 2020), those who can exert levels of control or who can focus on elements of the pandemic situation that they can control (Dijkstra & Homan, 2016), and those who are capable of exercising acceptance (Coyne et al., 2020) report lower levels of perceived stress and anxiety and better mood than their peers. As such, while many of the primary sources of assistance might be unavailable to parents during this pandemic, they are in a much more powerful position than their children to adapt and develop these to match their evolving situation. A parent's stress is heavily influenced by their children's behaviors and as such parents have the capacity to reduce the stressors impacting themselves by aiding their children to adapt to the "COVID-19 normal" lifestyle. For instance, providing structured daily routines (Szabo et al., 2020), modeling psychological flexibility and self-care (Coyne et al., 2020), encouraging outdoor activities and involvement in physical play (Wang et al., 2020), and providing the opportunity for positive social interactions, even if limited to online or virtual settings, with friends and extended family members (Coyne et al., 2020; Prime et al., 2020; Szabo et al., 2020). Parents can also aid their children emotionally by providing opportunities for their children to speak with them about the pandemic and by encouraging their children to discuss their emotions and the ways that they are attempting to manage during this time (Prime et al., 2020).

Of course, as mentioned earlier in this chapter the presence of stressors, no matter their magnitude nor number, automatically confers the negative outcomes discussed thus far. In fact, a good number of studies highlight that periods of stress can engender resilience in individuals (Calhoun & Tedeschi, 1998) and even among families (Szabo et al., 2020; Wang et al., 2020). The development of resilience is dependent upon exposure to a given challenge (or stressor) and the capacity to call to arms any number of coping strategies at one's disposal, or indeed engineer an entirely new approach. A number of models speak to this process of facing a stressor, meeting it existing emotional (e.g., motivation) or physical (e.g., assistance from others) resources, the recovery following this challenge-resource balance, and emerging from this challenge unchanged or more capable than before. For instance, Fredrickson's (2001) Broaden and Build Theory highlighted how resilience could be developed through the gradual exposure to a stressor, the mapping or creation of coping strategies to allow resolution of the stressor, and how the individual arises more capable of handling a more difficult challenge on the next occasion. Certainly the COVID-19 environment is a time that call on all the coping resources individuals already have at their disposal but it is critical to recognize that this is truly a period calling for creativity regarding these resources and many of the most useful pre-COVID-19 strategies (e.g., taking time out to exercise at a gym, going out for coffee with friends, calling on extended family for assistance, or even accessing a general practitioner) are no longer available or accessible in the same way.

Parent-led posttraumatic growth

While in this chapter we have shied away from delineating the COVID-19 pandemic as a trauma (that is a whole other debate right there—see Reference) there are good reasons to at least be open minded to this position. Certainly, many of the psychological disturbances reported by individuals in the aftermath of an event which simply/cleaning/maps to the trauma nosology as detailed in the DSM5 and ICD10 are being documented around the world during this period to a much higher rate than is typically documented on a year-by-year basis. For instance, individuals are reporting a loss of predictability about the world, a sense of detachment from self and others, a loss of identity, and even a lost sense of time (Fontanesi et al., 2020). For others there is evidence of hypervigilant states associated with preventing contact with the virus, avoidance of people and places that might signal a risk of infection, negative mood states accompanying the isolation of quarantine and cognitions consistent with a sense of helplessness and hopelessness about the now, and about the future (Horesh & Brown, 2018). For this reason some authors have gone so far as to recognize the pandemic period as a an "ongoing cardiac stress test" (Horesh & Brown, 2018), or a "chronic trauma" (Fontanesi et al., 2020), wherein individuals are faced with an uncertain future, where the "end" is undetermined and where the pathway forward lacks direction and even momentum. With respect to children, recent research has even demonstrated that children who have been quarantined as a result of the pandemic have posttraumatic stress scores four times higher than for their nonquarantined peers (Sprang & Silman, 2013).

Given the parallels between the experiences commonly reported with respect to exposure to a readily accepted trauma and the experiences reported by many during the pandemic (Horesh & Brown, 2018) it is worthwhile considering a related outcome of trauma exposure—posttraumatic growth (Calhoun & Tedeschi, 1998). As noted before not all parents and families throughout the world are displaying outcomes reminiscent of the negative effects of trauma. Some parents appear to be traversing the COVID-19 period remarkably well according to many self-reports of their own wellbeing, their children's wellbeing, and indeed with respect to family functioning (Brown et al., 2020; Morris, 2020). Some authors have even reported on families that appear to be thriving in the face of the apparent adversity of the pandemic (Humphreys et al., 2020).

A recent news story emanating from Australia in the midst of their lockdown and social isolation measures for combatting COVID-19 suggested that for some couples, an increase in awareness and appreciation of their significant other was actually improving their marital satisfaction (Morris, 2020). This in part was as a result of "role renegotiation" in the home. Seemingly some of the more traditional gendered roles around child-rearing have been challenged as parents are both spending more equal amounts of time at home with their children (Morris, 2020). Parents are also reporting an enjoyment of the home time afforded by the quarantine measures with the constant travels for the school, extracurricular and social activities of their children no longer impinging on family time (Wang et al., 2020). Several information studies undertaken in the United Kingdom (Childcare.co.UK, 2020) and the United States (Mtetwa, 2020) suggest somewhere between 25 and 40% of parents are considering ongoing home-schooling options in the postpandemic period. Indeed in Australia parents are reporting a "surprising" enjoyment out of the quarantine home-schooling and had developed a confidence in their capacity to support their children's academic development (Morris, 2020). Children too have reported increasing levels of respect had been developed during the pandemic as both they and their parents were provided an opportunity in perspective tasking (Szabo et al., 2020).

These positive outcomes, borne out of adaptation and resiliency at the family level, to the many challenges the individual family members and the family unit had experienced during the COVID-19 pandemic. Such familial posttraumatic growth sees parents and children managing to draw together under a belief that the family could overcome the challenges it was facing (Morris, 2020). Those families best placed to experience such growth are those led by parents, typically with an authoritarian parenting style provided within a context of warmth (Horesh & Brown, 2018) that are able to establish a collective value and belief system that all family members invest in (Evans, Boustead, & Owens, 2008).

Conclusion

The COVID-19 pandemic has undoubtedly impacted the roles, practices, and wellbeing of parents, and, inherently the larger family unit. The extraordinary times that parents are traversing through are without close parallel and with little to no warning parents have found themselves navigating some truly stressful circumstances that are affecting them directly and indirectly, via their children (and partners). Unsurprisingly these stressors, by way of their number and uniqueness, do pose a significant risk to parents' mental health leading to the reality of increasing levels of parental burnout and familial neglect and abuse. However, this period of challenge has also been a time of growth and resilience for some families on the back of facing and overcoming the pandemic challenges together. As the chief executive officers of their households, parents hold significant responsibility for wellbeing outcomes of their family unit during the COVID-19 pandemic. As such, benefits will be found from enabling families to minimize the stressors they are facing and to learn strategies in psychological flexibility and adaptability. This will place them in a better position to cope with the shifting landscape that currently affords no time course for its conclusion.

Finally, it is critical that families who do find themselves in circumstances they are unable to control are provided with meaningful support to avoid the family slipping into patterns of neglect and/or violence. The outcomes of the COVID-19 pandemic for parents are not inevitably negative and moving toward outcomes of remarkable positivity and growth is equally possible during this remarkable COVID-19 pandemic period.

References

'Yotti' Kingsley, J., Townsend, M., Phillips, R., & Aldous, D. (2009). "If the land is healthy … it makes the people healthy": The relationship between caring for Country and health for the Yorta Yorta Nation, Boonwurrung and Bangerang Tribes. *Health & Place*, *15*(1), 291–299. https://doi.org/10.1016/j.healthplace.2008.05.009.

Ackerman, B. P., Kogos, J., Youngstrom, E., Schoff, K., & Izard, C. (1999). Family instability and the problem behaviors of children from economically disadvantaged families. *Developmental Psychology*, *35*(1), 258–268. https://doi.org/10.1037//0012-1649.35.1.258.

Ahmed, M., Advani, S., Moreira, A., Zoretic, S., Martinez, J., Chorath, K., et al. (2020). Multisystem inflammatory syndrome in children: A systematic review. *EClinicalMedicine*. https://doi.org/10.1016/j.eclinm.2020.100527, 100527.

American Psychological Association. (2020). High stress related to coronavirus is the new normal for many parents, says new APA survey. *Mental Health Weekly Digest*, *256*.

Barsom, E. Z., Feenstra, T. M., Bemelman, W. A., Bonjer, J. H., & Schijven, M. P. (2020). Coping with COVID-19: Scaling up virtual care to standard practice. *Nature Medicine*, *26*(5), 632–634. https://doi.org/10.1038/s41591-020-0845-0.

Beckerman, M., van Berkel, S. R., Mesman, J., & Alink, L. R. A. (2016). The role of negative parental attributions in the associations between daily stressors, maltreatment history, and harsh and abusive discipline. *Child Abuse & Neglect*, *64*, 109–116. https://doi.org/10.1016/j.chiabu.2016.12.015.

Bengtson, V. L. (2001). Beyond the nuclear family: The increasing importance of multigenerational bonds. *Journal of Marriage and Family*, *63*(1), 1–16. https://doi.org/10.1111/j.1741-3737.2001.00001.x.

Biggs, A., Brough, P., & Drummond, S. (2017). *Lazarus and Folkman's psychological stress and coping theory* (pp. 349–364). Chichester, UK: John Wiley & Sons, Ltd.

Boston University. (2017). Researchers from Boston University report details of new studies and findings in the area of pediatrics (modifiable resilience factors to childhood adversity for clinical pediatric practice). *Health & Medicine Week*, *554*.

Bowen, M. (1966). The use of family theory in clinical practice. *Comprehensive Psychiatry*, *7*(5), 345–374. https://doi.org/10.1016/s0010-440x(66)80065-2.

Bronfenbrenner, U. (1981). *The ecology of human development: Experiments by nature and design*. Cambridge: Harvard University Press.

Brown, S. M., Doom, J. R., Lechuga-Peña, S., Watamura, S. E., & Koppels, T. (2020). Stress and parenting during the global COVID-19 pandemic. *Child Abuse & Neglect*. https://doi.org/10.1016/j.chiabu.2020.104699, 104699.

Buitron, V., Hill, R. M., Pettit, J. W., Green, K. L., Hatkevich, C., & Sharp, C. (2016). Interpersonal stress and suicidal ideation in adolescence: An indirect association through perceived burdensomeness toward others. *Journal of Affective Disorders*, *190*, 143–149. https://doi.org/10.1016/j.jad.2015.09.077.

Calhoun, L. G., & Tedeschi, R. G. (1998). Beyond recovery from trauma: Implications for clinical practice and research. *Journal of Social Issues*, *54*(2), 357–371. https://doi.org/10.1111/0022-4537.701998070.

Campbell, A. M. (2020). An increasing risk of family violence during the Covid-19 pandemic: Strengthening community collaborations to save lives. *Forensic Science International: Reports*, *2*, 100089. https://doi.org/10.1016/j.fsir.2020.100089.

Carr, A. (2016). *The evolution of systems theory* (1st ed., pp. 13–29). Routledge.

Chary, M., McQuillan, M. E., Bates, J. E., & Deater-Deckard, K. (2018). Maternal executive function and sleep interact in the prediction of negative parenting. *Behavioral Sleep Medicine*, *18*(2), 203–216. https://doi.org/10.1080/15402002.2018.1549042.

Childcare.co.UK. (2020). *Nearly 1 in 4 parents say they are more likely to home school their children after the Coronavirus pandemic is over*. Retrieved from: https://www.childcare.co.uk/news/homeschool.

Colbert, S., Wilkinson, C., Thornton, L., & Richmond, R. (2020). COVID-19 and alcohol in Australia: Industry changes and public health impacts. *Drug and Alcohol Review*, *39*(5), 435–440. https://doi.org/10.1111/dar.13092.

Coleman, L., & Glenn, F. (2010). The varied impact of couple relationship breakdown on children: Implications for practice and policy. *Children & Society*, *24*(3), 238–249. https://doi.org/10.1111/j.1099-0860.2009.00289.x.

Cooklin, A. R., Giallo, R., & Rose, N. (2012). Parental fatigue and parenting practices during early childhood: An Australian community survey. *Child: Care, Health and Development*, *38*(5), 654–664. https://doi.org/10.1111/j.1365-2214.2011.01333.x.

Coyne, L. W., Gould, E. R., Grimaldi, M., Wilson, K. G., Baffuto, G., & Biglan, A. (2020). First things first: Parent psychological flexibility and self-compassion during COVID-19. *Behavior Analysis in Practice*, *1*. https://doi.org/10.1007/s40617-020-00435-w.

Dijkstra, M. T. M., & Homan, A. C. (2016). Engaging in rather than disengaging from stress: Effective coping and perceived control. *Frontiers in Psychology*, *7*. https://doi.org/10.3389/fpsyg.2016.01415.

Doyle, O. (2020). *COVID-19: Exacerbating educational inequalities?*. Retrieved from: http://publicpolicy.ie/papers/covid-19-exacerbating-educational-inequalities/.

Duxbury, L., Higgins, C., & Lee, C. (1994). Work-family conflict: A comparison by gender, family type, and perceived control. *Journal of Family Issues*, *15*(3), 449–466. https://doi.org/10.1177/019251394015003006.

Eastin, C., & Eastin, T. (2020). Epidemiological characteristics of 2143 pediatric patients with 2019 coronavirus disease in China: Dong Y, Mo X, Hu Y, et al. *The Journal of Emergency Medicine*, *58*(4), 712–713. https://doi.org/10.1016/j.jemermed.2020.04.006.

Evans, C., Boustead, R., & Owens, C. (2008). Expressions of spirituality in parents with at-risk children. *Families in Society: The Journal of Contemporary Social Services*, *89*(2), 245–252. https://doi.org/10.1606/1044-3894.3740.

Fave, A. D. (2004). Well-being. Positive development across the life course. In M. H. Bronstein, L. Davidson, C. L. M. Keyes, K. A. Moore, & The Centre for Child Well-Being (Eds.), *Infant and child development* (pp. 361–362). Mahwah, NJ: Lawrence Erlbaum Associates.

Feldman, R. (2016). Parent–infant synchrony. *Current Directions in Psychological Science: A Journal of the American Psychological Society*, *16*(6), 340–345. https://doi.org/10.1111/j.1467-8721.2007.00532.x.

Fontanesi, L., Marchetti, D., Mazza, C., Di Giandomenico, S., Roma, P., & Verrocchio, M. C. (2020). The effect of the COVID-19 lockdown on parents: A call to adopt urgent measures. *Psychological Trauma*, *12*(S1), S79–S81. https://doi.org/10.1037/tra0000672.

Fortier-Brochu, É., Beaulieu-Bonneau, S., Ivers, H., & Morin, C. M. (2012). Insomnia and daytime cognitive performance: A meta-analysis. *Sleep Medicine Reviews*, *16*(1), 83–94. https://doi.org/10.1016/j.smrv.2011.03.008.

Fredrickson, B. L. (2001). The role of positive emotions in positive psychology. The broaden-and-build theory of positive emotions. *The American Psychologist*, *56*(3), 218–226. https://doi.org/10.1037//0003-066X.56.3.218.

Gardner, F., Shaw, D. S., Dishion, T. J., Burton, J., & Supplee, L. (2007). Randomized prevention trial for early conduct problems: Effects on proactive parenting and links to toddler disruptive behavior. *Journal of Family Psychology*, *21*(3), 398–406. https://doi.org/10.1037/0893-3200.21.3.398.

Ghosh, R., Dubey, M. J., Chatterjee, S., & Dubey, S. (2020). Impact of COVID-19 on children: Special focus on psychosocial aspect. *Minerva Pediatricia*, *72*(3), 226–235.

Griffith, A. (2020). Parental burnout and child maltreatment during the COVID-19 pandemic. *Journal of Family Violence*, *23*, 1–7.

Grose, M. (2010). *Thriving! Raising confident kids with confidence, character and resilience*. Sydney: Random House Australia.

Haig-Ferguson, A., Cooper, K., Cartwright, E., Loades, M. E., & Daniels, J. (2020). Practitioner review: Health anxiety in children and young people in the context of the COVID-19 pandemic. *Behavioural and Cognitive Psychotherapy*, 1–34. https://doi.org/10.1017/S1352465820000636.

Heffernan, E. B., Andersen, K. C., Dev, A., & Kinner, S. (2012). Prevalence of mental illness among Aboriginal and Torres Strait Islander people in Queensland prisons. *Medical Journal of Australia*, *197*(1), 37–41. https://doi.org/10.5694/mja11.11352.

Hertz, R., & Marshall, N. L. (2001). *Working families: The transformation of the American home*. Berkeley: University of California Press.

Horesh, D., & Brown, A. D. (2018). Editorial: Post-traumatic stress in the family. *Frontiers in Psychology*, *9*, 40. https://doi.org/10.3389/fpsyg.2018.00040.

Howard, M. (2020). Coffee catch-ups. *Planning News*, *46*(5), 26.

Huang, Y., & Zhao, N. (2020). Generalized anxiety disorder, depressive symptoms and sleep quality during COVID-19 outbreak in China: A web-based cross-sectional survey. *Psychiatry Research*, *288*, 112954. https://doi.org/10.1016/j.psychres.2020.112954.

Humphreys, K., Myint, M. T., & Zeanah, C. H. (2020). Increased risk for family violence during the COVID-19 pandemic. *Pediatrics*, *146*(1), e20200982.

Hurley, D. (2020). Sleep neurologists call it 'COVID-Somnia'—Increased sleep disturbances linked to the pandemic. *Neurology Today*, *20*(13), 1–27. https://doi.org/10.1097/01.NT.0000694012.58759.9c.

Isumi, A., Doi, S., Yamaoka, Y., Takahashi, K., & Fujiwara, T. (2020). Do suicide rates in children and adolescents change during school closure in Japan? The acute effect of the first wave of COVID-19 pandemic on child and adolescent mental health. *Child Abuse & Neglect*. https://doi.org/10.1016/j.chiabu.2020.104680, 104680.

Johnston, K. (2020). *Covid 19 coronavirus: Domestic violence is the second, silent epidemic amid lockdown*. Retrieved from: https://www.nzherald.co.nz/nz/news/article.cfm?c_id=1&objectid=12324237.

Kagi, J. (2020). *Crime rate in WA plunges amid coronavirus social distancing lockdown measures*. Retrieved from: https://www.abc.net.au/news/2020-04-08/coronavirus-shutdown-sees-crime-rate-drop-in-wa/12132410.

Kawamoto, T., Furutani, K., & Alimardani, M. (2018). Preliminary validation of japanese version of the parental burnout inventory and its relationship with perfectionism. *Frontiers in Psychology*, *9*. https://doi.org/10.3389/fpsyg.2018.00970.

Kelley, M. L., Self-Brown, S., Le, B., Bosson, J. V., Hernandez, B. C., & Gordon, A. T. (2010). Predicting posttraumatic stress symptoms in children following Hurricane Katrina: A prospective analysis of the effect of parental distress and parenting practices. *Journal of Traumatic Stress*, *23*(5), 582–590. https://doi.org/10.1002/jts.20573.

Kilroy, S. J., Egan, J., Maliszewska, A., & Sarma, K. M. (2014). "Systemic trauma": The impact on parents whose children have experienced sexual abuse. *Journal of Child Sexual Abuse*, *23*(5), 481–503. https://doi.org/10.1080/10538712.2014.920458.

Kliewer, W., Parrish, K. A., Taylor, K. W., Jackson, K., Walker, J. M., & Shivy, V. A. (2006). Socialization of coping with community violence: Influences of caregiver coaching, modeling, and family context. *Child Development*, *77*(3), 605–623. https://doi.org/10.1111/j.1467-8624.2006.00893.x.

Lazarus, R. S. (1984). *Stress, appraisal, and coping*. New York: Springer.

Lee, P.-I., Hu, Y.-L., Chen, P.-Y., Huang, Y.-C., & Hsueh, P.-R. (2020). Are children less susceptible to COVID-19? *Journal of Microbiology, Immunology and Infection*, *53*(3), 371–372. https://doi.org/10.1016/j.jmii.2020.02.011.

Lindstrom, C., Aman, J., & Norberg, A. L. (2010). Increased prevalence of burnout symptoms in parents of chronically ill children. *Acta Paediatrica*, *99*(3), 427–432. https://doi.org/10.1111/j.1651-2227.2009.01586.x.

Liu, J. J., Bao, Y., Huang, X., Shi, J., & Lu, L. (2020). Mental health considerations for children quarantined because of COVID-19. *Lancet Child and Adolescent*, *4*, 347–349.

Loades, M. E., Chatburn, E., Higson-Sweeney, N., Reynolds, S., Shafran, R., Brigden, A., et al. (2020). Rapid systematic review: The impact of social isolation and loneliness on the mental health of children and adolescents in the context of COVID-19. *Journal of the American Academy of Child and Adolescent Psychiatry*. https://doi.org/10.1016/j.jaac.2020.05.009.

Ludvigsson, J. F. (2020). Systematic review of COVID-19 in children shows milder cases and a better prognosis than adults. *Acta Paediatrica (Oslo)*, *109*(6), 1088–1095. https://doi.org/10.1111/apa.15270.

Marques, E. S., Moraes, C. L.d., Hasselmann, M. H., Deslandes, S. F., & Reichenheim, M. E. (2020). Violence against women, children, and adolescents during the COVID-19 pandemic: Overview, contributing factors, and mitigating measures. *Cadernos de Saúde Pública*, *36*(4), e00074420.

McCann, D., Bull, R., & Winzenberg, T. (2015). Sleep deprivation in parents caring for children with complex needs at home: A mixed methods systematic review. *Journal of Family Nursing*, *21*(1), 86–118. https://doi.org/10.1177/1074840714562026.

Meadows, S. (2018). *Understanding child development: Psychological perspectives and applications* (1st ed.). Milton: Routledge.

Meltzer, L. J. P., & Montgomery-Downs, H. E. P. (2011). Sleep in the family. *Pediatric Clinics of North America*, *58*(3), 765–774. https://doi.org/10.1016/j.pcl.2011.03.010.

Mikolajczak, M., Brianda, M. E., Avalosse, H., & Roskam, I. (2018). Consequences of parental burnout: Its specific effect on child neglect and violence. *Child Abuse & Neglect*, *80*, 134–145. https://doi.org/10.1016/j.chiabu.2018.03.025.

Mikolajczak, M., Gross, J. J., & Roskam, I. (2019). Parental burnout: What is it, and why does it matter? *Clinical Psychological Science*, *7*(6). https://doi.org/10.1177/2167702619858430. 216770261985843-216770261981329.

Mikolajczak, M., Gross, J. J., Stinglhamber, F., Lindahl Norberg, A., & Roskam, I. (2020). Is parental burnout distinct from job burnout and depressive symptoms? *Clinical Psychological Science*, *8*(4). https://doi.org/10.1177/2167702620917447. 216770262091744-216770262091689.

Miles, M. S., Carter, M. C., Spicher, C., & Hassanein, R. (1984). Maternal and paternal stress reactions when a child is hospitalized in a pediatric intensive care unit. *Issues in Comprehensive Pediatric Nursing*, *7*(6), 333–342. https://doi.org/10.3109/01460868409009770.

Morris, E. (2020). *How families are closer after time together in coronavirus isolation*. Retrieved from: https://www.abc.net.au/life/how-families-are-even-closer-after-coronavirus-isolation/12262812.

Morrow, M. R. (2019). *How many hours do you homeschool?*. Retrieved from: https://www.homeschoolingdownunder.com/how_many_hours_do_you_homeschool/.

Mtetwa, D. (2020). *Survey shows up to 40% of parents will continue to homeschool after lockdown ends*. Retrieved from: https://www.moms.com/parents-will-continue-to-homeschool-after-lockdown-ends-survey/.

Mueller, C., Rowe, M. L., & Zuckerman, B. (2017). Mindset matters for parents and adolescents. *JAMA Pediatrics*, *171*(5), 415–416. https://doi.org/10.1001/jamapediatrics.2016.5160.

Murray, M. (2003). Treading water: Self-reflections on generalized anxiety disorder. *Human Architecture*, *2*(1), 50.

Newland, R. P., & Crnic, K. A. (2017). Developmental risk and goodness of fit in the mother–child relationship: Links to parenting stress and children's behaviour problems. *Infant and Child Development*, *26*(2). https://doi.org/10.1002/icd.1980.

Pai, A. L. H., Greenley, R. N., Lewandowski, A., Drotar, D., Youngstrom, E., & Peterson, C. C. (2007). A meta-analytic review of the influence of pediatric cancer on parent and family functioning. *Journal of Family Psychology*, *21*(3), 407–415. https://doi.org/10.1037/0893-3200.21.3.407.

Parczewska, T. (2020). Difficult situations and ways of coping with them in the experiences of parents homeschooling their children during the COVID-19 pandemic in Poland. *Education, 3-13*, 1–12. https://doi.org/10.1080/03004279.2020.1812689.

Paster, A., Brandwein, D., & Walsh, J. (2009). A comparison of coping strategies used by parents of children with disabilities and parents of children without disabilities. *Research in Developmental Disabilities*, *30*(6), 1337–1342. https://doi.org/10.1016/j.ridd.2009.05.010.

Patrick, S. W., Henkhaus, L. E., Zickafoose, J. S., Lovell, K., Halvorson, A., Loch, S., et al. (2020). Well-being of parents and children during the COVID-19 pandemic: A national survey. *Pediatrics*, *146*(4).

Patterson, J. M. (2002). Integrating family resilience and family stress theory. *Journal of Marriage and Family*, *64*(2), 349–360. https://doi.org/10.1111/j.1741-3737.2002.00349.x.

Pelham, W. E., & Lang, A. R. (1999). Can your children drive you to drink? *Alcohol Research & Health*, *23*(4), 292.

Pew Research Centre. (2015). *Parenting in America: Outlook, worries, aspirations are strongly linked to financial situation*. United States: Pew Research Centre.

Pew Research Centre. (2020). *Most Americans say coronavirus outbreak has impacted their lives*. Retrieved from: https://www.pewsocialtrends.org/wp-content/uploads/sites/3/2020/03/PSDT_03.30.20_W64-COVID-19.Personal-impact-FULL-REPORT.pdf.

Poate, S. (2020). *75% increase in domestic violence searches since coronavirus*. Retrieved from: https://www.nbnnews.com.au/2020/03/31/dvsearches-coronavirus/.

Poole-Boykin, C. (2020). *Homeschooling during COVID-19: Why all kids may not need eight hours of instruction a day at home*. Retrieved from: https://www.goodmorningamerica.com/family/story/parents-teachers-tips-homeschooling-covid-19-kids-hours-69774140.

Portrie, T., & Hill, N. R. (2016). Blended families: A critical review of the current research. *The Family Journal (Alexandria, VA)*, *13*(4), 445–451. https://doi.org/10.1177/1066480705279014.

Prime, H., Wade, M., & Browne, D. T. (2020). Risk and resilience in family well-being during the COVID-19 pandemic. *The American Psychologist*, *75*(5), 631–643. https://doi.org/10.1037/amp0000660.

Qouta, S., Punamäki, R.-L., & El Sarraj, E. (2008). Child development and family mental health in war and military violence: The Palestinian experience. *International Journal of Behavioral Development*, *32*(4), 310–321. https://doi.org/10.1177/0165025408090973.

Rolland, J. S. (2020). COVID-19 pandemic: Applying a multi-systemic lens. *Family Process*. https://doi.org/10.1111/famp.12584.

Ruggles, S. (1994). The transformation of American family structure. *The American Historical Review*, *99*(1), 103–128. https://doi.org/10.1086/ahr/99.1.103.

Schrodt, P., Witt, P. L., & Messersmith, A. S. (2008). A meta-analytical review of family communication patterns and their associations with information processing, behavioral, and psychosocial outcomes. *Communication Monographs*, *75*(3), 248–269. https://doi.org/10.1080/03637750802256318.

Spinelli, M., Lionetti, F., Pastore, M., & Fasolo, M. (2020). Parents' stress and children's psychological problems in families facing the COVID-19 outbreak in Italy. *Frontiers in Psychology*, *11*. https://doi.org/10.3389/fpsyg.2020.01713.

Sprang, G., & Silman, M. (2013). Posttraumatic stress disorder in parents and youth after health-related disasters. *Disaster Medicine and Public Health Preparedness*, *7*, 105–110.

Stanke, C., Murray, V., Amlôt, R., Nurse, J., & Williams, R. (2012). The effects of flooding on mental health: Outcomes and recommendations from a review of the literature. *PLoS Currents*, *4*. https://doi.org/10.1371/4f9f1fa9c3cae, e4f9f1fa9c3cae.

Strohschein, L., & Gauthier, A. H. (2017). Poverty dynamics, parenting, and child mental health in Canada. *Society and Mental Health*, *8*(3), 231–247. https://doi.org/10.1177/2156869317731603.

Szabo, T. G., Richling, S., Embry, D. D., Biglan, A., & Wilson, K. G. (2020). From helpless to hero: Promoting values-based behavior and positive family interaction in the midst of COVID-19. *Behavior Analysis in Practice*, *13*(3), 568–576. https://doi.org/10.1007/s40617-020-00431-0.

Taylor, D. J., Lichstein, K. L., & Durrence, H. H. (2003). Insomnia as a health risk factor. *Behavioral Sleep Medicine*, *1*(4), 227–247. https://doi.org/10.1207/s15402010bsm0104_5.

The National Inquiry Into the Separation of Aboriginal, & Torres Strait Islander Children From Their Families. (1997). *Bringing them home: Report of the national inquiry into the separation of aboriginal and torres strait islander children from their families*. Sydney: Human Rights and Equal Opportunity Commission.

Usher, K., Bhullar, N., Durkin, J., Gyamfi, N., & Jackson, D. (2020). Family violence and COVID-19: Increased vulnerability and reduced options for support. *International Journal of Mental Health Nursing*, *29*(4), 549–552. https://doi.org/10.1111/inm.12735.

Vaala, S. E., & Bleakley, A. (2015). Monitoring, mediating, and modeling: Parental influence on adolescent computer and internet use in the United States. *Journal of Children and Media: Children and Media in the Family Context*, *9*(1), 40–57. https://doi.org/10.1080/17482798.2015.997103.

Van Baval, J., Baiker, K., Boggio, P. S., Capraro, V., Cichocka, A., Cikara, M., et al. (2020). Using social and behavioural science to support COVID-19 pandemic response. *Nature Human Behaviour*, *4*(5), 460–471. https://doi.org/10.1038/s41562-020-0884-z.

van Gelder, N., Peterman, A., Potts, A., O'Donnell, M., Thompson, K., Shah, N., et al. (2020). COVID-19: Reducing the risk of infection might increase the risk of intimate partner violence. *EClinicalMedicine*, *21*, 100348. https://doi.org/10.1016/j.eclinm.2020.100348.

Wang, G., Zhang, Y., Zhao, J., Zhang, J., & Jiang, F. (2020). Mitigate the effects of home confinement on children during the COVID-19 outbreak. *The Lancet (British Edition)*, *395*(10228), 945–947. https://doi.org/10.1016/s0140-6736(20)30547-x.

Webster, P. (2020). Virtual health care in the era of COVID-19. *The Lancet (British Edition), 395*(10231), 1180–1181. https://doi.org/10.1016/S0140-6736(20)30818-7.

Willmott, M., Nicholson, A., Busse, H., MacArthur, G. J., Brookes, S., & Campbell, R. (2016). Effectiveness of hand hygiene interventions in reducing illness absence among children in educational settings: A systematic review and meta-analysis. *Archives of Disease in Childhood, 101*(1), 42–50. https://doi.org/10.1136/archdischild-2015-308875.

World Health Organisation. (1994). *Global strategy on occupational health for all: The way to health at work.* Beijing, China: WHO.

Xiang, Y.-T., Yang, Y., Li, W., Zhang, L., Zhang, Q., Cheung, T., et al. (2020). Timely mental health care for the 2019 novel coronavirus outbreak is urgently needed. *The Lancet Psychiatry, 7*(3), 228–229. https://doi.org/10.1016/s2215-0366(20)30046-8.

Chapter 15

Compliance with health-protective behaviors in relation to COVID-19: The roles of health-related misinformation, perceived vulnerability, and personality traits

Zahir Vally

Department of Clinical Psychology, United Arab Emirates University, Al Ain, United Arab Emirates; Nuffield Department of Population Health, University of Oxford, Oxford, United Kingdom

Introduction

The year 2019 witnessed the emergence of the novel coronavirus disease which precipitated extraordinary challenges for humankind. People across the globe and across all segments of society were called upon to work collectively in restraining the spread of the disease. In an attempt to do so, countless governments implemented a range of measures that variously included the imposition of curfews limiting movement of their residents, both within and between countries, mandated home quarantine, closure of public spaces, social distancing requirements, and isolation of those infected or suspected of infection. Moreover, governments also commensurately recommended, and at varying times, required of their residents, strict adherence to a number of behaviors (e.g., handwashing and mask wearing being the most common) directed at suppressing the spread of the disease, controlling the number of infections at any given point in time, and therefore buffering the consequent strain that would inevitably be placed on health services.

Alongside the work of ensuring that health facilities could meet the task of completing the requisite testing for the virus and the fervent race to develop a vaccine and/or treatment, social scientists and public health professionals have been challenged to understand how best to ensure that the public comply with

Mental Health Effects of COVID-19. https://doi.org/10.1016/B978-0-12-824289-6.00001-5

these health-protective behaviors and continue to cooperate with official directives over time. During previous public health crises, the mobilization of public support for official health-protective guidance was most likely when communication about the disease and the strategies residents should employ to protect themselves and others was clear and understandable (Rubin, Amlot, Page, & Wessely, 2009). The general rationale in relation to the provision of clear and transparent information is that the public must understand the magnitude of the challenge that their society is facing and thus be persuaded of the value of compliance. This is a sensible course of action, especially where the recommended behaviors such as social distancing and self-quarantine, as is the case for COVID-19, may be perceived as being burdensome and laborious. Coercion is unlikely to prove successful particularly in democratic societies. During the lockdown period of 2020, some countries imposed exorbitant fines for infringement of the required behaviors. In the United Arab Emirates, for example, the Dubai Police used radar surveillance systems to monitor motorists violating the imposed curfew, introduced fines for infringements, and published the identities of violators in the media (Vally, 2020). In the United Kingdom, September 2020 saw the introduction of harsh penalties for refusing to self-isolate. The prime minister announced that if individuals test positive for COVID-19 or are instructed to self-isolate by the National Health Service, they are legally obliged to self-isolate, refusal to do so could carry a fine of up to £10,000.

In an attempt to explain which beliefs and attitudes are associated with the adoption of health-protective behaviors, the Health Beliefs Model (Janz & Becker, 1984; Rosenstock, Strecher, & Becker, 1994) is a frequently cited framework and has been applied to examine a range of health-related issues such as smoking (Mohammadi et al., 2017), vaccination (Vermandere et al., 2016), HIV risk behaviors (Zhao et al., 2012), adherence to exercise regimens (Soleymanian, Niknami, Hajizadeh, Shojaeizadeh, & Montazeri, 2014), and engagement in dietary behaviors (Khoramabadi et al., 2015). The Health Beliefs Model regards the following five factors as being instrumental in accounting for the adoption of health-protective behaviors: 1. Threat perceptions, 2. Response efficacy beliefs, 3. Self-efficacy, 4. Cues to action, and 5. Individual characteristics. Factors 1, 2, and 3 are most relevant to the present review. Threat perceptions consist of two components, perceived vulnerability and perceived severity, which collectively capture an individual's subjective belief about their perceived degree of vulnerability to a given illness and the perceived level of severity of the consequences of becoming infected. Response efficacy beliefs and self-efficacy refer to the individual's perception of the likely efficacy of the recommended health-protective behaviors and their confidence in their capacity to enact them successfully (Janz & Becker, 1984; Rosenstock et al., 1994). The evidence in support of this model's contentions suggests that where individuals perceive themselves to be at greater risk of infection and that the consequences of infection would be substantially severe, individuals are more likely to exact compliance with behaviors designed to protect themselves from these deleterious consequences. Moreover, where the recommended behaviors are perceived to be effective and individuals perceive themselves to be capable of deploying them, rates of compliance similarly increase (Clark, Davila, Regis, & Kraus, 2020).

A review of the literature that has proliferated over the course of 2020 has revealed that these factors may indeed also be relevant in understanding the public's level of compliance with health-protective behaviors toward COVID-19. This chapter reviews the current literature relating to three principal predictive variables that the literature suggests may be related to compliance: the tendency to believe and propagate health-related misinformation (commonly referred to as conspiracy theories), varying perceptions/beliefs relating to threat or vulnerability to the disease, and personality traits, both those regarded as socially desirable and the dark traits. These three factors are reviewed in turn below.

Health-related misinformation

Some individuals hold the belief that major public events, including public health crises, are secretly masterminded by nefarious entities within society or at the governmental level to serve some malicious or self-serving purpose. The prevailing tendency to believe in conspiracy theories and its resultant impact in shaping social reality were captured in Popper's (1969) "conspiracy theory of society" and Hofstadter's (1964) "conspirational fantasies." Five decades later, within the context of the COVID-19 pandemic, conspiracy theories relating to the purported origin of the virus abound online. The pandemic is an ideal context for the proliferation of conspiracy theories as this crisis situation is fraught with uncertainty. Indeed, a range of theories have surfaced online that propose that the COVID-19 virus was developed as a bioweapon by China, or the CIA, that a vaccine exists but is being withheld to incite panic and profit off the pandemic, or that the virus is caused by exposure to the 5G mobile network (Ahmed, Vidal-Alaball, Downing, & López Seguí, 2020; Conspiracy Watch, 2020).

Belief in conspiracy theories appears to be common. For example, 43% of French respondents believe that health authorities are concealing the negative effects of vaccinations and 27% of the population believe in the existence of the Illuminati, a supposed secret society whose membership includes influential people from government and industry that operates in the shadows manipulating political and socioeconomic events (Ifop, 2019). The consistent finding that individuals who endorse a conspiracy theory are also likely to endorse a range of additional, sometimes mutually exclusive theories, have prompted some scholars to suggest that a general worldview may underlie conspiracy beliefs which Bruder, Haffke, Neave, Nouripanah, and Imhoff (2013) refer to as a *conspiracy mentality*. Subscribing to conspiracy beliefs has frequently been shown to relate to less engagement in health-protective behaviors in relation to HIV, childhood vaccination, or the practice of safe sex (Dunn et al., 2017; Goertzel, 2010; Grebe & Nattrass, 2011; Jolley & Douglas, 2014; Thorburn & Bogart, 2005;

Zimmerman et al., 2005). Similarly, Lamberty and Imhoff (2018) report that the presence of a conspiracy mentality was associated with the preferred use of alternative therapies as opposed to the recommended biomedical treatment. These studies collectively suggest that people who subscribe to conspiracy beliefs tend to engage in nonnormative preventive behaviors (i.e., those not promoted or required by the government), because, as Marinthe, Brown, Delouvée, and Jolley (2020) suggest, these behaviors are typically endorsed by the low-power rather than high-power entities in society. This is a particularly troublesome finding when one considers the typical response that followed the WHO's declaration of COVID-19 as a pandemic. Most governments across the globe instituted mandated measures that significantly impacted the lives of its residents. These measures were often substantial, restricting work, schooling, and the normalcy of life but were intended to impede the spread of the virus. Some individuals clearly experienced adherence to these measures as an onerous task and this may indeed have impacted the consistency with which they adhered to the recommended behaviors to prevent infection (Vally, 2020). An additional and reasonable prediction would be that individuals who espouse a conspiracy mentality would actively resist adherence to these imposed measures, whether recommended or mandatory, as the information flowed directly from governments and public health agencies, entities that represent "untrusted" sources of information for individuals who hold a conspiracy mentality. But this skepticism and mistrust would place both themselves and others at risk of infection. A burgeoning body of literature conducted in the midst of this pandemic suggests that this may very well be the case. These studies linking a conspiracy mentality and its ensuing impact on the adoption of normative preventive behaviors are reviewed later in this chapter.

The propagation of health-related misinformation on social media

Conspiracy theories are frequently propagated across social media platforms but also, to a lesser extent, in mainstream broadcast and print media. Social media is described as being the home of conflicting information, misinformation, and manipulated information with some arguing that this phenomenon should be regarded as a serious threat to global public health (Larson, 2018). A plethora of studies spanning a diverse range of world regions have found that social media platforms, specifically, Facebook, Twitter, and YouTube are significant mechanisms for the dispersal of misinformation related to medical issues. For example, during the H1N1 influenza outbreak, researchers found that YouTube contained a substantial amount of useful information about the pandemic, 61.3% of the videos examined contained useful information about the disease, much of which originated from the Centers for Disease Control and Prevention, however, 23% of the uploaded videos contained misleading information (Pandey, Patni, Sing, Sood, & Singh, 2010). Researchers recently conducted a similar video analysis of YouTube content in relation to COVID-19 information and found that over one-quarter of the most viewed videos about COVID-19 contained inaccurate information and had been viewed, at the time of analysis, more than 62 million times (Oi-Yee Li, Bailey, Huynh, & Chan, 2020). A similar pattern of misinformation has been found on Twitter. Kouzy et al. (2020) examined tweets using 14 different trending hashtags and keywords about COVID-19 and found that 24.8% contained clear misinformation and a further 17.4% included information that was unverifiable.

Broadcast and print media tend to be closely regulated while social media content remains largely unregulated. Misinformation about COVID-19 was recently broadcast on the London Live television station to which the broadcast regulator in the United Kingdom responded by sanctioning the owner of the station for broadcasting content that posed harmful consequences to viewers (Ofcom, 2020). In contrast, similar content continues to be distributed on social media with some platforms exercising occasional and/or inconsistent editorial monitoring (Brennen, Simon, Howard, & Nielsen, 2020). This lack of active monitoring and control is precisely what conspiracy theorists capitalize upon in propagating their misinformation.

Factors associated with the sharing of COVID-19 misinformation

An interesting area of research that has recently emerged has sought to determine which psychological factors are associated with the increased likelihood to share, upload, or retweet COVID-19 misinformation on social media. The results of this line of study indicate that individuals who are experiencing social media fatigue or information overload and those who exhibit a deficiency in their capacity for self-regulation are more prone to share unverified COVID-19 information while individuals who are driven by the need for self-promotion are less likely to do so (Islam, Laato, Talukder, & Sutinen, 2020; Laato, Islam, Islam, & Whelan, 2020). These three factors are discussed in turn.

Social media fatigue (SMF) has variously been defined as "persistent impulses to back away from social media due to information and communication overload" (Bright, Kleiser, & Grau, 2015) and "a subjective and self-evaluated feeling of tiredness from social media use" (Lee, Son, & Kim, 2016). Cognitive Load Theory (CLT) postulates that human beings possess a limited capacity for working memory and, if presented with information that exceeds this capacity, information overload occurs (Sweller, 2011). When overloaded, the evolutionary protective mechanism is to retreat and avoid the source of the incoming information (Sweller, 2011). Within the context of social media and COVID-19, this is certainly relevant. Given the scale of the pandemic and its rapidly evolving nature, information detailing its progression, the virus' spread across the globe, rates of infection and mortality and, of course, postulations about its origin were being generated and broadcast at an exponential rate. Thus, if the proposition of CLT is to be believed, any individual experiencing SMF (communication and information overload) would possess less cognitive resources to process this onslaught of information and which would consequently inhibit their ability to verify any of the information and further increasing the likelihood of them sharing this potential misinformation. Similar findings in previous research also demonstrate a connection between SMF and the tendency to share fake news which suggests that, when users become fatigued, they do not disengage from the platform, but rather they become less cognizant of interrogating the authenticity of the content they have viewed and shared (Talwar, Dhir, Kaur, Zafar, & Alrasheedy, 2019).

Individuals who possess deficient self-regulation (DSR) skills are typically unable to exert thoughtful control and planning over their actions but are rather driven by impulse and habit (Whelan, Islam, & Brooks, 2020). Empirical evidence has linked DSR to engagement in maladaptive behaviors, diminished levels of psychological wellbeing, and an increased likelihood for the development of behavioral addictions (Laato et al., 2020; LaRose, Lin, & Eastin, 2003; Lee & Perry, 2004; Vally & Ahmed, 2020). The finding of a demonstrated association between DSR and internet addiction is especially relevant given that internet addiction, in turn, is typically associated with a substantial increase in social media use (LaRose et al., 2003). At the height of the pandemic, during the imposed lockdown across globe, the normative routine of daily life was disrupted. Individuals engaged in spatial isolation, commenced remote working and schooling, and some individuals became unemployed as a result of the economic impact of the lockdown (Barbieri, Basso, & Scicchitano, 2020). This dramatic and sudden change to the routine of daily life would be experienced as being especially challenging for individuals with DSR as they are reliant on the structure provided by routine. Concurrently, it has been reported that social media use increased, exponentially, during the lockdown (Cellini, Canale, Mioni, & Costa, 2020). Islam et al.'s (2020) findings suggest that individuals deficient in self-regulation skills experienced difficulty in modulating their behaviors during the imposed lockdown as conditions that lack structure are especially problematic for these individuals. They were therefore more likely to share unverified and potentially inaccurate information about the pandemic. The notable increase in social media use may also be related to SMF in that the increased time spent perusing information and engaging with others about the pandemic invariably results in an prodigious increase in incoming information (i.e., information overload) which, as reviewed earlier, has been demonstrated to be associated with an increased tendency to share unverified COVID-19 information (Islam et al., 2020).

It appears that for those individuals who place importance on the development of a positive self-image and self-promotion, their behaviors in the online realm are directed toward building social capital with others so that the overly positive image that they have created for themselves is carefully maintained (Islam, Mäntymäki, & Benbasat, 2019). This is relevant when considering

Thompson, Wang, and Daya's (2019) finding that status-seeking, a construct closely related to self-promotion, was associated with the intention to share news and information. Thus, when an individual's reputation (and self-image) may be compromised by their online actions, they are likely to exercise caution when selecting the content they share.

Evidence of the association between belief in conspiracy theories and COVID-19 health-protective behaviors

There is now empirical evidence of the association between the preferred use of social media and the tendency to espouse conspiracy theories as well as of the deleterious impact of conspiracy beliefs and adherence to health-protective behaviors during the COVID-19 pandemic. For example, Allington, Duffy, Wessely, Dhavan, and Rubin (2020) conducted a large-scale survey of UK residents at the height of the pandemic and found a highly significant negative relationship between holding one or more conspiracy beliefs about COVID-19 (i.e., the virus that causes COVID-19 was probably created in a laboratory; the symptoms of COVID-19 seem to be connected to 5G mobile network radiation; the COVID-19 pandemic was planned by certain pharmaceutical corporations and government agencies) and engagement in health-protective behaviors to mitigate infection (i.e., spending as little time as possible outside your home; staying at least 2 m apart from anyone outside of your household; washing your hands more often, for 20 s). Individuals who held conspiracy beliefs were less likely to protect themselves from infection. Interestingly, the belief that evidenced the strongest statistical association was the belief that COVID-19 symptoms resulted from the 5G mobile network. This particular conspiracy theory about the origin of COVID-19 was extremely popular on social media. In Ahmed et al.'s (2020) content analysis of Twitter data in which the #5GCoronavirus hashtag was trending in the United Kingdom, a third of the sampled tweets expressed the view that the virus was the result of 5G. The risk to public health posed by the spread of COVID-19 misinformation and conspiracy theories is further highlighted by research that demonstrates that individuals who received misinformation about the pandemic from their social media accounts, and believed it, possessed less knowledge of the virus and its prevention strategies and also consequently engaged in fewer health-protective strategies (Lee et al., 2020).

While the presence of a conspiracy mentality inhibits engagement in normative preventive behaviors, the individuals' perception of their degree of personal risk appears to mediate this effect. A number of factors could potentially explain this effect. Previous research shows that individuals who believe in conspiracy theories tend to be motivated by their own self-interest and therefore tend to adopt behaviors that are in their best interests (Cichocka, Marchlewska, & de Zavala, 2016; Jolley, Douglas, Leite, & Schrader, 2019). Similarly, conspiracy theorists have also been shown to demonstrate high levels of paranoia (Bruder et al., 2013). This is a construct that could potentially increase one's sense of personal risk, as a key feature of paranoid individuals is the perception that others or situations may be hostile toward the self. They also tend to formulate negative and threatening interpretations when faced with an ambiguous situation (Combs, Finn, Wohlfahrt, Penn, & Basso, 2013). Research also indicates that individuals high in narcissistic traits tend to find conspiracy theories appealing (Cichocka et al., 2016). Individuals high in narcissism place self-preservation as their primary priority, they tend to express little empathy toward others, and regard their own lives and wellbeing as superseding that of others (Campbell & Foster, 2007; Watson & Morris, 1991). The proposition then is that individuals who hold a conspiracy mentality, as a function of the aforementioned psychological factors, may perceive themselves to be at great risk within the context of a pandemic and, as such, will more than likely take precautionary measures to protect themselves from infection. These findings also suggest that individuals who hold a conspiracy mentality may only be motivated to take preventive action against COVID-19 infection if they perceive *themselves* to be at risk, rather than the risk posed to the larger society in which they reside.

The preliminary evidence suggests that this proposition may indeed be valid. Marinthe et al. (2020) examined the links between conspiracy mentality, perceived risk of contamination and death associated with COVID-19, and adherence to nonnormative preventive behaviors in a nationally representative sample of French residents. A conspiracy mentality was indeed positively associated with the adoption of nonnormative preventive behaviors during the pandemic (talking to people, using public transportation, eating in a restaurant, attending gatherings in closed or open spaces), although the effect size was small, as well as with a greater perception of risk. Moreover, this evidence supports the proposition that an indirect association between conspiracy mentality and preventive behaviors resulting from self-perceived personal risk is likely valid. In other words, the stronger an individuals' conspiracy mentality is, the more likely they are to take preventive action, particularly when they perceive themselves to be at risk of contamination or death. With regard to compliance to confinement orders imposed by the government, a similar relationship was evident. French residents with a conspiracy mentality were less likely to respect the confinement and lockdown order, thus confirming the contention that these individuals are unlikely to adhere to normative prevention strategies that originate from a government source. However, this effect was similarly mediated by a self-perceived risk of death and therefore acted as motivator for adherence to normative behaviors (Marinthe et al., 2020).

These findings support previous work which demonstrates that the normative context of the recommended behaviors during a pandemic determines conspiracy theorists' adherence. In other words, conspiracy theorists will gladly and willingly engage in behaviors to protect themselves from infection during an outbreak of disease, but if these same behaviors become part of the official advice disseminated by government or public health agencies, conspiracy theorists are likely to disengage from using these behaviors. The finding that the motivation to protect oneself was especially salient for this group of individuals is a valuable tool for public health officials. It is typical for public health agencies, during the context of a public health crisis, to promote the importance of adopting health-protective behaviors to reduce the risk one poses for others in one's community and society (Pechmann, Zhao, Goldberg, & Reibling, 2003). This prosocial motivation has been linked to effective antismoking campaigns in which the messaging has focused on death and the social impact to others (Martin & Kamins, 2019).

Perceived risk and health-protective behaviors

Perceived risk refers to an individual's subjective perception of the extent to which they are vulnerable to contracting an illness. Perceived risk is relevant not just in relation to conspiracy theorists and those who propagate or believe misinformation but also in relation to the general public. Indeed, it appears that people across the world have been, and still are, exceptionally concerned about the health risks, and the potential impact to other areas of their lives, posed by the COVID-19 pandemic. Governmental responses to the pandemic have included requiring residents to social distance, engage in numerous hygiene behaviors, and, at various stages of the pandemic, to adhere to the imposition of lockdown measures but research conducted in the context of previous pandemics indicates that the success of such governmental policies to impede the spread of the disease is reliant, to some extent, on the public's access to and awareness of accurate information about the disease, specifically information relating to personal and societal risk factors (Epstein, Parker, Cummings, & Hammond, 2008; Funk, Gilad, Watkins, & Jansen, 2009; Reluga, 2010; Van Bavel et al., 2020).

Dryhurst et al. (2020) sought to map cross-country levels of risk perception related to COVID-19 in 10 countries and found that residents of Australia, Germany, Spain, Italy, South Korea, Japan, Mexico, Sweden, United Kingdom, and the United States uniformly reported elevated perceptions of risk and that several psychological factors consistently emerged as significant predictors of perceived risk across all 10 nations. Experiential and sociocultural factors more strongly predicted perceived risk than any sociodemographic characteristic. More specifically, social amplification, operationalized as having heard about the virus from friends or family, and direct experience with the virus proved particularly important (Dryhurst et al., 2020). These findings are consistent with the wider literature (Leiserowitz, 2006; Loewenstein, Weber, Hsee, & Welch, 2001; Slovic, Finucane, Peters, & MacGregor, 2004; Weber, 2006) which suggests that "having had visceral contact with the virus strongly encourages the affective experiential system which is known to be more dominant in the processing of risk under these conditions" (Dryhurst et al., 2020). Scholars have also suggested that contact with a virus, both having been infected oneself or secondary contact via a friend or family member, may concretize the situation for the individual bringing it closer to the self and thus elevating the perception of risk at a construal level (Trope & Liberman, 2010).

These findings are especially important given the plethora of research that emphasizes the motivating action that risk perception plays in the promotion of health-protective behaviors, including within the context of major outbreaks of disease (Bish & Michie, 2010; Floyd, Prentice-Dunn, & Rogers, 2000; Rudisill, 2013; van der Weerd, Timmermans, Beaujean, Oudhoff, & van Steenbergen, 2011; Wise, Zbozinek, Michelini, & Hagan, 2020). Indeed, Dryhurst et al.'s (2020) assessment of COVID-19 risk perception concurs with the preceding research evidence; risk perception was significantly and positively associated with the adoption of preventive health-behaviors (handwashing, wearing face-mask, and social distancing); however, previous research in the context of other outbreaks suggests that this relationship may be more nuanced. Elevated and diminished levels of risk perceptions may impact adherence to health-protective behaviors differently across time. While the perception of higher personal risk may promote the adoption of such behaviors (Wise et al., 2020; Yıldırım, Geçer, & Akgül, 2020), some individuals who have taken the necessary precautionary actions to protect themselves from infection may evidence a commensurate reduction in their perception of risk and therefore discard continued adherence to the protective behaviors during later stages of the pandemic (Brewer, Weinstein, Cuite, & Herrington, 2004; Leppin & Aro, 2009).

An additional and related issue is that of the government's role in ensuring that the public have access to reliable and accurate information about the risks posed by a given disease. Certainly, preliminary research indicates that trust in the government is essential in promoting the perception among the public that the government can control the COVID-19 pandemic. Han et al. (2020) sampled residents of 23 nations and consistently found that governments that were perceived as being fair, well organized, and disseminating clear and understandable information about COVID-19 were consequently perceived as being more trustworthy. Where individuals hold higher levels of trust in their governments, they appear to be more likely to adopt health-protective behaviors and adhere to the imposed government measures (Han et al., 2020; Vally, 2020). Governments were required to play an integral role during COVID-19 pandemic, especially during the early stages of the disease where much uncertainty existed about its origin, means of infection, and the strategies that one could employ to protect oneself from infection. Where governments did not respond timeously with the flow of public health information, uncertainty and misconceptions were common. For example, one-third of Australian respondents sampled by Faasse and Newby (2020) reported uncertainty about whether people were likely to have natural or existing immunity to the illness, whether home remedies (e.g., saline rinses, vitamins) might be useful in preventing infection, or whether the virus was deliberately created in a laboratory and released to the public for some nefarious purpose. Such uncertainty should be the target of public health interventions so as to allay the public's misconceptions and ensure their adherence to bona fide preventive strategies. Where the public have reported access to clear and understandable public health messaging about COVID-19, their reported adherence has equally been high (Vally, 2020).

The role of personality traits in the adoption of health-protective behaviors

During the imposition of governmental restrictions directed at reducing the spread of the virus, researchers were also interested in assessing whether a particular set of personality traits could be implicated in individuals' decision to adopt and comply with government-mandated health-protective behaviors.

The lens of the Big Five traits provides the most immediate framework for examining the association of personality traits and compliance as they provide a broad cross-section of individual differences, some of which are particularly relevant as potential predictors of compliance. First, neuroticism has been shown to be related to the avoidance of personal risk (Jonason & Sherman, 2020) and, as such, these individuals may be more likely to adopt behaviors that reduce their perceived sense of risk and maximize personal safety. Second, individuals high in agreeableness are generally prosocial in their view of the world (Wilkowski, Robinson, & Meier, 2006) and may adopt health-protective behaviors to protect others from infection. Third, a public health crisis such as the COVID-19 pandemic may elicit greater compliance in individuals who rate highly on the conscientiousness trait as avoidance of germs and the pursuit of an organized life are important for these individuals (McRae & Costa, 2008). Moreover, conscientious individuals tend to frequent fewer places/spaces during a given day; therefore, the task of social isolation, a primary restrictive measure imposed by most governments, may be less taxing in comparison to extraverted individuals who have been shown to visit a comparably larger number of places/spaces in a given day (Ai, Liu, & Zhao, 2019).

Research conducted by Zajenkowski, Jonason, Leniarska, and Kozakiewicz (2020) in Poland, when restrictions were at their most stringent in this country (middle April 2020) found that, among the Big Five traits, agreeableness was indeed associated with an increased tendency to comply with government recommendations, a finding that has similarly been replicated and is uniformly present across multicountry samples of English, French, Italian, and Spanish-speaking individuals (Clark et al., 2020). This finding is understandable given the characteristics that are typical of agreeable individuals. Compliance to government-imposed restrictions during the pandemic was an onerous task for many. Individuals were required to sacrifice the normalcy of their lives for a greater good, both the protection of their health but also the safeguarding of the health of their communities. Agreeable individuals tend to be socially conscious, value compassion for others, and are willing to sacrifice their own needs for the betterment of their societies, despite incurring a personal cost in doing so (Matthews, Deary, & Whiteman, 2009; McRae & Costa, 2008).

Much of the research relating to the connection between personality and preventive behaviors has elected to measure socially desirable personality traits (i.e., the Big Five personality traits of agreeableness, conscientiousness, emotional stability, extraversion, and openness) but a burgeoning body of research conducted in the context of the COVID-19 pandemic suggests that the Dark Triad personality traits may also be relevant, particularly in relation to impeding adherence to preventive behaviors. The Dark Triad traits encompass Machiavellianism, narcissism, and psychopathy (Paulhus & Williams, 2002). Two recent studies conducted in Poland that collectively sampled more than 1000 respondents indicate that individuals with Dark Triad personality traits, particularly those scoring highly on Machiavellianism, callous and manipulative use of others, and narcissistic rivalry, were less likely to adhere to the government restrictions (Nowak et al., 2020; Zajenkowski et al., 2020). However, additionally, these results also suggest that how individuals perceive the COVID-19 situation is more instrumental than personality traits in determining compliance to health-protective behaviors. In Zajenkowski et al. (2020), perception variables accounted for more variance in relation to individual differences in compliance (5.7%) compared to both Dark Triad traits (2.9%) and Big Five traits (2.4%). These findings provide support for the "strong situation hypothesis" (Snyder & Ickes, 1985). The novel and unpredictable nature of the COVID-19 pandemic, its global and overarching impact, and the range of deleterious ramifications for peoples' lives render it a particularly salient experience for most individuals. It is an experience (or situation) that is emotionally charged, and this is invariably amplified by the continued onslaught of information relating to infections, mortality rates, and the race for a vaccine. Zajenkowski et al. (2020) and Nowak et al.'s (2020) results suggest that, within the context of a "strong situation," dispositional tendencies such as personality traits play less of a role in accounting for an individual's behavior. In relation to COVID-19, people who perceived the situation as driven by *duty* and *negativity* were more likely to comply (Zajenkowski et al., 2020). When one's behavior is driven by a sense of duty and moral obligation toward others, the required behavior is enacted despite personal sacrifice or discomfort because this is viewed as a contribution to the protection of society to whom one feels a sense of duty—this perhaps explains why some individuals are motivated to comply with government restrictions. Where a perception of negativity pervades and the situation is perceived as being a threat, this perception is often accompanied by feelings of dread, fear, and anxiety, which has certainly been the case for the current pandemic (Ahorsu et al., 2020). These negative emotions that result from the perception of negativity promote compliance with protective behaviors (Zajenkowski et al., 2020).

The Dark traits of Machiavellianism, psychopathy, and narcissism can be regarded as person-focused traits; they are traits that are relevant to the self rather than the larger group and revolve around maximizing one's individual benefit (Sedikides, Gaertner, Luke, O'Mara, & Gebauer, 2013). Nowak et al. (2020) proposed that group-focused Dark traits may also be relevant in accounting for the adoption of COVID-19 health-protective behaviors as the pandemic poses a risk not just to the self but also to one's larger group. To investigate this proposition, they assessed individuals' sense of collective narcissism which refers to an overwhelmingly strong identification with one's in-group and unrealistic positive beliefs about the group's level of communality and communal value (Sternisko, Cichocka, Cislak, & Van Bavel, 2020) but assessed its association, not only with preventive behaviors, but also in relation to maladaptive behavioral responses to the pandemic. In short, collective narcissism was not associated with the adoption of health-protective behaviors but collective narcissists were more likely to engage in hoarding behavior (i.e., stockpiling food, hygiene, and protective products) and so too were those high in Dark Triad personality traits. It has been suggested that collective narcissists employ this strategy as an attempt to compensate for the presence of a fragile sense of self as well as a hypersensitivity to external threats (Golec de Zavala, 2018). In the presence of the COVID-19 pandemic, which represents a clear threat to both the self and the larger group, the engagement in hoarding behavior is an egoistic and self-serving manifestation of the desire to maximize the self-interest of one's in-group to the clear detriment of others whom such individuals likely regard as being comparably less superior to their own or whose needs and welfare are deemed to be less meaningful than their own.

Summary and conclusion

The literature overwhelmingly points to the consistent finding that access to information that is both clear and understandable within the context of the COVID-19 pandemic is more frequently associated with a greater uptake of health-protective behaviors. A number of factors, however, impinge upon the public's access to information that meet these requirements. Social media, and to a lesser extent, mainstream media are frequently implicated in the proliferation of misinformation about the pandemic. While the majority of the information available on social media appears to be valid and legitimate, a worryingly large proportion of content (a third of the sampled data, in some cases) contains unverifiable or clearly inaccurate information.

This inevitably contributes to a proportion of the public in any given region not fully understanding the severity of the pandemic, nor the risks associated with particular behaviors, and therefore the magnitude of the need to protect themselves and others from infection. Even if they felt the need to act, they may not be aware of how to go about doing so. Public health agencies have an integral role to play in the promotion of campaigns to educate the public. Information that is clear and concrete and communicates the risks and behaviors as simply as possible is essential. In addition, public health messaging that highlights the effectiveness of the recommended behaviors will likely improve compliance as the public's perception of efficacy is paramount and also serves the secondary purpose of promoting the publics' sense of self-efficacy.

Where individuals believe behaviors will be effective and believe themselves capable of enacting them, compliance generally improves. The issue of the avenues through which public health information is disseminated to the public may be an additional issue to reflect upon as well as the degree of trust that the public holds in the prevailing governmental body. In locations where governments have maintained consistent messaging, and multiple mechanisms have been used to disseminate the information, the public tend to report high levels of familiarity with the relevant information, a factor that is related to greater compliance and adherence to health-protective behaviors (Vally, 2020). Conversely, in locations where the public report little access to information about COVID-19, levels of health-related information among participants are uniformly low, and this appears to be related to a greater mistrust of government messaging, and a diminished likelihood to actively seek out relevant information or to engage in precautionary behaviors (Shiina et al., 2020).

Of note, despite the following factors being present, clear concrete information, combating misinformation on social media, instilling an accurate perception of risk in the public eye, promotion of the public's self-efficacy, and highlighting the efficacy of the recommended behaviors, some individuals may still be resistant to do so as a result of their predisposing personality. There are therefore some individuals for whom public health messaging, regardless of its content and design, will be entirely ineffective. Individuals who possess any of the Dark Triad traits will be more likely to engage in maladaptive behaviors in response to a pandemic (e.g., hoarding and stockpiling) and unlikely to employ health-protective behaviors. However, despite there being evidence of such associations, the magnitude of these statistical associations tends to be small. Therefore, over and above these personality factors, it is individuals' perceptions and beliefs about both themselves and the pandemic itself that appears to exert greater predictive value in relation to health-protective behavior. Individuals' perceptions relating to personal risk and vulnerability, the severity of the disease and the consequences of infection, which would be particularly elevated if no treatment or vaccine exists as is the case for COVID-19 at present, and the perception of one's capacity to protect oneself appear to be primarily pivotal.

References

Ahmed, W., Vidal-Alaball, J., Downing, J., & López Seguí, F. (2020). COVID-19 and the 5G conspiracy theory: Social network analysis of twitter data. *Journal of Medical Internet Research, 22*(5), e19458.

Ahorsu, D. K., Lin, C. Y., Imani, V., Saffari, M., Griffiths, M. D., & Pakpour, A. H. (2020). The fear of COVID-19 scale: Development and initial validation. *International Journal of Mental Health and Addiction*. https://doi.org/10.1007/s11469-020-00270-8. Advance online publication.

Ai, P., Liu, Y., & Zhao, X. (2019). Big Five personality traits predict daily spatial behavior: Evidence from smartphone data. *Personality and Individual Differences, 147*, 285–291.

Allington, D., Duffy, B., Wessely, S., Dhavan, N., & Rubin, J. (2020). Health-protective behaviour, social media usage and conspiracy belief during the COVID-19 public health emergency. *Psychological Medicine*, 1–7. https://doi.org/10.1017/S003329172000224X.

Barbieri, T., Basso, G., & Scicchitano, S. (2020). *Italian workers at risk during the Covid-19 epidemic*. Available at SSRN 3572065.

Bish, A., & Michie, S. (2010). Demographic and attitudinal determinants of protective behaviours during a pandemic: A review. *British Journal of Health Psychology*, *15*(4), 797–824.

Brennen, J. S., Simon, F., Howard, P. N., & Nielsen, R. K. (2020). *Types, sources, and claims of COVID-19 misinformation*. Oxford: Report published by the Reuters Institute for the Study of Journalism. Retrieved from https://reutersinstitute.politics.ox.ac.uk/types-sources-and-claims-covid-19-misinformation.

Brewer, N. T., Weinstein, N. D., Cuite, C. L., & Herrington, J. E. (2004). Risk perceptions and their relation to risk behavior. *Annals of Behavioral Medicine*, *27*(2), 125–130.

Bright, L. F., Kleiser, S. B., & Grau, S. L. (2015). Too much Facebook? An exploratory examination of social media fatigue. *Computers in Human Behavior*, *44*, 148–155.

Bruder, M., Haffke, P., Neave, N., Nouripanah, N., & Imhoff, R. (2013). Measuring individual differences in generic beliefs in conspiracy theories across cultures: Conspiracy mentality questionnaire. *Frontiers in Psychology*, *4*, 225.

Campbell, W. K., & Foster, J. D. (2007). The narcissistic self: Background, an extended agency model, and ongoing controversies. In C. Sedikides, & S. Spencer (Eds.), *Frontiers in social psychology: The self* (pp. 115–138). Philadelphia, PA: Psychology Press.

Cellini, N., Canale, N., Mioni, G., & Costa, S. (2020). Changes in sleep pattern, sense of time and digital media use during COVID-19 lockdown in Italy. *Journal of Sleep Research*, *29*, e13074.

Cichocka, A., Marchlewska, M., & de Zavala, A. G. (2016). Does self-love or self-hate predict conspiracy beliefs? Narcissism, self-esteem, and the endorsement of conspiracy theories. *Social Psychological and Personality Science*, *7*, 157–166.

Combs, D. R., Finn, J. A., Wohlfahrt, W., Penn, D. L., & Basso, M. R. (2013). Social cognition and social functioning in nonclinical paranoia. *Cognitive Neuropsychiatry*, *18*(6), 531–548. https://doi.org/10.1080/13546805.2013.766595.

Conspiracy Watch. (2020). *La carte des théories du complot sur le coronavirus* [The coronavirus conspiracy theory map]. Conspiracy Watch | L'Observatoire du conspirationnisme. https://www.lemonde.fr/planete/article/2020/03/05/lutte-contre-le-coronavirus-le-point-sur-les-recommandations-officielles_6031938_3244.html.

Dryhurst, S., Schneider, C. R., Kerr, J., Freeman, A. L. J., Recchia, G., Marthe van der Bles, A., … van der Linden, S. (2020). Risk perceptions of COVID-19 around the world. *Journal of Risk Research*. https://doi.org/10.1080/13669877.2020.1758193.

Dunn, A. G., Surian, D., Leask, J., Dey, A., Mandl, K. D., & Coiera, E. (2017). Mapping information exposure on social media to explain differences in HPV vaccine coverage in the United States. *Vaccine*, *35*, 3033–3040.

Epstein, J. M., Parker, J., Cummings, D., & Hammond, R. A. (2008). Coupled contagion dynamics of fear and disease: Mathematical and computational explorations. *PLoS One*, *3*(12), e3955. https://doi.org/10.1371/journal.pone. 0003955.

Faasse, K., & Newby, J. M. (2020). Public perceptions of COVID-19 in Australia: Perceived risk, knowledge, health-protective behaviours, and vaccine intentions. *medRxiv*. https://doi.org/10.1101/2020.04.25.20079996.

Floyd, D. L., Prentice-Dunn, S., & Rogers, R. W. (2000). A meta-analysis of research on protection motivation theory. *Journal of Applied Social Psychology*, *30*(2), 407–429.

Funk, S., Gilad, E., Watkins, C., & Jansen, V. A. A. (2009). The spread of awareness and its impact on epidemic outbreaks. *Proceedings of the National Academy of Sciences*, *106*(16), 6872–6877.

Goertzel, T. (2010). Conspiracy theories in science. *European Molecular Biology Organization Reports*, *11*, 493–499.

Golec de Zavala, A. (2018). Collective narcissism: antecedents and consequences of exaggeration of the in-group image. In A. Hermann, A. Brunell, & J. Foster (Eds.), *Handbook of trait narcissism*. Cham: Springer.

Grebe, E., & Nattrass, N. (2011). AIDS conspiracy beliefs and unsafe sex in Cape Town. *AIDS and Behavior*, *16*(3), 761–773.

Han, Q., Zheng, B., Cristea, M., et al. (2020). Trust in government and its associations with health behaviour and prosocial behaviour during the COVID-19 pandemic. *OSF Preprints*. https://doi.org/10.31234/osf.io.

Hofstadter, R. (1964). The paranoid style in American politics. *Harper's Magazine*, 77–86 (November).

Ifop. (2019). *Enquête sur le complotisme—Vague 2*. https://www.ifop.com/publication/enquete-sur-le-complotisme-vague-2/.

Janz, N. K., & Becker, M. H. (1984). The health belief model: A decade later. *Health Education Quarterly*, *11*(1), 1–47.

Jolley, D., & Douglas, K. M. (2014). The effects of anti-vaccine conspiracy theories on vaccination intentions. *PLoS One*, *9*(2), e89177.

Jolley, D., Douglas, K. M., Leite, A. C., & Schrader, T. (2019). Belief in conspiracy theories and intentions to engage in everyday crime. *British Journal of Social Psychology*, *58*, 534–549.

Jonason, P. K., & Sherman, R. A. (2020). Personality and the perception of situations: The Big Five and Dark Triad traits. *Personality and Individual Differences*, *163*, 110081.

Khoramabadi, M., Dolatian, M., Hajian, S., Zamanian, M., Taheripanah, R., Sheikhan, Z., … Seyedi-Moghadam, A. (2015). Effects of education based on health belief model on dietary behaviors of Iranian pregnant women. *Global Journal of Health Science*, *8*(2), 230–239.

Kouzy, R., Jaoude, J. A., Kraitem, A., El Alam, M. B., Karam, B., Adib, E., … Baddour, K. (2020). Coronavirus goes viral: Quantifying the COVID-19 misinformation epidemic on Twitter. *Cureus*, *12*(3), e7255.

Laato, S., Islam, A. K. M. N., Islam, M. N., & Whelan, E. (2020). What drives unverified information sharing and cyberchondria during the COVID-19 pandemic? *European Journal of Information Systems*, 1–18.

Lamberty, P., & Imhoff, R. (2018). Powerful pharma and its marginalized alternatives? Effects of individual differences in conspiracy mentality on attitudes toward medical approaches. *Social Psychology*, *49*, 255–270.

LaRose, R., Lin, C. A., & Eastin, M. S. (2003). Unregulated Internet usage: Addiction, habit, or deficient self-regulation? *Media Psychology*, *5*(3), 225–253.

Larson, H. J. (2018). The biggest pandemic risk? Viral misinformation. *Nature*, *562*(7727), 309.

Lee, A. R., Son, S. M., & Kim, K. K. (2016). Information and communication technology overload and social networking service fatigue: A stress perspective. *Computers in Human Behavior*, *55*, 51–61.

Lee, J. J., Kang, K. A., Wang, M. P., Wong, J. Y. H., O'Connor, S., & Shin, S. H. (2020). Associations of COVID-19 misinformation exposure and belief with COVID-19 knowledge and preventive behaviours: A population-based study. *JMIR Preprints*, 22205. https://doi.org/10.2196/preprints.22205.

Lee, K. C., & Perry, S. D. (2004). Student instant message use in a ubiquitous computing environment: Effects of deficient self-regulation. *Journal of Broadcasting and Electronic Media*, *48*(3), 399–420.

Leiserowitz, A. (2006). Climate change risk perception and policy preferences: The role of affect, imagery, and values. *Climatic Change*, *77*(1–2), 45–72. https://doi.org/10.1007/s10584-006-9059-9.

Leppin, A., & Aro, A. R. (2009). Risk perceptions related to SARS and avian influenza: Theoretical foundations of current empirical research. *International Journal of Behavioral Medicine*, *16*(1), 7–29.

Loewenstein, G., Weber, E., Hsee, C., & Welch, N. (2001). Risk as feelings. *Psychological Bulletin*, *127*(2), 267–286. https://doi.org/10.1037/0033-2909.127.2.267.

Marinthe, G., Brown, G., Delouvée, S., & Jolley, D. (2020). Looking out for myself: Exploring the relationship between conspiracy mentality, perceived personal risk, and COVID-19 prevention measures. *British Journal of Health Psychology*. https://doi.org/10.1111/bjhp.12449.

Martin, I. M., & Kamins, M. A. (2019). Effectively using death in health messages: Social loss versus physical mortality salience. *Journal of Consumer Behaviour*, *18*, 205–218.

Matthews, G., Deary, I. J., & Whiteman, M. C. (2009). *Personality traits* (3rd ed.). Cambridge University Press.

McRae, R. R., & Costa, P. T. (2008). The five-factor theory of personality. In O. P. John, R. W. Robins, & L. A. Pervin (Eds.), *Handbook of personality: Theory and research* (3rd ed., pp. 159–181). New York, NY: Guilford.

Mohammadi, S., Ghajari, H., Valizade, R., Ghaderi, N., Yousefi, F., Taymoori, P., & Nouri, B. (2017). Predictors of smoking among the secondary high school boy students based on the health belief model. *International Journal of Preventive Medicine*, *8*, 24.

Ofcom. (2020). *London real: Covid-19. Ofcom broadcast and on demand bulletin*. Retrieved from https://www.ofcom.org.uk/__data/assets/pdf_file/0020/194402/sanction-decision-estv.pdf.

Oi-Yee Li, H., Bailey, A., Huynh, D., & Chan, J. (2020). Youtube as a source of information on COVID-19: A pandemic of misinformation? *BMJ Global Health*, *5*, e002604.

Pandey, A., Patni, N., Sing, M., Sood, A., & Singh, G. (2010). Youtube as a source of information on the H1N1 influenza pandemic. *American Journal of Preventative Medicine*, *38*(3), e1–e3.

Paulhus, D. L., & Williams, K. M. (2002). The Dark Triad of personality: Narcissism, Machiavellianism, and psychopathy. *Journal of Research in Personality*, *36*, 556–563.

Pechmann, C., Zhao, G., Goldberg, M. E., & Reibling, E. T. (2003). What to convey in antismoking advertisements for adolescents: The use of protection motivation theory to identify effective message themes. *Journal of Marketing*, *67*(2), 1–18.

Popper, K. (1969). *Conjectures and refutations: The growth of scientific knowledge*. London: Routledge & Kegan Paul.

Reluga, T. C. (2010). Game theory of social distancing in response to an epidemic. *PLoS Computational Biology*, *6*(5), e1000793–e1000799. https://doi.org/10.1371/journal.pcbi.1000793.

Rosenstock, I. M., Strecher, V. J., & Becker, M. H. (1994). The health belief model and HIV risk behavior change. In R. J. DiClemente, & J. L. Peterson (Eds.), *Preventing AIDS*. Boston, MA: AIDS Prevention and Mental Health. Springer. https://doi.org/10.1007/978-1-4899-1193-3_2.

Rubin, G. J., Amlot, R., Page, L., & Wessely, S. (2009). Public perceptions, anxiety, and behaviour change in relation to the swine flu outbreak: Cross sectional telephone survey. *British Medical Journal*, *339*, b2651.

Rudisill, C. (2013). How do we handle new health risks? Risk perception, optimism, and behaviors regarding the H1N1 virus. *Journal of Risk Research*, *16*(8), 959–980.

Sedikides, C., Gaertner, L., Luke, M. A., O'Mara, E. M., & Gebauer, J. (2013). A three-tier hierarchy of motivational self-potency: Individual self, relational self, collective self. *Advances in Experimental Social Psychology*, *48*, 235–295.

Shiina, A., Niitsu, T., Kobori, O., et al. (2020). Relationship between perception and anxiety about COVID-19 infection and risk behaviors for spreading infection: A national survey in Japan. *Brain, Behavior & Immunity – Health*, *6*, 100101.

Slovic, P., Finucane, M. L., Peters, E., & MacGregor, D. G. (2004). Risk as analysis and risk as feelings: Some thoughts about affect, reason, risk, and rationality. *Risk Analysis*, *24*(2), 311–322.

Soleymanian, A., Niknami, S., Hajizadeh, E., Shojaeizadeh, D., & Montazeri, A. (2014). Development and validation of a health belief model based instrument for measuring factors influencing exercise behaviors to prevent osteoporosis in pre-menopausal women (HOPE). *BMC Musculoskeletal Disorders*, *15*, 61.

Sternisko, A., Cichocka, A., Cislak, A., & Van Bavel, J. J. (2020). *Collective narcissism predicts the belief and dissemination of conspiracy theories during the COVID-19 pandemic*. https://doi.org/10.31234/osf.io/4c6av.

Sweller, J. (2011). *Cognitive load theory* (pp. 37–76). Academic Press.

Talwar, S., Dhir, A., Kaur, P., Zafar, N., & Alrasheedy, M. (2019). Why do people share fake news? Associations between the dark side of social media use and fake news sharing behavior. *Journal of Retailing and Consumer Services*, *51*, 72–82.

Thompson, N., Wang, X., & Daya, P. (2019). Determinants of news sharing behavior on social media. *Journal of Computer Information Systems*, 1–9.

Thorburn, S., & Bogart, L. M. (2005). Conspiracy beliefs about birth control: Barriers to pregnancy prevention among African Americans of reproductive age. *Health Education & Behavior*, *32*, 474–487.

Trope, Y., & Liberman, N. (2010). Construal theory. *Psychological Review*, *117*(2), 440–463.

Vally, Z. (2020). Public perceptions, anxiety and the perceived efficacy of health-protective behaviours to mitigate the spread of the SARS-Cov-2/COVID-19 pandemic. *Public Health*, *187*, 67–73.

Vally, Z., & Ahmed, K. (2020). Emotion regulation strategies and psychological wellbeing: Examining cognitive reappraisal and expressive suppression in an Emirati college sample. *Neurology, Psychiatry, and Brain Research*, *38*, 27–32.Van Bavel et al., 2020Van Bavel, J. J., Boggio, P., Capraro, V., Cichocka, A., Cikara, M., Crockett, M., … Ellemers, N. (2020). Using social and behavioural science to support COVID-19 pandemic response. *Nature Human Behaviour*, *4*, 460–471.

van der Weerd, W., Timmermans, D. R., Beaujean, D. J., Oudhoff, J., & van Steenbergen, J. E. (2011). Monitoring the level of government trust, risk perception and intention of the general public to adopt protective measures during the influenza A (H1N1) pandemic in the Netherlands. *BMC Public Health*, *11*(1), 575.

Vermandere, H., van Stam, M., Naanyu, V., Michielsen, K., Degomme, O., & Oort, F. (2016). Uptake of the human papillomavirus vaccine in Kenya: Testing the health belief model through pathway modeling on cohort data. *Globalization and Health*, *12*, 72.

Watson, P. J., & Morris, R. J. (1991). Narcissism, empathy and social desirability. *Personality and Individual Differences*, *12*, 575–579. https://doi.org/10.1016/0191-8869(91)90253-8.

Weber, E. U. (2006). Experience-based and description-based perceptions of long-term risk: Why global warming does not scare us (yet). *Climatic Change*, *77*(1/2), 103–120.

Whelan, E., Islam, A. N., & Brooks, S. (2020). Is boredom proneness related to social media overload and fatigue? A stress–strain–outcome approach. *Internet Research*, *30*(3), 869–887.

Wilkowski, B. M., Robinson, M. D., & Meier, B. P. (2006). Agreeableness and the prolonged spatial processing of antisocial and prosocial information. *Journal of Research in Personality*, *40*, 1152–1168.

Wise, T., Zbozinek, T. D., Michelini, G., & Hagan, C. C. (2020). *Changes in risk perception and protective behavior during the first week of the COVID-19 pandemic in the United States*. PsyArXiv Preprints. https://psyarxiv.com/dz428/.

Yıldırım, M., Geçer, E., & Akgül, Ö. (2020). The impacts of vulnerability, perceived risk, and fear on preventive behaviours against COVID-19. *Psychology, Health & Medicine*. https://doi.org/10.1080/13548506.2020.1776891.

Zajenkowski, M., Jonason, P. K., Leniarska, M., & Kozakiewicz, Z. (2020). Who complies with the restrictions to reduce the spread of COVID-19? Personality and perceptions of the COVID-19 situation. *Personality and Individual Differences*, *166*, 110199.

Zhao, J., Song, F., Ren, S., Wang, Y., Wang, L., et al. (2012). Predictors of condom use behaviors based on the health belief model (HBM) among female sex workers: A cross-sectional study in Hubei Province, China. *PLoS One*, *7*(11), e49542. https://doi.org/10.1371/journal.pone.0049542.

Zimmerman, R. K., Wolfe, R. M., Fox, D. E., Fox, J. R., Nowalk, M. P., Troy, J. A., & Sharp, L. K. (2005). Vaccine criticism on the world wide web. *Journal of Medical Internet Research*, *7*(2), e17.

Clark, C., Davila, A., Regis, M., & Kraus, S. (2020). Predictors of COVID-19 voluntary compliance behaviors: An international investigation. *Global Transitions*, *2*, 76–82. https://doi.org/10.1016/j.glt.2020.06.003.

Islam, A., Laato, S., Talukder, S., & Sutinen, E. (2020). Misinformation sharing and social media fatigue during COVID-19: An affordance and cognitive load perspective. *Technological Forecasting and Social Change*, *159*, 120201. https://doi.org/10.1016/j.techfore.2020.120201.

Islam, A. K. M. N., Mäntymäki, M., & Benbasat, I. (2019). Duality of self-promotion on social networking sites. *Information Technology & People*, *32*(2), 269–296.

Nowak, B., Brzóska, P., Piotrowski, J., Sedikides, C., Żemojtel-Piotrowska, M., & Jonason, P. K. (2020). Adaptive and maladaptive behavior during the COVID-19 pandemic: The roles of Dark Triad traits, collective narcissism, and health beliefs. *Personality and Individual Differences*, *167*, 110232. https://doi.org/10.1016/j.paid.2020.110232.

Snyder, M., & Ickes, W. (1985). Personality and social behavior. In G. Lindzey, & E. Aronson (Eds.), *Handbook of social psychology* (pp. 883–947). New York, NY: Random House.

Chapter 16

Social media use, experiences of social connectedness and wellbeing during COVID-19

Jacqui Taylor-Jackson[a], Imogen Abba[a], Alessandra Baradel[a], Jeremy Lay[a], Jasmin Herewini[a], and Amber Taylor[b]
[a]*School of Psychology, Western Sydney University, Sydney, NSW, Australia,* [b]*Division of Psychology and Language Science, University College London, London, United Kingdom*

Literature review

The increasing use of social media platforms globally has led some researchers to explore and discuss their many benefits in bringing people closer and extending relationships across distance (Bayer, Triệu, & Ellison, 2020). In contrast to these benefits, other researchers have investigated and highlighted the potentially damaging outcomes that using social media can have on mental health and wellbeing for some of its users. Broadly, social media are defined as online channels of communication that allow for synchronous and asynchronous interpersonal engagement among users. These interactions, which are based on user-generated content (e.g., posts, comments, and virtual "reactions"), can be to a wide audience or at a one-to-one level between individuals (Carr & Hayes, 2015). A subcategory of social media, Social Networking Sites (SNSs) enable users to create a more personalized and wide-reaching online social environment. SNSs are regarded as distinct from other social media platforms due to three central elements—the profile, the network, and the feed (Bayer et al., 2020). A profile is a user-developed and maintained space that contains the user's personal details and platform-specific contributions (e.g., posts); a network is the user's curated collection of social contacts for that platform; a feed is an ongoing display of user-generated content created by each user's social network. These elements, among others, have allowed sites such as Facebook, LinkedIn, Instagram, Pinterest, YouTube, Twitter, and Snapchat to create a complex online social world, in which people can interact more quickly, more widely, and more regularly than ever before.

In Australia where the data was collected, there were approximately 18 million social media users in 2019, with people aged between 18 and 26 using social media the most frequently (We Are Social, 2019). This date is similar to other Western countries (Statista, 2020) and globally internet users spend

Mental Health Effects of COVID-19. https://doi.org/10.1016/B978-0-12-824289-6.00013-1

2 h and 23 min on social media per day (Statista, 2020). As social media has become intimately connected with the lives of young people in Australia, concern has arisen regarding the possible impact that online social media use may have on wellbeing. This concern has given rise to an ever-expanding body of literature producing evidence of both positive and negative psychological effects associated with social media use. However, there remains little consensus regarding the cause of these effects and what can be done to mitigate risks to wellbeing (Casale, 2020). By considering the complexities associated with online communication technologies, research has begun to shift toward looking at interactions between social media use, social connectedness, and psychological wellbeing (Bayer et al., 2020). Such complexities include the context of social media use, the experiences and perceptions of the users, and the capacity for social media to be used as a tool for social enhancement rather than purely an impediment to social wellbeing.

This review will explore how social media use, social connectedness, and psychological wellbeing are interrelated. Globally, government responses to the COVID-19 pandemic have included house and hotel quarantines, physical distancing, and reducing opportunities to eat or socialize in commercial areas to reduce its spread and impact. These responses are naturally affecting individual's patterns of communications. Most of the research reviewed took place before COVID-19; however, there were a small number of articles published during the first 3 months[a] since the virus was identified which discuss these factors. For example, in a discussion of social isolation during the first 3 months of COVID-19 in China Banerjee and Rai (2020) highlight the impact of loneliness. They recommended that mental health professionals be sensitive to the personal and psychological needs of individuals with (or suspected of having) COVID-19 isolated in quarantine, specifically stating that "digital communication needs to be maintained with their loved ones ... social connectedness matters" (p. 527). Most articles are review articles and therefore there exists a gap in the research regarding the experiences of social media users during the COVID-19 pandemic and whether changes to offline and online social connection have affected young people.

A recent market research survey (Kantar Group and Affiliates, 2020) using a sample of 25,000 consumers found that social media use increased by 61% during the first months of the COVID-19 pandemic, with the largest increases coming from WhatsApp and then Facebook. Similarly, Microsoft reported a 500% increase in the use of their Microsoft Teams collaboration software (Microsoft, 2020). The videoconferencing platform Zoom now has around 265,400 customers with more than 10 employees, a number that's grown 354% in 3 months when it added 175,000 licenses for new company customers. At its peak in April 2020, usage grew to 300 million meeting participants each day, up from just 10 million in December (Kastrenakes, 2020).

a This study was conducted in May 2020 after the first 3 months. Research conducted since this study was analyzed from May to August 2020 is presented in the Discussion.

Social connectedness and psychological wellbeing

Belonginess theory (Baumeister & Leary, 1995) suggests that people develop and maintain gratifying social relationships to experience a sense of relatedness with others. Such relatedness needs are met through social connection with members of one's social network. Social connectedness has been traditionally measured based on the number of social ties an individual has (Goswami, Köbler, Leimeister, & Krcmar, 2010) or the frequency with which an individual interacts with their social network or participates in social activities (Shankar, Rafnsson, & Steptoe, 2015). The existence of a social network alone cannot meet these relatedness needs, as individuals require both high quality and meaningful engagement (Baumeister & Leary, 1995). As such, social connectedness can be conceptualized as the perceived experience of *meaningful* social connection with others, and it is this kind of social engagement that has been consistently associated with positive psychological outcomes (Wu, Outley, Matarrita-Cascante, & Murphrey, 2016). In a longitudinal survey study of New Zealand adolescents, participants who reported higher levels of real-life connectedness in family and school contexts also reported higher levels of wellbeing in areas such as life satisfaction, positive affect, and self-confidence (Jose, Ryan, & Pryor, 2012). In a survey study of undergraduate women in the United States, real-life social connectedness was negatively associated with anxiety and positively associated with self-esteem (Lee & Robbins, 1998). In a study of an adventure holiday program for boys, participants who reported a greater sense of belongingness within their adventure group scored more highly on a measure of resilience at the end of the program (Scarf et al., 2017). Notably, social support did not contribute to the improvement in resilience, suggesting that it was the sense of social connectedness, rather than just group membership, that was associated with positive outcomes.

Social media and social connectedness

Face-to-face communication has traditionally been viewed as the most effective and efficient way to satisfy one's need for social connectedness (Grieve, Indian, Witteveen, Tolan, & Marrington, 2013). Like its communication technology predecessors, however, social media platforms have increasingly been used to enhance and satisfy these same connectedness needs. Social media have been found to provide a range of benefits to users in relation to social connectedness, including relationship development, relationship maintenance, social capital building, and social support seeking behaviors (Allen, Ryan, Gray, McInerney, & Waters, 2014). For example, in a series of interviews with adolescents, Davis (2012) found that those who engaged in casual interactions with others on Facebook reported experiencing an increased sense of belonging. This sense of belongingness stemmed from the enhanced connection with friends and other networks made possible by social media. In a qualitative study of young adults on Snapchat, participants reported that social media platforms enabled them to strengthen their existing relationships by providing a more intimate way of communicating, for example through pictures and text (Vaterlaus, Barnett, Roche, & Young, 2016). Further, a study on loneliness and social media use found a positive impact on the psychological wellbeing and sense of social connectedness for individuals who used social media specifically for relationship building and maintenance (Nowland, Necka, & Cacioppo, 2018). Notably, a mixed-methods study using a survey and interviews with South Australian high school students found that adolescents who reported higher levels of online social connection were more likely to cope actively when they were cyberbullied, as it facilitated help-seeking and in turn led to more positive mental health outcomes (McLouglin, Spears, & Taddeo, 2018). The uses and gratifications model suggests that individuals actively participate in the selection and consumption of specific media as a means of satisfying specific needs (Lichtenstein & Rosenfeld, 1983). Previous research has identified a range of uses and gratifications of social media relevant to social connection, such as maintaining existing relationships, developing new relationships, information sharing, social interaction with others, support seeking, and self-presentation or personal expression (see Wang, Tchernev, & Solloway, 2012).

Unimpeded by physical distance and time, social media has also facilitated connectedness for those who may otherwise be unable to connect through face-to-face engagement. For example, Tiwari, Lane, and Alam (2019) investigated the role of SNS use in social capital building and maintenance in rural communities. Surveyed participants with higher SNS use were able to build and maintain a larger network of connections through these online platforms. This provided rural communities with broader support networks and resources from which they could draw on more effectively, compared to their offline connections. In addition, a survey study of older adults found that social connectedness could be derived from Facebook use and was an important source of interpersonal engagement for users in this demographic (Sinclair & Grieve, 2017).

Research on the role of social media in enhancing social connectedness for those who are unable to connect face to face has found positive outcomes for the social and psychological wellbeing of individuals with intellectual disabilities, communication difficulties, chronic illness, and physical disability. For example, Chadwick and Fullwood (2018) interviewed adults with intellectual disabilities regarding their experiences of using social media and using thematic network analysis highlighted the positive potential of social media in helping to develop and maintain social bonds, and feelings of enjoyment, autonomy, and self-worth. Raghavendra, Newman, Grace, and Wood (2015) investigated the effectiveness of an intervention which involved social media training for young people with disabilities and communication difficulties based in two Australian rural towns. Following the intervention, interviews with participants and parents identified increased social connections, improved communication frequency and nature, and speech intelligibility and literacy. Lee and Cho (2019) used hierarchical regression analyses to examine the relationships between social media use, social support, and depression for a sample of 91 individuals with movement or mobility disabilities in Korea. They found that that intensity of SNS use significantly predicted different types of perceived support and also led to lower levels of depression through the mediation of support. As such, in a world where one's social network can and often is made up of people outside one's immediate physical vicinity, online communication tools have enabled interpersonal connection in a manner and capacity unseen before (Davis, 2012). These findings offer a positive view of the way social media may affect users positively during COVID-19 times when physical interaction is limited.

Social media and negative impacts on psychological wellbeing

While the accessibility and ease of interaction associated with social media may facilitate a range of positive outcomes for wellbeing, the constantly connected social world may also exacerbate social stressors that undermine the capacity of these platforms to facilitate relatedness and belonginess with others (Taylor-Jackson & Mustafa, in press). Unlike previously discussed studies, the use of social media has been associated with poorer subjective wellbeing, such as increased loneliness (Twenge, Spitzberg, & Campbell, 2019), depression and anxiety (Woods & Scott, 2016), and social isolation (Primack et al., 2017). Using social media can also undermine social connectedness, where it leads to less face-to-face interaction (Abeele, Antheunis, & Schouten, 2016) or opportunities for in-person engagement are reduced (Kushlev, Proulx, & Dunn, 2017).

Methodological limitations of research relating to social media use and wellbeing

The large variability in findings relating the impacts of social media on mental health can be attributed, in part, to the way wellbeing and social media use are measured and conceptualized. For example, Ekström and Östman (2015) propose that social media use can be categorized by the engagement of the individual with the platform. Active engagement refers to usage that facilitates direct interaction with others (e.g., posting photos, commenting, messaging), whereas passive engagement refers to consuming information without active interaction with the content (e.g., lurking, scrolling, viewing but not commenting). Passive rather than active social media use has been associated with a reduction in subjective wellbeing (Verduyn et al., 2015). This suggests that it is not social media use in general but specific kinds of use that may be associated with negative outcomes for wellbeing. Similarly, while some studies have found social media use to be associated with negative social experiences, a qualitative study by Clark and Green (2018) found social media use to produce positive social experiences when online communication was perceived as a real and meaningful social tool. Again, the conceptualization of the platform and the use appears to directly impact the findings, with more nuanced conceptualizations producing more nuanced findings.

The primarily quantitative literature relating social media use and wellbeing has repeatedly used survey-based studies and correlational and cross-sectional analysis methods. These approaches often miss the context and individual experiences of social media users, which may provide a depth and breadth of understanding regarding wellbeing outcomes that survey studies cannot provide alone.

It is clear, then, that the primarily quantitative body of social media research has failed to produce meaningful consensus regarding the efficacy of social media as a social connection tool and its impact on psychological wellbeing in young adults. As such, research that specifically explores the perceptions and experiences of young adults' social media use and the changes that have occurred in their social media use may provide valuable insight into the evolving relationship they experience with the online world. By moving toward a focus on individual experiences, qualitative study designs may also provide more generalizable and culturally specific insight.

Rationale

Researchers face a "moving-target" problem when investigating the psychological effects of online communication technology (Bayer et al., 2020). The research conducted and reported in this chapter therefore presents a snapshot of the way social media is used during a specific time period. The findings will be generalizable to other instances where users are suddenly unable to interact face to face, e.g., due to illness or security-based lockdowns, but also for other pandemic-like situations in the future. The current impact of social media use on wellbeing and connectedness may be highly distinct to that found in previous research, and so warrants considered and reconceptualized focus during the COVID-19 pandemic.

There is a gap in understanding the experiences of social media users regarding the impacts of COVID-19 on changing levels of engagement with social media and the effects of this on their wellbeing. The following overarching question will be explored through collecting and analyzing qualitative data: How do young adults perceive and use social media for social connection during COVID-19, and has engagement with social media during COVID-19 impacted on wellbeing?

Method

An online survey was completed by 377 students aged 18–28 years between May and June 2020. An open-ended question was asked and it is the responses to this question that are reported in this chapter. The question was, "What ways (if any) has COVID-19 and its physical distancing and social gathering restrictions changed your social media habits?"

Results

Quantitative data analysis

Initially, the responses were categorized into whether participants gave some indication as to whether they used social media more or less compared to before COVD-19, to provide an overview of the quantitative impact of COVID-19 on social media usage. This was completed by using content analysis and producing a tally of the responses relating to changes in quantity of social media use. The frequencies are presented in Table 1, where it can be seen that the majority of participants used social media more during COVID-19.

Qualitative data analysis

Qualitative responses were then analyzed through thematic analysis, and participants were assigned individual numbers (e.g., P1) to achieve anonymity. Data was analyzed based on the thematic analysis procedure outlined by Braun and Clarke (2006), which consists of six stages. First, one of the coauthors (JTJ) made reflexive notes to familiarize the researcher with data. Second, responses were reread and initial recurring themes identified. Third, a second researcher (ATJ) individually coded each response according to these initial themes and introduced new themes where a response could not be coded. Next, sensitivity of the themes was assessed again against the data to ensure they are explanatory of the participant's responses. A theme table was created to describe the themes and any subthemes that may have also been descriptive of the data; validity of the themes was ensured by adding example words from the participants (in vivo).

There were five main themes reflecting changes in the use of social media and the impacts of these changes: (1) using social media for relationship maintenance and initiation; (2) passive social media use; (3) mental health impacts;

TABLE 1 Frequency count.

More use of social media	251
Less use of social media	24
Both (more and less) usage	10
Same use of social media	61
Missing data	31

(4) using social media to relieve boredom, procrastinate, or entertain; and (5) related to COVID-19 news or discussion. Subthemes can be seen as follows within each main theme.

Theme 1: Using social media for relationship maintenance and initiation

Forty-five participants made comments within this theme and they were divided into two subthemes.

1.1 Relationship maintenance

There was a lot of evidence of participants connecting more and the following three examples are indicative of the many comments in this subtheme. As can be seen, most comments relate to increased usage and connectedness, with only one comment relating the quality of communication with enhanced connectedness (P211):

> *social media use as it is now the primary way for me to connect with loved ones (P55)*
>
> *I've increased my social media usage in order to feel more connected with my friends (P96)*
>
> *to feel connected and keep up relationships with my friends (P144)*
>
> *I am posting more meaningful and sentimental kind of content (P211)*

1.2 Relationship initiation

Two participants specifically mentioned that they had initiated new relationships and had interacted with strangers (which they wouldn't have done before COVID-19), for example:

> *I'm more active online. I responded to strangers (P228)*
>
> *I reply to strangers (P293)*

Theme 2: Passive social media use and less connectionRegarding the quality of communications, many participants indicated that social media use was related to less meaningful connections with others. The type of usage was commented on frequently, where participants differentiated between three main activities: scrolling, messaging individuals, and posting updates. Comments within this theme were divided into three subthemes.

2.1. More scrolling and less one-to-one messaging

A number of participants expressed that they were using social media more, but not messaging others. A common sentiment expressed by P127 is, "On it more, connecting less."

A common comment was that participants were scrolling more or browsing on social media, suggesting they aren't being social, rather just looking at social media. This relates to the differentiation between active and passive use and the following examples are reflective of this:

> *It has both increased and decreased my time spent on social media. I spend more time scrolling through FB (before I rarely did) and less time talking on Messenger as there is not much to talk about (P10)*

I spend more time in bed on social media and less time interacting with other people. In particular, I use TikTok much more than I used to (P252)

It's made me less interested with talking to people but more interested in keeping up on instagram/facebook/tiktok (P25)

often I find myself scrolling mindlessly through my feeds more than once within the same hour (P350)

Scrolling over the same thing more often (P190)

I find myself opening the apps without even thinking about it, and often I find myself scrolling mindlessly through my feeds more than once within the same hour (P350)

I spend more time than often browsing through social media even if there is nothing there (P276)

2.2. Reduced social media use due to partaking in less offline social activities
Some participants reported using social media less as they are not going out and so have nothing to post about.

Use has decreased. This is mainly because not many people are posting or are active on social media due to going out restrictions (P50)

It has limited myself on posting images during my daily lifestyle as I rarely go out anymore (P76)

I am less on social media, as not many people are much are posting nor am I posting due to not going out (P279)

I spend more time scrolling through FB (before I rarely did) and less time talking on Messenger as there is not much to talk about (P10)

i don't post as often because i haven't been out as often (P227)

2.3. Fear of Missing Out (FOMO)
Related to subtheme 2.2, 18 participants related their use of social media with catching up on what everyone is doing and are indicative of FOMO, for example:

a new habit is constant and late night checking for anything new -like new ideas, opinions and so forth (P208)

In the beginning there was an increase in engaging in other posts. But now it's just watching from the sidelines (P177)

looking through instagram wishing I could do the things I used to do (P234)

Theme 3: Mental health impactsComments within this theme were divided into three subthemes.
3.1 Overuse of social media
This subtheme included a number of comments relating to those thinking it was more acceptable to overuse social media, to those who recognized overuse as a problem and addressed it. Many participants provided examples that they

were aware of the negative impacts of overuse of social media or described it as overwhelming or bad for mental health.
Some participants felt that it had now become "more acceptable" to be on SM (suggesting an assumption that SM is unhealthy), for example:

It only made it more acceptable (P351)

It hasn't changed it just made it more acceptable to be on socials more (P145)

I used to take breaks from social media but now I feel too lonely without it because not having that in-person contact (P6)

[social media usage] has lessened as it became overwhelming (P254)

There were some examples of participants mentioning, or implying, that they were addicted:

Cant seem to put my phone down at times (P367)

I used social media more frequently, and feel as though i am addicted to my phone. I find that i cannot concentrate or get through my day without checking social media. I do believe it did get worse during the pandemic and i have an addiction to my phone (P156)

I find myself on my phone most of the day, switching between different social medias (P153)

i am constantly on social media due to always being at home (P240)

I feel that I am on social media too much but I don't do anything to stop it or change it (P198)

i think its benifit me in a way that i don't look at social media as often as i used to which is an eye opener for me when things start going back to how they were to not get caught up in my phone (P26)

Three participants went as far as to disable their social media accounts, rejoining only when they felt they could cope:

I took it upon myself to deactivate and delete most of my social media accounts, and have realised the amount of time I have wasted on social media (P366)

At first, I was on social media more often. I realised that it was having a negative impact on my life so I disabled my FB account for a few weeks until things settles and I was better able to deal with the situation and I reactivated when I received news that a family member had a baby and since then, I'm happy with my use (P66)

it had a very negative impact on me so I disabled my facebook account for a few weeks until things settled down and I was able to make decisions that were best for my family. Then when I was in a better frame of mind I reactivated my account and i'm now using it to catch up with friends and family (P222)

3.2 Negative socioemotional changes

Five participants related their changes in social media use to negative impacts on their thoughts or behavior:

> *I have become more reserved and introverted (P344)*

> *Made me lazy and sad (P355)*

> *i use it more frequently because im stressed (P87)*

> *I do not feel as anxious now that I have avoided it [covid coverage] online (P129)*

> *Sometimes, I notice that that I am on social media longer when I'm alone/isolated (P70)*

3.3 Positive socioemotional changes

In contrast to the comments in subtheme 3.2, some participants related their changes in social media use to positive impacts on their behavior. This subtheme is closely linked to subtheme 4.3 "entertainment."

> *I also find funny apps and memes to put me in a better mood and therefore resort to social media to lift my mood (P241)*

> *it has allowed me to appreciate nature a lot more and social media does keep you entertained and happy but it is only temporary whereas admiring nature, colours and other things it really makes you think about life and the meaning of It allowing you to be happy for a longer period of time (P221)*

> *social media does keep you entertained and happy but it is only temporary (P221)*

Theme 4: Using social media to relieve boredom, procrastinate, or entertain

Forty-three participants provided comments which were categorized within this theme and they were divided into three subthemes.

4.1 Procrastination

Nine participants related their use to procrastination, for example:

> *I have been on my phone and laptop way more than usual. I use my social media as a way of procrastinating university work (P202)*

> *For me personally I haven't noticed a huge change in my social media habits, My social media use has increased slightly but i can contribute most of that time to procrastination (P29)*

> *Covid-19 has increased by screentime on social media apps as well as procrastination (P32)*

> *Social media is the only thing I do, I'm always on it and it is the reason for why I procrastinate so much (P271)*

4.2 Boredom

There were 19 responses which mentioned boredom, some examples follow:

> *I am feeling constantly bored at home and the only way to enlighten my mood is through the use of social media more (P20)*

It has increased my habits, such as habitually clicking on social media when I am bored or if there's something I do not want to do (e.g. chores, studying etc.) (P22)

I have gone on social more now as I want to find ways to cure my boredom (P52)

I find myself more bored than I usually am (before COVID19) (P136)

4.3 Entertainment

There were 15 responses which linked social media to a form of entertainment, for example:

it is my only source of entertainment other than talking to friends as family thought phone calls (P154)

I am much more inclined to use social media now as it feels like my only source of entertainment and connection to the outside world (P206)

Theme 5: Related to COVID-19 news or discussion

5.1 Avoiding news about COVID-19

This was reflected by seven participants:

I avoid anything on social media related to Covid-19 (P322)

all I hear about is coronavirus, which kind of annoyed me into staying off social media, unless it's for social contacts (P136)

I am now also very selective in the content I allow myself to see/read as alot of it is negative surrounding Covid and I do not feel as anxious now that I have avoided it online (P129)

I found in the beginning I was on social a lot looking at news and opinions surrounding COVID-19 and it had a very negative impact on me (P222)

lessened them due to negative news impacts (P258)

I use social media a lot less than before as it has been full of hype and fear, and it has been better for me to avoid it (P322)

I use social media a lot less than before as it has been full of hype and fear, and it has been better for me to avoid it (P326)

5.2 Seeking news about COVID-19

Although in contrast to Theme 5.1, five participants reported using social media more to stay updated with the news about COVID-19:

I have been using social media platforms more often to gather news upon COVID-19 (P381)

also look at the authenticity of health information more than before (P326)

i spend quite a while per day reading the news from news apps, which is time i probably would have spent on social media before (P237)

I am a lot more interactive and aware on social media to stay updated with news (P170)

Discussion

The comments coded under Theme 1, "using social media for relationship maintenance and initiation" support much of the research reviewed in the Introduction relating social media use to enhanced connectedness in terms of quantity of connections (Allen et al., 2014; Davis, 2012; Wang et al., 2012) and enhanced quality of connections (Vaterlaus et al., 2016). Nowland et al. (2018) found a positive impact on the psychological wellbeing and sense of social connectedness for those individuals who used social media specifically for relationship building and maintenance. So, it may be that the impacts are differential depending on how individuals normally use social media and whether they perceive it as a tool for relationship building and maintenance, rather than a tool to portray their online identity or a tool for keeping up with current crazes, news, and generally entertainment. An interesting question to explore in the next stage of research is to explore whether those individuals already using social media for enhancing connectedness or introverts experience less impact due to COVID-19, while those not using social media to enhance connectedness prior to COVID-19 or extraverts may be more affected. Differences in personality will be explored in further research.

In contrast to research reviewed in the Introduction, the comments coded under Theme 2 "passive social media use" indicate that many participants perceived there being less meaningful use of social media, rather than more meaningful connections. There were many comments relating passive use (such as scrolling) with lower quality of interactions; this supports the differentiation of the impacts depending on whether use is regarded as active or passive highlighted by Ekström and Östman (2015). Escobar-Viera et al. (2018) have also suggested that the way in which an individual participates and interacts with social media can influence their wellbeing. The authors utilized a scale created by Li (2016) which measures an individual's passive and active social media use. Participants were asked how much they engage in a number of behaviors on any social media site, and these behaviors were either defined as being passive or active. Participants were asked to respond on a seven-point scale ranging from "never" to "constantly/all the time." A factor analysis revealed active and passive items to be distinct and robust variables. Escobar-Viera et al. (2018) found a positive correlation between passive social media use and depressive symptoms, and conversely a negative correlation between active social media use and depressive symptoms. These findings support those of Deters and Mehl (2013), who found a reduction of loneliness through an intervention that required active engagement on Facebook. Further research will investigate the influence of active and passive use during the continuing COVID-19 restrictions.

Theme 3 identified positive and negative "mental health impacts," where the majority of comments within this theme related to the subtheme "over-use of social media." An article published since this data was analyzed provides support for the link between overuse of social media during the COVID-19 restrictions. In an article aiming to provide consensus guidance, Király et al. (2020) state that although the majority of use of information and communications technology during COVID-19 is directed at achieving work and social goals and should not be pathologized, there exists a group of already vulnerable individuals who are at risk of developing problematic usage patterns. Király et al. (2020) go on to make some practical recommendations to help reduce these risks for vulnerable individuals.

It seems that permanent connectedness may produce ambiguous and complex feelings for social media users, similar to those found in a cross-sectional mixed methods study by Thomas, Azmitia, and Whittaker (2016) of attitudes toward "unplugging" from social media. In the Thomas et al. (2016) study, participants reported feelings of anxiety in response to unplugging from social media, due to FOMO; however interestingly, participants also reported feelings of freedom and a sense of relief from the perceived pressure to always be available to others. Similarly, in our study there were examples of individuals recognizing that avoiding social media could lead to better wellbeing by reducing negative psychological outcomes. It is clear then that social media use and its impact on social connection and wellbeing is complex, as incongruent experiences of connectedness and disconnectedness may occur simultaneously when engaging with others on social media. It is possible that individual differences in personality may play a mediating or moderating role here and this will be investigated in further research.

Linking the comments coded within Themes 2 and 3, it seems that participants were more likely to experience negative wellbeing outcomes when their lack of offline connectedness became disruptive to their connections online. For example, there was more passive use of social media and reduced online commenting due to less offline socializing and both link to a FOMO. The findings of this research provided some insight into the negotiation between connectedness needs and the permanently connected nature of online communication technologies. The bidirectional nature of the impacts on behavior and perception confirms some previous research showing similar impacts. A cross-sectional survey study by Dhir, Yossatorn, Kaur, and Chen (2018) of social media fatigue[b] and psychological wellbeing found an association between mental exhaustion from social media overload and increased levels of anxiety and depression. However, Dhir et al. (2018) found that the need to be permanently connected was driven in part by a fear of missing out on social engagement with others, which itself was driven by the permanently online nature of the platforms. Similarly, a survey study investigating online vigilance found that those who were constantly monitoring and responding to social media cues reported less life satisfaction and affective wellbeing (Johannes et al., 2018). However, this was only the case for those who experienced a corresponding reduction in mindfulness (i.e., feeling unable

b According to Techopedia (2017), social media fatigue refers to, "social media users' tendency to pull back from social media when they become overwhelmed with too many social media sites, too many friends and followers and too much time spent online maintaining these connections."

to attend fully to the present moment due to online vigilance behaviors). This suggested that participants were more likely to experience negative wellbeing outcomes when their online connectedness became disruptive to their ability to connect in real life.

Conclusions and further research

This research contributes to an understanding of how perceptions and experiences are related to individual's social media use during COVID-19 and indicates some impacts on their psychological wellbeing. The findings can be used in educational campaigns aimed at helping individuals engage with social media platforms in a positive and socially productive way. The results may also inform policy aimed at enhancing online mental health in socially at-risk groups (i.e., chronically ill, or homebound people) who have less opportunity for offline interactions.

The findings will inform the next stage of research which involves conducting semistructured interviews with 15 participants to explore in more depth the lived experiences of young people during the extended COVID-19 restriction period. In addition to a qualitative study, a quantitative study will explore individual differences and their role as potential mediators for the relationships between social media use and wellbeing. Personality could be a potential mediating factor influencing a reduction in wellbeing as a result of increasing social media use. Attrill (2015) proposed that certain individuals are more susceptible to the negative or positive effects of social media. However, there has been little research to investigate personality, with research instead exploring the role of self-esteem in social media use. For example, Paramboukis, Skues, and Wise (2016) found a weak correlation associating higher narcissism and lower self-esteem with more Instagram use. Woods and Scott (2016) found a negative relationship between trait self-esteem and social media use, whereby lower self-esteem scores were associated with higher levels of social media use, and emotional investment in social media. The findings of further research could be used in personalizing education campaigns aimed at helping individuals to manage their social media use.

References

Abeele, M. M. V., Antheunis, M. L., & Schouten, A. P. (2016). The effect of mobile messaging during a conversation on impression formation and interaction quality. *Computers in Human Behavior*, *62*, 562–569. https://doi.org/10.1016/j.chb.2016.04.005.

Allen, K. A., Ryan, T., Gray, D. L., McInerney, D. M., & Waters, L. (2014). Social media use and social connectedness in adolescents: The positives and the potential pitfalls. *Australian Educational and Developmental Psychologist*, *31*(1), 18–31. https://doi.org/10.1017/edp.2014.2.

Attrill, A. (2015). *Cyberpsychology*. Oxford: Oxford University Press.

Banerjee, D., & Rai, M. (2020). Social isolation in Covid-19: The impact of loneliness. *International Journal of Social Psychiatry*, *66*(6), 525–527. https://doi.org/10.1177/0020764020922269.

Baumeister, R. F., & Leary, M. R. (1995). The need to belong: Desire for interpersonal attachments as a fundamental human motivation. *Psychological Bulletin*, *117*(3), 497–529. https://doi.org/10.1037/0033-2909.117.3.497.

Bayer, J. B., Triệu, P., & Ellison, N. B. (2020). Social media elements, ecologies, and effects. *Annual Review of Psychology*, *71*, 471–497. https://doi.org/10.1146/annurev-psych-010419-050944.

Braun, V., & Clarke, V. (2006). Using thematic analysis in psychology. *Qualitative Research in Psychology*, *3*(2), 77–101. https://doi.org/10.1191/1478088706qp063oa.

Carr, C. T., & Hayes, R. A. (2015). Social media: Defining, developing, and divining. *Atlantic Journal of Communication*, *23*(1), 46–65. https://doi.org/10.1080/15456870.2015.972282.

Casale, S. (2020). Problematic social media use: Conceptualization, assessment and trends in scientific literature. *Addictive Behaviors Reports*, *12*, 100281. https://doi.org/10.1016/j.abrep.2020.100281.

Chadwick, D. D., & Fullwood, C. (2018). An online life like any other: Identity, self-determination, and social networking among adults with intellectual disabilities. *Cyberpsychology, Behavior and Social Networking*, *21*(1), 56–64. https://doi.org/10.1089/cyber.2016.0689.

Clark, J. L., & Green, M. C. (2018). Self-fulfilling prophecies: Perceived reality of online interaction drives expected outcomes of online communication. *Personality and Individual Differences*, *133*, 73–76. https://doi.org/10.1016/j.paid.2017.08.031.

Davis, K. (2012). Friendship 2.0: Adolescents' experiences of belonging and self-disclosure online. *Journal of Adolescence*, *35*(6), 1527–1536. https://doi.org/10.1016/j.adolescence.2012.02.013.

Deters, F. G., & Mehl, M. R. (2013). Does posting Facebook status updates increase or decrease loneliness? An online social networking experiment. *Social Psychological and Personality Science*, *4*(5), 579–586. https://doi.org/10.1177/1948550612469233.

Dhir, A., Yossatorn, Y., Kaur, P., & Chen, S. (2018). Online social media fatigue and psychological wellbeing—A study of compulsive use, fear of missing out, fatigue, anxiety and depression. *International Journal of Information Management*, *40*, 141–152. https://doi.org/10.1016/j.ijinfomgt.2018.01.012.

Ekström, M., & Östman, J. (2015). Information, interaction, and creative production: The effects of three forms of internet use on youth democratic engagement. *Communication Research*, *42*(6), 796–818. https://doi.org/10.1177/0093650213476295.

Escobar-Viera, C. G., Shensa, A., Bowman, N. D., Sidani, J. E., Knight, J., James, A. E., & Primack, B. A. (2018). Passive and active social media use and depressive symptoms among United States adults. *Cyberpsychology, Behavior and Social Networking*, *21*(7), 437–443. https://doi.org/10.1089/cyber.2017.0668.

Goswami, S., Köbler, F., Leimeister, J. M., & Krcmar, H. (2010). *Using online social networking to enhance social connectedness and social support for the elderly. 109*. Association for Information Systems. https://aisel.aisnet.org/cgi/viewcontent.cgi?article=1106&context=icis2010_submissions.

Grieve, R., Indian, M., Witteveen, K., Tolan, G. A., & Marrington, J. (2013). Face-to-face or Facebook: Can social connectedness be derived online? *Computers in Human Behavior*, *29*(3), 604–609. https://doi.org/10.1016/j.chb.2012.11.017.

Johannes, N., Veling, H., Dora, J., Meier, A., Reinecke, L., & Buijzen, M. (2018). Mind-wandering and mindfulness as mediators of the relationship between online vigilance and well-being. *Cyberpsychology, Behavior and Social Networking*, *21*(12), 761–767. https://doi.org/10.1089/cyber.2018.0373.

Jose, P. E., Ryan, N., & Pryor, J. (2012). Does social connectedness promote a greater sense of well-being in adolescence over time? *Journal of Research on Adolescence*, *22*(2), 235–251. https://doi.org/10.1111/j.1532-7795.2012.00783.x.

Kantar Group and Affiliates. (2020). *COVID-19 barometer: Consumer attitudes, media habits and expectations*. Retrieved on 3 April 2020 from https://www.kantar.com/Inspiration/Coronavirus/COVID-19-Barometer-Consumerattitudes-media-habits-and-expectations.

Kastrenakes, J. (2020). *Zoom saw a huge increase in subscribers—and revenue—thanks to the pandemic*. Retrieved on 10 August 2020 from https://www.theverge.com/2020/6/2/21277006/zoom-q1-2021-earnings-coronavirus-pandemic-work-from-home.

Király, O., Potenza, M. N., Stein, D. J., King, D. L., Hodgins, D. C., Saunders, J. B., … Abbott, M. W. (2020). Preventing problematic internet use during the COVID-19 pandemic: Consensus guidance. *Comprehensive Psychiatry*, *100*, 152180. https://www.sciencedirect.com/science/article/pii/S0010440X20300225.

Kushlev, K., Proulx, J. D., & Dunn, E. W. (2017). Digitally connected, socially disconnected: The effects of relying on technology rather than other people. *Computers in Human Behavior*, *76*, 68–74. https://doi.org/10.1016/j.chb.2017.07.001.

Lee, H. E., & Cho, J. (2019). Social media use and well-being in people with physical disabilities: Influence of SNS and online community uses on social support, depression, and psychological disposition. *Health Communication*, *34*(9), 1043–1052. https://doi.org/10.1080/10410236.2018.1455138.

Lee, R. M., & Robbins, S. B. (1998). The relationship between social connectedness and anxiety, self-esteem, and social identity. *Journal of Counseling Psychology*, *45*(3), 338–345. https://doi.org/10.1037/0022-0167.45.3.338.

Li, Z. (2016). Psychological empowerment on social media: Who are the empowered users? *Public Relations Review*, *42*(1), 49–59. https://doi.org/10.1016/j.pubrev.2015.09.001.

Lichtenstein, A., & Rosenfeld, L. B. (1983). Uses and misuses of gratifications research: An explication of media functions. *Communication Research*, *10*(1), 97–109. https://doi.org/10.1177/009365083010001005.

McLouglin, L., Spears, B., & Taddeo, C. (2018). The importance of social connection for cybervictims: How connectedness and technology could promote mental health and wellbeing in young people. *International Journal of Emotional Education*, *10*(1), 5–24. https://www.um.edu.mt/library/oar//handle/123456789/29667.

Microsoft. (2020). *Our commitment to customers during COVID-19 by Jared Spataro, Corporate Vice President for Microsoft 365*. Blog published on March 5, 2020 https://www.microsoft.com/en-us/microsoft-365/blog/2020/03/05/our-commitment-to-customers-during-covid-19/.

Nowland, R., Necka, E. A., & Cacioppo, J. T. (2018). Loneliness and social internet use: Pathways to reconnection in a digital world? *Perspectives on Psychological Science*, *13*(1), 70–87. https://doi.org/10.1177/1745691617713052.

Paramboukis, O., Skues, J., & Wise, L. (2016). An exploratory study of the relationships between narcissism, self-esteem and Instagram use. *Social Networking*, *5*, 82–92. https://doi.org/10.4236/sn.2016.52009.

Primack, B. A., Shensa, A., Sidani, J. E., Whaite, E. O., Lin, L. Y., Rosen, D., … Miller, E. (2017). Social media use and perceived social isolation among young adults in the US. *American Journal of Preventive Medicine*, *53*(1), 1–8. https://doi.org/10.1016/j.amepre.2017.01.010.

Raghavendra, P., Newman, L., Grace, E., & Wood, D. (2015). Enhancing social participation in young people with communication disabilities living in rural Australia: Outcomes of a home-based intervention for using social media. *Disability and Rehabilitation*, *37*(17), 1576–1590. https://doi.org/10.3109/09638288.2015.1052578.

Scarf, D., Hayhurst, J. G., Riordan, B. C., Boyes, M., Ruffman, T., & Hunter, J. A. (2017). Increasing resilience in adolescents: The importance of social connectedness in adventure education programmes. *Australasian Psychiatry*, *25*(2), 154–156. https://doi.org/10.1177/1039856216671668.

Shankar, A., Rafnsson, S. B., & Steptoe, A. (2015). Longitudinal associations between social connections and subjective wellbeing in the English longitudinal study of ageing. *Psychology & Health, 30*(6), 686–698. https://doi.org/10.1080/08870446.2014.979823.

Sinclair, T. J., & Grieve, R. (2017). Facebook as a source of social connectedness in older adults. *Computers in Human Behavior, 66*, 363–369. https://doi.org/10.1016/j.chb.2016.10.003.

Statista. (2020). Accessed on 12 August 2020 from https://www.statista.com/chart/18983/time-spent-on-social-media/.

J. Taylor-Jackson & A. Mustafa. The relationships between social media use and factors relating to depression. Depression. in A. Mustafa (eds) in press. Elsevier.

Techopedia. (2017). *Accessed on 17 August 2020*. https://www.techopedia.com/definition/27372/social-media-fatigue.

Thomas, V., Azmitia, M., & Whittaker, S. (2016). Unplugged: Exploring the costs and benefits of constant connection. *Computers in Human Behavior, 63*, 540–548. https://doi.org/10.1016/j.chb.2016.05.078.

Tiwari, S., Lane, M., & Alam, K. (2019). Do social networking sites build and maintain social capital online in rural communities? *Journal of Rural Studies, 66*, 1–10. https://doi.org/10.1016/j.jrurstud.2019.01.029.

Twenge, J. M., Spitzberg, B. H., & Campbell, W. K. (2019). Less in-person social interaction with peers among US adolescents in the 21st century and links to loneliness. *Journal of Social and Personal Relationships, 36*(6), 1892–1913. https://doi.org/10.1177/0265407519836170.

Vaterlaus, J. M., Barnett, K., Roche, C., & Young, J. A. (2016). "Snapchat is more personal": An exploratory study on Snapchat behaviors and young adult interpersonal relationships. *Computers in Human Behavior, 62*, 594–601. https://doi.org/10.1016/j.chb.2016.04.029.

Verduyn, P., Lee, D. S., Park, J., Shablack, H., Orvell, A., Bayer, J., … Kross, E. (2015). Passive Facebook usage undermines affective well-being: Experimental and longitudinal evidence. *Journal of Experimental Psychology: General, 144*(2), 480–488. https://doi.org/10.1037/xge0000057.

Wang, Z., Tchernev, J. M., & Solloway, T. (2012). A dynamic longitudinal examination of social media use, needs, and gratifications among college students. *Computers in Human Behavior, 28*(5), 1829–1839. https://doi.org/10.1016/j.chb.2012.05.001.

We Are Social. (2019). *Digital in Australia 2019*. https://wearesocial.com/au/digital-2019-australia.

Woods, H. C., & Scott, H. (2016). #Sleepyteens: Social media use in adolescence is associated with poor sleep quality, anxiety, depression and low self-esteem. *Journal of Adolescence, 51*, 41–49. https://doi.org/10.1016/j.adolescence.2016.05.008.

Wu, Y. J., Outley, C., Matarrita-Cascante, D., & Murphrey, T. P. (2016). A systematic review of recent research on adolescent social connectedness and mental health with internet technology use. *Adolescent Research Review, 1*(2), 153–162. https://doi.org/10.1007/s40894-015-0013-9.

Chapter 17

Cognitive behavior therapy for COVID-19 related distress

Karen Moses[a] and Bethany M. Wootton[b]
[a]*School of Psychology, Western Sydney University, Sydney, NSW, Australia,* [b]*Graduate School of Health, University of Technology Sydney, Sydney, NSW, Australia*

COVID-19 and distress

The COVID-19 pandemic has had a profound mental health impact with several studies demonstrating that the pandemic has resulted in increased incidence of anxiety, depression, sleep disorders, posttraumatic stress disorders, and substance use disorders in both those who have been infected with the illness and those who have been impacted by restrictions in place as a consequence of the illness (Luo, Guo, Yu, & Wang, 2020; Rajkumar, 2020; Rogers et al., 2020). The COVID-19 pandemic has also resulted in an increased demand for mental health services (Titov et al., 2020), and it appears that the mental health effects of the COVID-19 pandemic are particularly pronounced for those who had a preexisting mental health condition prior to the onset of the pandemic (Asmundson et al., 2020; González-Sanguino et al., 2020; Taylor et al., 2020a).

Taylor and colleagues have proposed the presence of a COVID stress syndrome which includes five symptom categories relating to (1) danger and contamination fears (i.e., worry about self or others catching COVID-19); (2) socioeconomic concerns (i.e., concerns about personal finances, job losses, and disruption to the supply chain); (3) xenophobic concerns about foreign travelers spreading the illness; (4) traumatic stress symptoms, such as intrusive thoughts or nightmares related to direct or indirect exposure to COVID-19 related trauma; and (5) compulsive checking/reassurance seeking (i.e., checking oneself for symptoms of COVID-19, seeking reassurance from friends or family, and frequently reviewing material or other information about COVID-19) (Taylor et al., 2020a). The first category, related to danger and contamination fears, appears to be the central feature of the syndrome (Taylor et al., 2020a), and there is now a sizeable literature demonstrating that many individuals in the community are concerned about becoming infected with COVID-19, or similarly, a close family member or friend becoming infected (Mertens, Gerritsen, Duijndam, Salemink, & Engelhard, 2020; Titov et al., 2020; Wahlund et al.,

Mental Health Effects of COVID-19. https://doi.org/10.1016/B978-0-12-824289-6.00007-6

2020; Wang et al., 2020). These concerns have been labeled as *coronaphobia* by some authors (Asmundson & Taylor, 2020). Understandably, older adults appear to have higher levels of concern (Titov et al., 2020), which likely reflects the higher mortality rate from COVID-19 in this population (Zhou et al., 2020).

Assessment of COVID-19 related distress

The completion of an evidence-based assessment is generally considered critical to the effective treatment of mental health problems (Hansen, Oerbeck, Skirbekk, & Kristensen, 2016; Jensen-Doss & Weisz, 2008; Moses, Gayed, Chuah, & Wootton, 2020; Pogge et al., 2001) and symptoms related to COVID-19 distress are considered no exception to this (Ahorsu et al., 2020). Research has shown that without a multimethod and multiinformant assessment, patient care and outcome may be comprised, particularly through the provision of an incorrect treatment plan (Croskerry, 2003; Jensen-Doss & Weisz, 2008; Jensen-Doss, Youngstrom, Youngstrom, Feeny, & Findling, 2014; Pogge et al., 2001). Multimethod assessment refers to the importance of using multiple methods to gather assessment information, including where relevant use of the clinical interview, semistructured diagnostic interview, self-report or clinician administered rating scales, and behavioral observation. A multiinformant approach refers to the collection of information from multiple individuals where relevant, such as from parents or partners. Specific to the COVID-19, an understanding of an individual's symptoms experienced as either a direct or indirect consequence of the pandemic, and a valid and reliable means of assessing this, is essential to the development of psychosocial treatment programs (Ahorsu et al., 2020).

The unstructured clinical interview is typically the first assessment tool used in clinical practice. While possessing many benefits, including aiding in rapport development, the clinical interview can be subject to clinician bias and is particularly susceptible to diagnostic error when used as a stand-alone assessment tool (Ollendick & Hersen, 1993; Silverman & Ollendick, 2005). To date, no clinician-administered assessment tools, either structured interview schedules or clinician-administered rating scales, have been developed to assess COVID-19 related distress. The development of these measures is critical to enhancing assessment objectivity and to reduce the bias that self-report measures are often prone to (Ransing et al., 2020). Until such COVID-19 specific measures are developed, clinicians may find the use of existing structured diagnostic interviews, such as the Diagnostic Interview for Anxiety, Mood, Obsessive-Compulsive and Related Neuropsychiatric Disorders (DIAMOND) (Tolin et al., 2018), as a useful adjunct to their clinical interview to highlight the presence of psychiatric disorders. The DIAMOND is consonant with the Diagnostic and Statistical Manual of Mental Disorders (5th Edition) (American Psychiatric Association, 2013) and demonstrates strong psychometric properties (Tolin et al., 2018).

Numerous empirically validated self-report scales have been developed to measure COVID-19 related symptoms; however, these tools vary in the variables of interest. Some of the more commonly used measures include the Coronavirus Anxiety Scale (Lee, 2020a); the Obsession with COVID-19 Scale (Lee, 2020b); the Fear of COVID-19 Scale (Ahorsu et al., 2020); the COVID Stress Scale (Taylor et al., 2020b); the COVID-19 Perceived Risk Scale (Yıldırım & Güler, 2020); the Coronavirus Stress Measure (Arslan, Yıldırım, Tanhan, Buluş, & Allen, 2020); the Fear of COVID-19 Familial Infection Scale (Mayer, Etgar, Shiffman, & Lurie, 2020); and the Coronavirus Reassurance-Seeking Behaviors Scale (Lee, Jobe, Mathis, & Gibbons, 2020). Of these self-report tools, the Fear of COVID-19 Scale (FCV-19S) has received considerable attention, with empirically validated translations in Italian (Soraci et al., 2020), Bangla (Sakib et al., 2020), Turkish (Satici, Gocet-Tekin, Deniz, & Satici, 2020), and Russian (Reznik, Gritsenko, Konstantinov, Khamenka, & Isralowitz, 2020). The FCV-19S (Ahorsu et al., 2020) is a unidimensional seven-item self-report scale designed to assess general fear of COVID-19. All items are rated on a 5-point Likert scale and scores range from 7 to 35, with higher scores indicating more severe symptoms. Internal consistency for this scale was found to be acceptable ($\alpha=0.82$) in previous studies (Ahorsu et al., 2020; Reznik, Gritsenko, Konstantinov, Khamenka, & Isralowitz, 2020; Sakib et al., 2020; Satici, Gocet-Tekin, Deniz, & Satici, 2020; Soraci et al., 2020).

The COVID Stress Scale (CSS; Taylor et al., 2020b) is a 36-item self-report scale designed to measure the severity of distress and anxiety symptoms associated with COVID-19. Specific subscales of the CSS include (1) danger and contamination fears, (2) fears about economic consequences, (3) xenophobia, (4) compulsive checking, and (5) traumatic stress symptoms. All items are rated on a 5-point Likert scale and scores range from 0 to 144, with higher scores indicating more severe symptoms. Internal consistency for this scale was reported as being good to excellent ($\alpha \geq 0.80$) (Taylor et al., 2020b). A major strength of the CSS is that it reflects the multidimensionality of responses to COVID-19, in turn potentially providing a broader or more comprehensive assessment of symptoms. Further research is required to establish the psychometric properties of this scale in populations outside of the United States and Canada.

During the pandemic, self-report measures will likely play an important role in the assessment of COVID-19 related distress, offering a cost-effective and easy to administer assessment tool, which can be delivered in a face-to-face setting or via online platforms. Given the diversity of symptoms related to COVID-19 distress may not yet fully be understood, and the high prevalence of symptoms of anxiety and depression in general population, it may be advantageous to include other commonly used measures of low mood and anxiety to supplement the COVID-19 specific measures. Self-report tools such as the Patient Health Questionnaire—9 item (Kroenke, Spitzer, & Williams, 2001) and the Generalized Anxiety Disorder Scale—7 item (Spitzer, Kroenke, Williams, & Löwe, 2006), which measure depressive symptoms and generalized anxiety symptoms, respectively, may be useful adjuncts.

It is important to highlight that the utility of these self-report measures in the development of interventions, as well as their ability to measure treatment response, remains unknown, and further research is required. Given this, it is recommended that clinicians consider the use of a multimodal assessment consisting of a clinical interview, multiple self-report scales, and observation during the assessment process to support the completion of a comprehensive assessment that can best inform intervention, and potentially monitor treatment outcomes. In addition, given there is evidence to suggest that individuals with preexisting mental health conditions are particularly susceptible to experiencing distress as a consequences of COVID-19 (Asmundson et al., 2020; González-Sanguino et al., 2020; Taylor et al., 2020a), a thorough psychiatric history should be considered essential to the assessment process. Of particular note is that those experiencing COVID-19 related distress may be at increased risk of suicide (Goyal, Chauhan, Chhikara, Gupta, & Singh, 2020; Mamun & Griffiths, 2020), highlighting the need for the inclusion of a risk assessment when assessing and treating patients presenting with COVID-19 related distress.

Cognitive behavior therapy for COVID-19 related distress

Cognitive behavior therapy (CBT) is a psychological intervention that has been shown to be effective for many mental health presentations including anxiety disorders, depressive disorders, and trauma and stress-related disorders, demonstrated in both clinical trials (Hunsley, Elliott, & Therrien, 2014; Norton & Price, 2007; Olatunji, Cisler, & Deacon, 2010), as well as real-world settings (Hollon & Ponniah, 2010; Stewart & Chambless, 2009). At its core, CBT identifies that unhelpful or maladaptive patterns in thinking and behavior cause and maintain mental illness (Beck & Haigh, 2014), patterns which can subsequently be altered through treatment. As an intervention, CBT tends to be a time limited, present oriented, collaborative, active (including within-session and between-session tasks for clients to complete), and goal oriented (Tolin, 2016). Ultimately, CBT teaches patients to become their own therapists, learning skills to change their own unhelpful thinking and behavioral patterns.

Individualized case formulation

Preliminary research suggests that symptoms of distress in response to COVID-19 are likely to be multidimensional in nature (Taylor et al., 2020a, 2020b). Thus it is important to note that symptom presentations in those presenting with COVID-19 distress may be extremely heterogeneous. For this reason, an individualized case formulation approach will be important for treatment planning. A case formulation method to CBT provides a framework for the development of CBT intervention that is designed to meet the individual patient's needs. Case formulation offers a means to apply empirically supported CBT interventions to patients in everyday clinical practice. Key components of the case formulation include the identification of a patient's symptoms, factors that have contributed to the development of, and maintain the patients' COVID-19 related distress (Persons, 2008). CBT intervention is then tailored based on factors identified within this case formulation, particularly maintaining factors. The following cognitive-behavioral interventions may be useful to consider when devising a treatment plan for individuals presenting with COVID-19 related distress. While there is much research to support the efficacy and effectiveness of CBT for the treatment of many mental health presentations, it is important to highlight that at this stage there is little empirical evidence supporting these interventions specifically for COVID-19 related distress, and further research is required.

Psychoeducation

There is a wealth of information currently available on the COVID-19 pandemic, particularly through social media. Unfortunately, not all of the information available to patients will be accurate. Preliminary research has found that access to accurate health information (e.g., advice on local transmission and treatment options) and hygiene measures (e.g., hand hygiene and social distancing) is associated with reduced impacts to mental health, including stress, anxiety, and depression (Wang et al., 2020). When working with clients experiencing symptoms of distress associated with COVID-19, it will be important to consider and discuss with patients the role that access to accurate information has on distress associated with COVID-19 and encourage access to information through reputable sources.

Situation selection

There is evidence to suggest that repeated exposure to media reports about the COVID-19 pandemic results in increased psychological distress (Garfin, Silver, & Holman, 2020; Mertens et al., 2020) and this phenomenon has been seen during other stressful events, such as the September 11 terrorist attacks in the United States of America (Silver et al., 2013). Situation selection involves choosing to avoid a specific trigger in order to avoid the emotions that follow it (Tolin, 2016). While it is essential for individuals to remain informed about the COVID-19 pandemic, it may be helpful for some patients presenting with COVID-19 related distress to limit their media and social media consumption of information related to the pandemic. The therapist and the patient may wish to collaboratively examine the relationship between their media/social media consumption and their distress and discuss whether limits on such consumption may be a simple approach to reducing distress.

Cognitive restructuring

Worry about COVID-19 has been highlighted as a key feature of distress during the current pandemic (Mertens et al., 2020; Taylor et al., 2020a; Wahlund et al., 2020). Such thoughts or worries are likely to include fears related to danger and contamination (Taylor et al., 2020a) such as "my family or I will catch COVID-19 or die" or "the government will not be able to effectively control the pandemic and prevent me from getting COVID-19." Other common worries may be related to supply chain issues, such as "the grocery stores will run out of food or other essential items," or xenophobic concerns, such as "I will be near a recently returned traveller who will give me COVID-19" (Mertens et al., 2020; Taylor et al., 2020a).

The cognitive model is based on the understanding that maladaptive emotional states, such as anxiety, distress, and mood disturbances, are maintained or exacerbated by maladaptive, exaggerated, or biased ways of thinking (Beck & Haigh, 2014). Therefore cognitive interventions aim to identify and challenge these irrational or maladaptive thoughts. Frequently used cognitive techniques include structured or unstructured thought challenging and behavioral experiments (Hofmann & Asmundson, 2008; Leahy, 2017). These techniques engage patients in scientific and rational thinking by asking individuals to identify negative or maladaptive thoughts, examine the validity of these thoughts through gathered evidence and, where appropriate, examine the meaning of the thought. Importantly, this technique does not aim to develop positive thoughts, but realistic thoughts or a pragmatic way of thinking about things. This will be an important consideration when working with patients who experience negative or maladaptive thoughts related to the COVID-19 pandemic. When considering common worries that have been reported by individuals with COVID-19 related distress, the aim should not be to develop such thoughts as "I will never catch COVID-19," but rather develop such thoughts as "if I follow hygiene and social distancing advice, I am significantly less likely to contract COVID-19."

In vivo exposure

Individuals with COVID-19 related distress may report a number of avoidance behaviors. For instance, individuals may avoid leaving the house due to fears of catching the virus, they may avoid conversations/discussions about the COVID-19 pandemic, they may avoid media/social media in order to avoid hearing about the COVID-19 pandemic, or they may avoid touching things or coming in to contact with people who they fear may have the illness (e.g., foreign travelers or individuals from COVID-19 "hotspots"). While these avoidance behaviors are understandable (and often protective and encouraged during the COVID-19 pandemic) some patients may present with avoidance behaviors that go above and beyond health advice and subsequently prevent them from accessing services or information that they need. While avoidance helps to reduce distress in the short term, many cognitive behavioral models emphasize that avoidance maintains distress in the long term (Salkovskis, 1985; Veale, 2004; Warwick & Salkovskis, 1990). In vivo exposure may be helpful for patients who present with maladaptive forms of avoidance and it involves gradually confronting feared situations in order to reduce avoidance behaviors. Habituation theory

(Groves & Thompson, 1970) proposes that the more an individual encounters a feared stimuli the less distress it will cause. Many treatment outcome trials conducted with disorders characterized by high levels of avoidance, such as obsessive-compulsive disorder and social anxiety disorder, highlight that in vivo exposure is a highly effective treatment (Bouchard et al., 2017; Foa et al., 2005).

Prior to conducting in vivo exposure the therapist and client must work collaboratively to develop an exposure hierarchy. This hierarchy is a list of feared (and avoided) stimuli, ranging from 0 (no distress confronting the stimuli/situation) to 100 (extreme distress confronting the stimuli/situation). The therapist and patient then work together to identify a good target to start the in vivo exposure process. Usually an appropriate target is one that is given a distress rating of around 50. The patient then goes in to that feared environment and stays in the situation for a predetermined length of time. The patient will expose themselves to that stimuli/situation until it no longer causes significant distress. After this, the patient will then confront the next item on their exposure hierarchy. Over time the patient then works their way through the rest of the exposure hierarchy until they reach and overcome their most feared stimuli/situation.

Imaginal exposure

Patients who have experienced a COVID-19 associated traumatic event may experience intrusive thoughts, images, or memories related to that event (Taylor et al., 2020a). Such intrusions are common in individuals who have experienced a traumatic incident (Michael, Ehlers, Halligan, & Clark, 2005) and many patients who experience a traumatic event recover without any intervention (Ehlers & Clark, 2003). However, if such intrusions and other symptoms of posttraumatic stress disorder persist beyond 2 months after the event (Ehlers & Clark, 2003), prolonged imaginal exposure may be helpful for patients. Prolonged imaginal exposure involves asking the patient to provide a detailed account of their traumatic event, recording it, and reviewing the recording repeatedly during session (as well as later for homework) (Tolin, 2016). The intervention has been demonstrated to be safe and effective treatment for individuals with posttraumatic stress disorder (Foa et al., 1999; Foa, Zoellner, Feeny, Hembree, & Alvarez-Conrad, 2002).

For individuals with ongoing and uncontrollable worries related to the COVID-19 pandemic, worry exposure may be helpful. Worry exposure is useful for treating worries about hypothetical feared events (van der Heiden & ten Broeke, 2009). Taylor et al. (2020a) and Mertens et al. (2020) highlighted that during the COVID-19 pandemic, individuals may present with excessive worries related to catching the virus, collapse of the health care system, and societal breakdown, among others. Worry exposure involves asking the patient to provide a detailed account of their worst-case fears, recording it, and reviewing the recording repeatedly during session (as well as later for homework) (Tolin, 2016). For individuals with multiple worries, these can be tackled using a graded approach. Worry exposure has been demonstrated to be a safe and effective treatment for individuals with generalized anxiety disorder (Hoyer et al., 2009) and nonclinical participants (Goldman, Dugas, Sexton, & Gervais, 2007) in previous trials.

Eliminating safety behaviors

Safety behaviors are behaviors that a patient completes in order to make them feel safer or less anxious, which in turn only serve to reinforce the symptoms of mental illness (Tolin, 2016). Taylor et al. (2020a) highlight that compulsive checking and reassurance seeking are part of the COVID stress syndrome and these are examples of safety behaviors. Possible compulsive behaviors that may be seen in individuals presenting with COVID-19 related distress may include repeatedly checking temperature or signs of the illness, reviewing information on COVID-19 symptoms, excessive handwashing or cleaning, or seeking reassurance from health professionals/others about the likelihood of having COVID. The Coronavirus Reassurance-Seeking Behaviors Scale (Lee et al., 2020) may assist therapists in the assessment and monitoring of such symptoms. Similar to avoidance, performing a safety behavior often leads to short-term reductions in distress, but maintains the problem in the long term (Tolin, 2016). Thus it is important to reduce these behaviors in individuals who engage in them excessively. Safety behaviors can be eliminated in a graded approach similar to that described before in the in vivo exposure section. Here, the patient and therapist work together to first identify the relevant maladaptive safety behaviors, and second devise a list from easiest (0 = not at all difficult to stop behavior) to most difficult (100 = extremely difficult to stop behavior) to cease engagement in safety behaviors. The patient then works to reduce all relevant safety behaviors over time using a graded approach. Reducing safety behaviors was one of the core interventions provided in a recent study focusing on reducing COVID-19 related distress (Wahlund et al., 2020), with good outcomes.

Structured problem solving

The COVID-19 pandemic has resulted in many psychosocial impacts, such as financial stressors, and child care disruption. Many of these psychosocial impacts will be solvable problems that can be worked through in a structured way to in order to identify solutions. Structured problem solving involves teaching patients who are experiencing such difficulties a structured process for working through solvable problems. Structured problem solving has been delivered as part of an evidence-based treatment package for a number of disorders including hoarding disorder, generalized anxiety disorder, and major depressive disorder (Cuijpers, van Straten, & Warmerdam, 2007b; Ladouceur et al., 2000; Tolin et al., 2019). Importantly, one study has trialed the use of this technique, within a broader CBT treatment package, with results finding significant reductions in

COVID-19 related worry (Wahlund et al., 2020). The intervention involves the patient and therapist working collaboratively through a number of steps including (1) defining the problem in concrete terms, (2) brainstorming many possible solutions to the problem, (3) evaluating the pros and cons of each possible solution, (4) deciding on an outcome, and (5) evaluating the effectiveness of the solution (D'zurilla & Goldfried, 1971).

Physiological arousal and stress reduction

The COVID-19 pandemic has seen increases of physiological arousal and stress in the general community. Mindfulness-based interventions, including mindfulness-based stress reduction, has been shown to reduce symptoms of anxiety, low mood, stress, and distress (Goldberg et al., 2018). This technique involves teaching individuals to focus on the present and accept experiences in a nonjudgmental fashion (Goldberg et al., 2018). This technique may be particularly useful in reducing COVID-19 related distress experienced by patients across the lifespan, irrespective of an experience or skill in mindfulness techniques (Behan, 2020).

Similarly, arousal reduction techniques may be useful in reducing somatic symptoms of anxiety. Such techniques include progressive muscle relaxation and breathing retraining. Breathing retraining reduces physiological arousal through engagement in deliberately slowed and relaxed breathing. This technique may be used to create immediate relief from physiological symptoms of anxiety or distress (Jaywant, Vanderlind, Boas, & Dickerman, 2020). Research has shown that the use of relaxation techniques can reduce symptoms of stress and anxiety (Manansingh, Tatum, & Morote, 2019). Importantly, progressive muscle relaxation has been shown to reduce anxiety and improve sleep quality in individuals diagnosed with COVID-19 (Liu et al., 2020).

Activity scheduling

Isolation and widespread restrictions on social activities outside of the home have resulted in more time spent by individuals and families at home, potentially leading to such symptoms as loneliness, low mood, and anxiety. Research demonstrates that activity scheduling is particularly useful for those experiencing symptoms of depression (Cuijpers, Van Straten, & Warmerdam, 2007a; Jacobson et al., 1996) and anxiety (Martinsen, 2008; Turner & Leach, 2010). Activity scheduling involves an individual planning activities across waking hours of a day, with the aim of increasing active behavioral engagement and positive interactions (Cuijpers et al., 2007a). These activities are typically either pleasant or of mastery in nature. Pleasant activities refer to those activities that give a sense of enjoyment. Mastery activities refer to those activities that provide a sense of achievement or accomplishment, and may include household chores. When considering the use of activity scheduling with client's experiencing low mood or anxiety as a consequence of COVID-19, it will be important to consider the patient's personal health circumstances and government restrictions on activity when identifying appropriate tasks for completion. Appropriate examples may include home-based exercise, cooking, engaging in craft activities, or online social groups. Activity scheduling has been demonstrated to show promise in reducing COVID-19 related distress in previous studies (Wahlund et al., 2020).

Sleep hygiene

Existing research suggests that sleep is likely to be impacted by the COVID-19 pandemic as a consequence of reduced physical activity due to isolation (Fuller, Gooley, & Saper, 2006), reduced exposure to daylight, change to or irregularity in meal times (Altena et al., 2020), a history of insomnia prior to COVID-19 (Gehrman et al., 2013), and stress (Åkerstedt, Kecklund, & Axelsson, 2007; Ellis, Gehrman, Espie, Riemann, & Perlis, 2012; Gehrman et al., 2013). Research demonstrates that sleep difficulties can be effectively treated using CBT for both chronic and acute onset presentations (Boullin, Ellwood, & Ellis, 2017; Randall, Nowakowski, & Ellis, 2019). Key components of a sleep intervention should include (Altena et al., 2020): (a) stimulus control, including, using the bed for sleep or sexual activity only and adhering to a regular time to get up every morning; (b) sleep hygiene, including avoiding exposure to bright light, the consumption of caffeinated products, the consumption of alcohol and engagement in exercise immediately before bed; ensuring an optimal sleep environment; engagement in relaxation strategies prior to bed; and managing negative thoughts prior to sleep; (c) sleep restriction, including initially restricting time spent in bed (based on average sleep time over the past week, but no less than 5.5 h) and gradual increase to time spent in bed, with the intention of reducing middle of the night awakenings.

Crisis support

As research has highlighted that individuals experiencing distress as a consequence of COVID-19 have been found to be at risk of suicide (Goyal et al., 2020; Mamun & Griffiths, 2020), it is imperative that clinicians continue to provide ongoing assessment of risk and include crisis support as required. An evidence-based crisis intervention should typically include psychoeducation, safety planning (Stanley & Brown, 2012) and, following stabilization, treatment for the underlying mental health symptoms leading to suicidality (Stanley et al., 2009). High levels of suicidality are likely to require restrictive interventions and possible inpatient intervention. In most cases, it will be useful to involve the family in any suicide intervention (DeBeer et al., 2019; Wharff et al., 2019).

While the abovementioned interventions are part of evidence-based treatment packages for a variety of disorders, it is important to highlight that at the time of writing there was limited evidence supporting these interventions in the treatment of COVID-19 related distress. As the field progresses, it is important for clinicians to publish treatment outcomes in order to best inform treatment efforts of clinicians worldwide. It is also crucial that the abovementioned interventions are always implemented in a way that is consistent with local health advice (i.e., maintaining social distancing and hand hygiene and/or any lockdown laws). This is particularly important for interventions that focus on in vivo exposure, reducing safety behaviors, and activity scheduling.

Remote CBT

While CBT is generally delivered in face-to-face settings, the COVID-19 pandemic has resulted in many clinicians providing treatment remotely, that is without the patient and therapist being in the same location. Remote CBT can be delivered in either a low- or high-intensity fashion (Wootton, 2016). Low-intensity treatment requires very little therapist time or patient resources and involves the patient working their way through evidence-based CBT techniques in a primarily self-help fashion. The treatment may be supplemented with clinician support (i.e., guided treatments) or may be entirely self-guided. The most commonly utilized low-intensity CBT treatment approaches are bibliotherapy-delivered CBT (BCBT) (i.e., reading written treatment materials provided by the therapist) and internet-delivered CBT (ICBT). There are numerous research studies demonstrating the efficacy of BCBT (Chung & Kwon, 2008; Lidren et al., 1994; Wootton et al., 2018; Wootton, Dear, Johnston, Terides, & Titov, 2013) and ICBT (Dear et al., 2015; Spence et al., 2011; Wootton, Karin, Titov, & Dear, 2019) in the treatment of a variety of mental health problems.

Preliminary data has demonstrated the efficacy of ICBT in the treatment of COVID-19 related distress (Wahlund et al., 2020). For instance, in the largest and most robust study conducted to date, Wahlund et al. (2020) randomized participants with dysfunctional COVID-19 distress to either a brief self-guided ICBT intervention or waitlist control. Preliminary results indicate that the ICBT intervention outperformed the waitlist control group, with a medium between group effect size (Wahlund et al., 2020). High levels of patient acceptability were also reported (Wahlund et al., 2020).

High-intensity remote CBT is analogous to face-to-face treatment; however, the treatment is delivered using a medium such as the telephone (telephone-delivered CBT; TCBT) or internet-videoconferencing (videoconferencing-delivered CBT; VCBT). Sessions are generally the same length (i.e., approximately 60 min in duration) and include the same treatment elements as face-to-face treatment. While the COVID-19 pandemic required clinicians to quickly adapt their treatment to high-intensity remote CBT, it is encouraging that numerous previous studies have demonstrated the efficacy of these treatment approaches. For instance, TCBT has been demonstrated to be effective for generalized anxiety disorder, obsessive-compulsive disorder, and depression

(Brenes, Danhauer, Lyles, Hogan, & Miller, 2015; Lovell et al., 2006; Mohr et al., 2012) and VCBT has been demonstrated to be effective for patients with mood disorders, as well as a variety of anxiety and related disorders (Bouchard et al., 2004; Goetter, Herbert, Forman, Yuen, & Thomas, 2014; Matsumoto et al., 2018; Stubbings, Rees, Roberts, & Kane, 2013). At this stage no studies have demonstrated the efficacy of high-intensity remote CBT for COVID-19 related distress.

Conclusion

The current COVID-19 pandemic has had a significant impact on the mental health of the international community and those impacts may not yet be fully understood. In the absence of research to guide evidence-based psychological interventions specific to COVID-19 related distress, the development of an individualized formulation and intervention is essential to effective client care. This formulation must be guided by a comprehensive multimethod and multiinformant assessment. CBT can be delivered remotely and such remote treatments have the potential to increase accessibility to evidence-based interventions during the COVID-19 pandemic.

References

Ahorsu, D. K., Lin, C.-Y., Imani, V., Saffari, M., Griffiths, M. D., & Pakpour, A. H. (2020). The fear of COVID-19 scale: Development and initial validation. *International Journal of Mental Health and Addiction*.

Åkerstedt, T., Kecklund, G., & Axelsson, J. (2007). Impaired sleep after bedtime stress and worries. *Biological Psychology*, *76*(3), 170–173.

Altena, E., Baglioni, C., Espie, C. A., Ellis, J., Gavriloff, D., Holzinger, B., et al. (2020). Dealing with sleep problems during home confinement due to the COVID-19 outbreak: Practical recommendations from a task force of the European CBT-I Academy. *Journal of Sleep Research*, *25*(4), e13052.

American Psychiatric Association. (2013). *Diagnostic and statistical manual of mental disorders* (5th ed.). American Psychiatric Association.

Arslan, G., Yıldırım, M., Tanhan, A., Buluş, M., & Allen, K.-A. (2020). Coronavirus stress, optimism-pessimism, psychological inflexibility, and psychological health: Psychometric properties of the Coronavirus Stress Measure. *International Journal of Mental Health and Addiction*, *18*, 1.

Asmundson, G. J. G., Paluszek, M. M., Landry, C. A., Rachor, G. S., McKay, D., & Taylor, S. (2020). Do pre-existing anxiety-related and mood disorders differentially impact COVID-19 stress responses and coping? *Journal of Anxiety Disorders*, *74*, 102271. https://doi.org/10.1016/j.janxdis.2020.102271.

Asmundson, G. J. G., & Taylor, S. (2020). Coronaphobia: Fear and the 2019-nCoV outbreak. *Journal of Anxiety Disorders*, *70*. https://doi.org/10.1016/j.janxdis.2020.102196. Article 102196.

Beck, A. T., & Haigh, E. A. (2014). Advances in cognitive theory and therapy: The generic cognitive model. *Annual Review of Clinical Psychology*, *10*, 1–24.

Behan, C. (2020). The benefits of meditation and mindfulness practices during times of crisis such as Covid-19. *Irish Journal of Psychological Medicine*, *37*, 1–8.

Bouchard, S., Dumoulin, S., Robillard, G., Guitard, T., Klinger, E., Forget, H., et al. (2017). Virtual reality compared with in vivo exposure in the treatment of social anxiety disorder: A three-arm randomised controlled trial. *British Journal of Psychiatry*, *210*(4), 276–283. https://doi.org/10.1192/bjp.bp.116.184234.

Bouchard, S., Paquin, B., Payeur, R., Allard, M., Rivard, V., Fournier, T., et al. (2004). Delivering cognitive-behavior therapy for panic disorder with agoraphobia in videoconference. *Telemedicine Journal and E-Health*, *10*(1), 13–25. http://www.scopus.com/inward/record.url?eid=2-s2.0-1842783565&partnerID=40&md5=9544cf309c49464125db830abf4fdef9.

Boullin, P., Ellwood, C., & Ellis, J. G. (2017). Group vs. individual treatment for acute insomnia: A pilot study evaluating a "One-Shot" treatment strategy. *Brain Sciences*, *7*(1), 1.

Brenes, G. A., Danhauer, S. C., Lyles, M. F., Hogan, P. E., & Miller, M. E. (2015). Telephone-delivered cognitive behavioral therapy and telephone-delivered nondirective supportive therapy for rural older adults with generalized anxiety disorder: A randomized clinical trial. *JAMA Psychiatry*, *72*(10), 1012–1020. https://doi.org/10.1001/jamapsychiatry.2015.1154.

Chung, Y. S., & Kwon, J. H. (2008). The efficacy of bibliotherapy for social phobia. *Brief Treatment and Crisis Intervention*, *8*(4), 390–401. http://www.scopus.com/inward/record.url?eid=2-s2.0-64049098549&partnerID=40&md5=6981d91acae58e2c5e19a88e2798b1f4.

Croskerry, P. (2003). The importance of cognitive errors in diagnosis and strategies to minimize them. *Academic Medicine*, *78*(8), 775–780.

Cuijpers, P., Van Straten, A., & Warmerdam, L. (2007a). Behavioral activation treatments of depression: A meta-analysis. *Clinical Psychology Review*, *27*(3), 318–326.

Cuijpers, P., van Straten, A., & Warmerdam, L. (2007b). Problem solving therapies for depression: A meta-analysis. *European Psychiatry*, *22*(1), 9–15.

Dear, B. F., Staples, L. G., Terides, M. D., Karin, E., Zou, J., Johnston, L., et al. (2015). Transdiagnostic versus disorder-specific and clinician-guided versus self-guided internet-delivered treatment for generalized anxiety disorder and comorbid disorders: A randomized controlled trial. *Journal of Anxiety Disorders*, *36*, 63–77. https://doi.org/10.1016/j.janxdis.2015.09.003.

DeBeer, B. B., Matthieu, M. M., Kittel, J. A., Degutis, L. C., Clafferty, S., Qualls, N., et al. (2019). Quality improvement evaluation of the feasibility and acceptability of adding a concerned significant other to safety planning for suicide prevention with veterans. *Journal of Mental Health Counseling*, *41*(1), 4–20.

D'zurilla, T. J., & Goldfried, M. R. (1971). Problem solving and behavior modification. *Journal of Abnormal Psychology*, *78*(1), 107.

Ehlers, A., & Clark, D. (2003). Early psychological interventions for adult survivors of trauma: A review. *Biological Psychiatry*, *53*(9), 817–826. https://doi.org/10.1016/S0006-3223(02)01812-7.

Ellis, J. G., Gehrman, P., Espie, C. A., Riemann, D., & Perlis, M. L. (2012). Acute insomnia: Current conceptualizations and future directions. *Sleep Medicine Reviews*, *16*(1), 5–14.

Foa, E. B., Dancu, C. V., Hembree, E. A., Jaycox, L. H., Meadows, E. A., & Street, G. P. (1999). A comparison of exposure therapy, stress inoculation training, and their combination for reducing posttraumatic stress disorder in female assault victims. *Journal of Consulting and Clinical Psychology*, *67*(2), 194–200. https://doi.org/10.1037/0022-006X.67.2.194.

Foa, E. B., Liebowitz, M. R., Kozak, M. J., Davies, S., Campeas, R., Franklin, M. E., et al. (2005). Randomized, placebo-controlled trial of exposure and ritual prevention, clomipramine, and their combination in the treatment of obsessive-compulsive disorder. *American Journal of Psychiatry*, *162*(1), 151–161. https://doi.org/10.1176/appi.ajp.162.1.151.

Foa, E. B., Zoellner, L. A., Feeny, N. C., Hembree, E. A., & Alvarez-Conrad, J. (2002). Does imaginal exposure exacerbate PTSD symptoms? *Journal of Consulting and Clinical Psychology*, *70*(4), 1022–1028. https://doi.org/10.1037/0022-006X.70.4.1022.

Fuller, P. M., Gooley, J. J., & Saper, C. B. (2006). Neurobiology of the sleep-wake cycle: Sleep architecture, circadian regulation, and regulatory feedback. *Journal of Biological Rhythms*, *21*(6), 482–493.

Garfin, D. R., Silver, R. C., & Holman, E. A. (2020). The novel coronavirus (COVID-2019) outbreak: Amplification of public health consequences by media exposure [note]. *Health Psychology*. https://doi.org/10.1037/hea0000875.

Gehrman, P., Seelig, A. D., Jacobson, I. G., Boyko, E. J., Hooper, T. I., Gackstetter, G. D., et al. (2013). Predeployment sleep duration and insomnia symptoms as risk factors for new-onset mental health disorders following military deployment. *Sleep*, *36*(7), 1009–1018.

Goetter, E. M., Herbert, J. D., Forman, E. M., Yuen, E. K., & Thomas, J. (2014). An open trial of videoconference-mediated exposure and ritual prevention for obsessive-compulsive disorder. *Journal of Anxiety Disorders*, *28*(5), 460–462. https://doi.org/10.1016/j.janxdis.2014.05.004.

Goldberg, S. B., Tucker, R. P., Greene, P. A., Davidson, R. J., Wampold, B. E., Kearney, D. J., et al. (2018). Mindfulness-based interventions for psychiatric disorders: A systematic review and meta-analysis. *Clinical Psychology Review*, *59*, 52–60. https://doi.org/10.1016/j.cpr.2017.10.011.

Goldman, N., Dugas, M. J., Sexton, K. A., & Gervais, N. J. (2007). The impact of written exposure on worry: A preliminary investigation. *Behavior Modification*, *31*(4), 512–538. https://doi.org/10.1177/0145445506298651.

González-Sanguino, C., Ausín, B., Castellanos, M.Á., Saiz, J., López-Gómez, A., Ugidos, C., et al. (2020). Mental health consequences during the initial stage of the 2020 coronavirus pandemic (COVID-19) in Spain. *Brain, Behavior, and Immunity*. https://doi.org/10.1016/j.bbi.2020.05.040.

Goyal, K., Chauhan, P., Chhikara, K., Gupta, P., & Singh, M. P. (2020). Fear of COVID 2019: First suicidal case in India! *Asian Journal of Psychiatry*, *49*, 101989.

Groves, P. M., & Thompson, R. F. (1970). Habituation: A dual-process theory. *Psychological Review*, *77*(5), 419–450. https://doi.org/10.1037/h0029810.

Hansen, B. H., Oerbeck, B., Skirbekk, B., & Kristensen, H. (2016). Non-obsessive–compulsive anxiety disorders in child and adolescent mental health services – Are they underdiagnosed, and how accurate is referral information? *Nordic Journal of Psychiatry*, *70*(2), 133–139.

Hofmann, S. G., & Asmundson, G. J. (2008). Acceptance and mindfulness-based therapy: New wave or old hat? *Clinical Psychology Review*, *28*(1), 1–16.

Hollon, S. D., & Ponniah, K. (2010). A review of empirically supported psychological therapies for mood disorders in adults. *Depression and Anxiety*, *27*(10), 891–932.

Hoyer, J., Beesdo, K., Gloster, A. T., Runge, J., Höfler, M., & Becker, E. S. (2009). Worry exposure versus applied relaxation in the treatment of generalized anxiety disorder. *Psychotherapy and Psychosomatics*, *78*(2), 106–115. https://doi.org/10.1159/000201936.

Hunsley, J., Elliott, K., & Therrien, Z. (2014). The efficacy and effectiveness of psychological treatments for mood, anxiety, and related disorders. *Canadian Psychology/Psychologie Canadienne*, *55*(3), 161.

Jacobson, N. S., Dobson, K. S., Truax, P. A., Addis, M. E., Koerner, K., Gollan, J. K., et al. (1996). A component analysis of cognitive-behavioral treatment for depression. *Journal of Consulting and Clinical Psychology*, *64*(2), 295.

Jaywant, A., Vanderlind, W. M., Boas, S. J., & Dickerman, A. L. (2020). Behavioral interventions in acute COVID-19 recovery: A new opportunity for integrated care. *General Hospital Psychiatry*. https://doi.org/10.1016/j.genhosppsych.2020.07.001.

Jensen-Doss, A., & Weisz, J. R. (2008). Diagnostic agreement predicts treatment process and outcomes in youth mental health clinics. *Journal of Consulting and Clinical Psychology*, *76*(5), 711.

Jensen-Doss, A., Youngstrom, E. A., Youngstrom, J. K., Feeny, N. C., & Findling, R. L. (2014). Predictors and moderators of agreement between clinical and research diagnoses for children and adolescents. *Journal of Consulting and Clinical Psychology*, *82*(6), 1151.

Kroenke, K., Spitzer, R. L., & Williams, J. B. W. (2001). The PHQ-9: Validity of a brief depression severity measure. *Journal of General Internal Medicine*, *16*(9), 606–613. https://doi.org/10.1046/j.1525-1497.2001.016009606.x.

Ladouceur, R., Dugas, M. J., Freeston, M. H., Léger, E., Gagnon, F., & Thibodeau, N. (2000). Efficacy of a cognitive-behavioral treatment for generalized anxiety disorder: Evaluation in a controlled clinical trial. *Journal of Consulting and Clinical Psychology*, *68*(6), 957–964. https://doi.org/10.1037/0022-006X.68.6.957.

Leahy, R. L. (2017). *Cognitive therapy techniques: A practitioner's guide*. Guilford Publications.

Lee, S. A. (2020a). Coronavirus anxiety scale: A brief mental health screener for COVID-19 related anxiety. *Death Studies*, *44*(7), 393–401. https://doi.org/10.1080/07481187.2020.1748481.

Lee, S. A. (2020b). How much "Thinking" about COVID-19 is clinically dysfunctional? *Brain, Behavior, and Immunity*, *87*, 97–98. https://doi.org/10.1016/j.bbi.2020.04.067.

Lee, S. A., Jobe, M. C., Mathis, A. A., & Gibbons, J. A. (2020). Incremental validity of coronaphobia: Coronavirus anxiety explains depression, generalized anxiety, and death anxiety. *Journal of Anxiety Disorders*, *74*. https://doi.org/10.1016/j.janxdis.2020.102268. Article 102268.

Lidren, D. M., Watkins, P. L., Gould, R. A., Clum, G. A., Asterino, M., & Tulloch, H. L. (1994). A comparison of bibliotherapy and group therapy in the treatment of panic disorder. *Journal of Consulting and Clinical Psychology*, *62*(4), 865–869. https://doi.org/10.1037//0022-006X.62.4.865.

Liu, K., Chen, Y., Wu, D., Lin, R., Wang, Z., & Pan, L. (2020). Effects of progressive muscle relaxation on anxiety and sleep quality in patients with COVID-19. *Complementary Therapies in Clinical Practice*, *39*. https://doi.org/10.1016/j.ctcp.2020.101132. Article 101132.

Lovell, K., Cox, D., Haddock, G., Jones, C., Raines, D., Garvey, R., et al. (2006). Telephone administered cognitive behaviour therapy for treatment of obsessive compulsive disorder: Randomised controlled non-inferiority trial. *British Medical Journal*, *333*(7574), 883–886. http://www.scopus.com/inward/record.url?eid=2-s2.0-33750590360&partnerID=40&md5=7dee254ee6f2f95bd84d31c548d9e6c6.

Luo, M., Guo, L., Yu, M., & Wang, H. (2020). The psychological and mental impact of coronavirus disease 2019 (COVID-19) on medical staff and general public – A systematic review and meta-analysis. *Psychiatry Research*, *291*. https://doi.org/10.1016/j.psychres.2020.113190. Article 113190.

Mamun, M. A., & Griffiths, M. D. (2020). First COVID-19 suicide case in Bangladesh due to fear of COVID-19 and xenophobia: Possible suicide prevention strategies. *Asian Journal of Psychiatry*, *51*, 102073.

Manansingh, S., Tatum, S. L., & Morote, E. S. (2019). Effects of relaxation techniques on nursing students' academic stress and test anxiety. *Journal of Nursing Education*, *58*(9), 534–537. https://doi.org/10.3928/01484834-20190819-07.

Martinsen, E. W. (2008). Physical activity in the prevention and treatment of anxiety and depression. *Nordic Journal of Psychiatry*, *62*(Suppl 47), 25–29.

Matsumoto, K., Sutoh, C., Asano, K., Seki, Y., Urao, Y., Yokoo, M., et al. (2018). Internet-based cognitive behavioral therapy with real-time therapist support via videoconference for patients with obsessive-compulsive disorder, panic disorder, and social anxiety disorder: Pilot single-arm trial. *Journal of Medical Internet Research*, *20*(12), e12091. https://doi.org/10.2196/12091.

Mayer, Y., Etgar, S., Shiffman, N., & Lurie, I. (2020). *The fear of COVID-19 familial infection scale: Initial psychometric examination*. PsyArXiv Reprints.

Mertens, G., Gerritsen, L., Duijndam, S., Salemink, E., & Engelhard, I. M. (2020). Fear of the coronavirus (COVID-19): Predictors in an online study conducted in March 2020. *Journal of Anxiety Disorders, 74*. https://doi.org/10.1016/j.janxdis.2020.102258. Article 102258.

Michael, T., Ehlers, A., Halligan, S. L., & Clark, D. M. (2005). Unwanted memories of assault: What intrusion characteristics are associated with PTSD? *Behaviour Research and Therapy, 43*(5), 613–628. https://doi.org/10.1016/j.brat.2004.04.006.

Mohr, D. C., Ho, J., Duffecy, J., Reifler, D., Sokol, L., Burns, M. N., et al. (2012). Effect of telephone-administered vs face-to-face cognitive behavioral therapy on adherence to therapy and depression outcomes among primary care patients: A randomized trial. *JAMA – Journal of the American Medical Association, 307*(21), 2278–2285. https://doi.org/10.1001/jama.2012.5588.

Moses, K., Gayed, M., Chuah, S., & Wootton, B. M. (2020). The use of evidence-based assessment for anxiety disorders in an Australian sample. *Journal of Anxiety Disorders, 75*, 102279. https://doi.org/10.1016/j.janxdis.2020.102279.

Norton, P. J., & Price, E. C. (2007). A meta-analytic review of adult cognitive-behavioral treatment outcome across the anxiety disorders. *Journal of Nervous and Mental Disease, 195*(6), 521–531.

Olatunji, B. O., Cisler, J. M., & Deacon, B. J. (2010). Efficacy of cognitive behavioral therapy for anxiety disorders: A review of meta-analytic findings. *Psychiatric Clinics of North America, 33*(3), 557–577. https://doi.org/10.1016/j.psc.2010.04.002.

Ollendick, T. H., & Hersen, M. (1993). Child and adolescent behavioral assessment. *Handbook of child and adolescent assessment*. New York: Pergamon.

Persons, J. (2008). *The case formulation approach to cognitive-behavior therapy (guides to individualized evidence-based treatment)*. New York: Guilford.

Pogge, D. L., Wayland-Smith, D., Zaccario, M., Borgaro, S., Stokes, J., & Harvey, P. D. (2001). Diagnosis of manic episodes in adolescent inpatients: Structured diagnostic procedures compared to clinical chart diagnoses. *Psychiatry Research, 101*(1), 47–54.

Rajkumar, R. P. (2020). COVID-19 and mental health: A review of the existing literature. *Asian Journal of Psychiatry, 52*. https://doi.org/10.1016/j.ajp.2020.102066. Article 102066.

Randall, C., Nowakowski, S., & Ellis, J. G. (2019). Managing acute insomnia in prison: Evaluation of a "one-shot" cognitive behavioral therapy for insomnia (CBT-I) intervention. *Behavioral Sleep Medicine, 6*, 827–836.

Ransing, R., Ramalho, R., Orsolini, L., Adiukwu, F., Gonzalez-Diaz, J. M., Larnaout, A., et al. (2020). Can COVID-19 related mental health issues be measured?: Assessment options for mental health professionals. *Brain, Behavior, and Immunity, 88*, 32–34.

Reznik, A., Gritsenko, V., Konstantinov, V., Khamenka, N., & Isralowitz, R. (2020). COVID-19 fear in Eastern Europe: Validation of the Fear of COVID-19 Scale. *International Journal of Mental Health and Addiction, 18*, 1–6.

Rogers, J. P., Chesney, E., Oliver, D., Pollak, T. A., McGuire, P., Fusar-Poli, P., et al. (2020). Psychiatric and neuropsychiatric presentations associated with severe coronavirus infections: A systematic review and meta-analysis with comparison to the COVID-19 pandemic. *The Lancet Psychiatry*. https://doi.org/10.1016/S2215-0366(20)30203-0.

Sakib, N., Bhuiyan, A. I., Hossain, S., Al Mamun, F., Hosen, I., Abdullah, A. H., et al. (2020). Psychometric validation of the Bangla Fear of COVID-19 Scale: Confirmatory factor analysis and Rasch analysis. *International Journal of Mental Health and Addiction, 18*, 1–12.

Salkovskis, P. M. (1985). Obsessional-compulsive problems: A cognitive-behavioural analysis. *Behaviour Research and Therapy, 23*(5), 571–583. https://doi.org/10.1016/0005-7967(85)90105-6.

Satici, B., Gocet-Tekin, E., Deniz, M. E., & Satici, S. A. (2020). Adaptation of the Fear of COVID-19 Scale: Its association with psychological distress and life satisfaction in Turkey. *International Journal of Mental Health and Addiction, 18*, 1–9.

Silver, R. C., Holman, E. A., Andersen, J. P., Poulin, M., McIntosh, D. N., & Gil-Rivas, V. (2013). Mental- and physical-health effects of acute exposure to media images of the September 11, 2001, attacks and the Iraq War. *Psychological Science*, *24*(9), 1623–1634. https://doi.org/10.1177/0956797612460406.

Silverman, W. K., & Ollendick, T. H. (2005). Evidence-based assessment of anxiety and its disorders in children and adolescents. *Journal of Clinical Child and Adolescent Psychology*, *34*(3), 380–411. https://doi.org/10.1207/s15374424jccp3403_2.

Soraci, P., Ferrari, A., Abbiati, F. A., Del Fante, E., De Pace, R., Urso, A., et al. (2020). Validation and psychometric evaluation of the Italian version of the Fear of COVID-19 Scale. *International Journal of Mental Health and Addiction*, *18*, 1–10.

Spence, J., Titov, N., Dear, B. F., Johnston, L., Solley, K., Lorian, C., et al. (2011). Randomized controlled trial of Internet-delivered cognitive behavioral therapy for posttraumatic stress disorder. *Depression and Anxiety*, *28*(7), 541–550. https://doi.org/10.1002/da.20835.

Spitzer, R. L., Kroenke, K., Williams, J. B. W., & Löwe, B. (2006). A brief measure for assessing generalized anxiety disorder: The GAD-7. *Archives of Internal Medicine*, *166*(10), 1092–1097. https://doi.org/10.1001/archinte.166.10.1092.

Stanley, B., & Brown, G. K. (2012). Safety planning intervention: A brief intervention to mitigate suicide risk. *Cognitive and Behavioral Practice*, *19*(2), 256–264.

Stanley, B., Brown, G., Brent, D. A., Wells, K., Poling, K., Curry, J., et al. (2009). Cognitive-behavioral therapy for suicide prevention (CBT-SP): Treatment model, feasibility, and acceptability. *Journal of the American Academy of Child & Adolescent Psychiatry*, *48*(10), 1005–1013.

Stewart, R. E., & Chambless, D. L. (2009). Cognitive–behavioral therapy for adult anxiety disorders in clinical practice: A meta-analysis of effectiveness studies. *Journal of Consulting and Clinical Psychology*, *77*(4), 595.

Stubbings, D. R., Rees, C. S., Roberts, L. D., & Kane, R. T. (2013). Comparing in-person to videoconference-based cognitive behavioral therapy for mood and anxiety disorders: Randomized controlled trial. *Journal of Medical Internet Research*, *15*(11). https://doi.org/10.2196/jmir.2564. Article e258.

Taylor, S., Landry, C. A., Paluszek, M. M., Fergus, T. A., McKay, D., & Asmundson, G. J. G. (2020a). COVID stress syndrome: Concept, structure, and correlates. *Depression and Anxiety*. https://doi.org/10.1002/da.23071.

Taylor, S., Landry, C. A., Paluszek, M. M., Fergus, T. A., McKay, D., & Asmundson, G. J. G. (2020b). Development and initial validation of the COVID Stress Scales. *Journal of Anxiety Disorders*, *72*. https://doi.org/10.1016/j.janxdis.2020.102232. Article 102232.

Titov, N., Staples, L., Kayrouz, R., Cross, S., Karin, E., Ryan, K., et al. (2020). Rapid report: Early demand, profiles and concerns of mental health users during the coronavirus (COVID-19) pandemic. *Internet Interventions*, *21*. https://doi.org/10.1016/j.invent.2020.100327. Article 100327.

Tolin, D. F. (2016). *Doing CBT: A comprehensive guide to working with behaviors, thoughts, and emotions*. Guilford Publications.

Tolin, D. F., Gilliam, C., Wootton, B. M., Bowe, W., Bragdon, L. B., Davis, E., et al. (2018). Psychometric properties of a structured diagnostic interview for DSM-5 anxiety, mood, and obsessive-compulsive and related disorders. *Assessment*, *25*(1), 3–13. https://doi.org/10.1177/1073191116638410.

Tolin, D. F., Wootton, B. M., Levy, H. C., Hallion, L. S., Worden, B. L., Diefenbach, G. J., et al. (2019). Efficacy and mediators of a group cognitive-behavioral therapy for hoarding disorder: A randomized trial. *Journal of Consulting and Clinical Psychology*, *87*(7), 590–602. https://doi.org/10.1037/ccp0000405.

Turner, J. S., & Leach, D. J. (2010). Experimental evaluation of behavioral activation treatment of anxiety (BATA) in three older adults. *International Journal of Behavioral Consultation and Therapy*, *6*(4), 373.

van der Heiden, C., & ten Broeke, E. (2009). The when, why, and how of worry exposure. *Cognitive and Behavioral Practice*, *16*(4), 386–393. https://doi.org/10.1016/j.cbpra.2008.11.003.

Veale, D. (2004). Advances in a cognitive behavioural model of body dysmorphic disorder. *Body Image*, *1*(1), 113–125. https://doi.org/10.1016/S1740-1445(03)00009-3.

Wahlund, T., Mataix-Cols, D., Lauri, K., de Schipper, E., Ljótsson, B., Aspvall, K., et al. (2020). *Brief online-delivered cognitive-behavioural therapy for dysfunctional worry related to the covid-19 pandemic: A randomised trial*. https://doi.org/10.31234/osf.io/rdka2.

Wang, C., Pan, R., Wan, X., Tan, Y., Xu, L., Ho, C. S., et al. (2020). Immediate psychological responses and associated factors during the initial stage of the 2019 coronavirus disease (COVID-19) epidemic among the general population in China. *International Journal of Environmental Research and Public Health*, *17*(5). https://doi.org/10.3390/ijerph17051729. Article 1729.

Warwick, H. M. C., & Salkovskis, P. M. (1990). Hypochondriasis. *Behaviour Research and Therapy*, *28*(2), 105–117. https://doi.org/10.1016/0005-7967(90)90023-C.

Wharff, E. A., Ginnis, K. B., Ross, A. M., White, E. M., White, M. T., & Forbes, P. W. (2019). Family-based crisis intervention with suicidal adolescents: A randomized clinical trial. *Pediatric Emergency Care*, *35*(3), 170–175.

Wootton, B. M. (2016). Remote cognitive-behavior therapy for obsessive-compulsive symptoms: A meta-analysis. *Clinical Psychology Review*, *43*, 103–113. https://doi.org/10.1016/j.cpr.2015.10.001.

Wootton, B. M., Dear, B. F., Johnston, L., Terides, M. D., & Titov, N. (2013). Remote treatment of obsessive-compulsive disorder: A randomized controlled trial. *Journal of Obsessive-Compulsive and Related Disorders*, *2*(4), 375–384. https://doi.org/10.1016/j.jocrd.2013.07.002.

Wootton, B. M., Karin, E., Titov, N., & Dear, B. F. (2019). Self-guided internet–delivered cognitive behavior therapy (ICBT) for obsessive-compulsive symptoms: A randomized controlled trial. *Journal of Anxiety Disorders*, *66*. https://doi.org/10.1016/j.janxdis.2019.102111. Article 102111.

Wootton, B. M., Steinman, S. A., Czerniawski, A., Norris, K., Baptie, C., Diefenbach, G., et al. (2018). An evaluation of the effectiveness of a transdiagnostic bibliotherapy program for anxiety and related disorders: Results from two studies using a benchmarking approach. *Cognitive Therapy and Research*. https://doi.org/10.1007/s10608-018-9921-x.

Yıldırım, M., & Güler, A. (2020). Factor analysis of the COVID-19 perceived risk scale: A preliminary study. *Death Studies*, *44*, 1–8.

Zhou, F., Yu, T., Du, R., Fan, G., Liu, Y., Liu, Z., et al. (2020). Clinical course and risk factors for mortality of adult inpatients with COVID-19 in Wuhan, China: A retrospective cohort study. *The Lancet*, *395*(10229), 1054–1062. https://doi.org/10.1016/S0140-6736(20)30566-3.

Index

Note: Page numbers followed by *f* indicate figures and *t* indicate tables.

A

Active engagement, 287–288
Activity scheduling, 309–310
Acute lower respiratory infection (ALRI), 193–194
Acute respiratory distress syndrome (ARDS), 190
Acute stress disorder, 91
Adaptive coping mechanisms, 159–160
Addictive disorders, 9–10
Adherence, 263–265, 270–271
Alzheimer's disease (AD), 153–154, 226
American College of Sports Medicine (ASCM), 219–220
American Heart Association, 220
Anger/irritability, 75–76
Anorexia nervosa, 160, 162
Antidepressant nutrients, 203–204
Anxiety, 28–29, 76–77, 90–91, 106–107, 301
Arousal reduction techniques, 309
Australian Psychological Society, 123
Australian Securities and Investments Commission (ASIC), 9
Autism spectrum disorder (ASD), 188–189, 222

B

Bacterial-induced sepsis, 190
Behavioral despair, 139
Belonginess theory, 285
Bibliotherapy-delivered cognitive behavioral therapy (BCBT), 311
Big Five traits, 273
Biomedical model, 111
Boredom, 142, 293
Buddy style, 54–55
Bulimia nervosa, 160

C

Calcifediol, 189–190
Care leaving
- challenges, 20–21
- coping mechanisms
  - changing/holding on known, 30–31
  - informal support systems, 32
  - optimistic position and accepting change, 31
  - religion, faith and prayer, 29
- data analysis, 23, 24–25*t*
- effects of COVID-19
  - disrupted social support systems, 27
  - employment and livelihood-related issues, 26–27
  - fear and anxiety, 28–29
  - strained relationships, 27
- informal care arrangements, 19–20
- informal economy, 33
- internal resources, 34
- less resilient/maladaptive coping strategies, 33
- mental health and psychosocial support services, 32–33
- parental care, 19
- purposive sampling, 21
- qualitative approach, 21
- social demographic data, 21, 22*t*
- social protection responses, 33–34
- unstructured interview, 23
- vocational training and entrepreneurship, 20

CBT. *See* Cognitive behavioral therapy (CBT)
Centers for Disease Control and Prevention (CDC), 171
CF. *See* Cystic fibrosis (CF)
Children's Yale-Brown Obsessive-Compulsive Scale (CYBOCS), 177–178
Chronic obstructive pulmonary disease (COPD), 195
Chronic trauma, 253
Clinical psychology, 105
Clinician-administered rating scales, 302
CLT. *See* Cognitive load theory (CLT)
Coercion, 263–264

Cognitive behavioral therapy (CBT), 167–168
activity scheduling, 309–310
cognitive restructuring, 305–306
crisis support, 310–311
eliminating safety behaviors, 308
imaginal exposure, 307–308
individualized case formulation, 304–305
in vivo exposure, 306–307
physiological arousal and stress reduction, 309
psychoeducation, 305
remote, 311–312
situation selection, 305
sleep hygiene, 310
structured problem solving, 308–309
Cognitive distortions, 175–176
Cognitive functioning, 154–155
Cognitive load theory (CLT), 267–268
Cognitive restructuring, 305–306
Cohesive emotional unit, 239–240
Community mobilizer, 72
Compliance, 263–265, 273
Compulsions, 172–174
Compulsive sexual behavior disorder, 10
Congolese, 71, 75
Conspiracy mentality, 265–266, 270
Conspiracy theories. *See* Health-related misinformation
Conspiracy theory of society, 265
Conspirational fantasies, 265
COPD. *See* Chronic obstructive pulmonary disease (COPD)
Coping mechanisms, 80–81, 84
Coronaphobia, 83
Coronavirus Anxiety Scale, 302–303
Coronavirus Reassurance-Seeking Behaviors Scale, 302–303, 308
Coronavirus Stress Measure, 302–303
COVID-19 health-protective behaviors, 269–271
COVID-19 Perceived Risk Scale, 302–303
COVID-19 response team formation, 63–64
COVID Stress Scale (CSS), 302–303
COVID stress syndrome, 301–302, 308
Crisis support, 310–311
Cystic fibrosis (CF), 198–199

D

Dark Triad traits, 274, 276
Data explication process, 23, 24–25*t*
Deficient self-regulation (DSR), 268
Department of Refugees (DOR), 69
Depression, 46, 90–91, 106–107, 117, 133–134, 301
Diagnostic Interview for Anxiety, Mood, Obsessive-Compulsive and Related Neuropsychiatric Disorders (DIAMOND), 302
Digital communication, 284
Digital divide, 123
Digital literacy, 124, 126
Disengagement theory, 106
Distress
assessment, 302–304
cognitive behavioral therapy (*see* Cognitive behavioral therapy (CBT))
COVID-19, 301–302
Dopamine, 6
Dopaminergic neurons, 141–142
DOR. *See* Department of Refugees (DOR)
Down syndrome
physical exercise, 225–226
SARS COV 2, 224–225
DSR. *See* Deficient self-regulation (DSR)

E

Eating disorders
clinical implications
face-to-face therapy, 166
guided self-help, 168–169
inpatient, 166–167
outpatient, 167
telehealth, 167–168
treatment as usual, 165–166
exercise limitations, 163–164
food access, 164
media impact, 162–163
mental health, 159–162
pathology, 160
physiological resilience, 160
psychiatric disturbances, 159–160
roles and family dynamics, 164–165
social distancing and self-quarantine measures, 159–160
social isolation and decreased social support, 165
symptomatology, 161
Ecological systems theory, 238–239, 239*f*
Emotional health
chronic disease illnesses, 47
expressions, 41
hemorrhagic fevers, 41–42
infection rates and deaths, 41–42
intensive care unit, 45

observation, 46
personal protective equipment, 42–43
psychologically traumatized, 48
response team, 42
stress, 44–45
surgical procedures, 43
swabbing, 44
Ugandan context, 43–44
Emotional wellbeing, 122
Emotion-focused coping strategies, 53
Emotion regulation, 121
Entertainment, 294
Epigallocatechin-3-gallate (EGCG), 191
Episodic memory, 154–155
European College of Neuropsychopharmacology (OCRN), 178–179
Eusociality, 134–135
Exposure and response prevention (ERP), 173–174, 176–177

F

Family-based therapy (FBT), 168
Family separation, 247
Family support, 57
Family System's Model, 239–241
Family violence, 249–250
Fear of COVID-19 Familial Infection Scale, 302–303
Fear of COVID-19 Scale, 302–303
Fear of missing out (FOMO), 291, 296
Financial burden, 246
Financial distress, 76
Fogg behavior model (FBM), 106–107
Functional Independence Measure (FIM), 205

G

Gambling disorder
COVID-19 impact, 7–10
gambling and, 4–5
vulnerability, 5–7
Generalized Anxiety Disorder Scale, 303
Genetic disorders, 224
Geriatric diseases, 117
Ghana, 19
COVID-19
lockdowns and restrictions, 104–105
sociocultural challenges, 105–107
health belief and health-seeking attitudes, 103
health problems and COVID-19 compliance, 109–113
individuals, restrictions and lockdowns on, 107–109
sociocultural life, 103
Global nutrition report, 188
Good healthcare system leadership, 55

H

HAART. *See* Highly active antiretroviral therapy (HAART)
Hallucinations
Alzheimer's disease (AD), 153–154
assessment and results, 155
cases, 154–155
cognitive and functional impairments, 153–154
communal dining, 155–156
neuropsychiatric symptoms, 156–157
nursing homes, 153–154
psychiatric symptoms, 154
social distancing and isolation, 155–156
social restrictions, 156–157
HBV. *See* Hepatitis B vaccine (HBV)
Health anxiety, 241–242
Health belief model, 109–110, 109*f*, 264–265
Healthcare professionals, 179–181
Health-protective behaviors
adoption, personality traits, 273–275
perceived risk, 271–273
Health-related misinformation
conspiracy mentality, 265–266
COVID-19 health-protective behaviors, 269–271
factors, 267–269
nonnormative preventive behaviors, 265–266
political and socioeconomic events, 265–266
public health crises, 265
social media, 266–267
Health-seeking behavior, 108–109, 109*f*
Health workers
appropriate scheduling of duties, 53–54
behavioral mental health challenges, 51–52
biological, physiological and psychological responses, 38
clinical and nonclinical, 38
coping mechanisms, 52–53
developed positive thinking, 59
developing mutual support, 54–55
emotional effects, 41–48
family support, 57
good healthcare system leadership, 55
infected returnees, 37
infection prevention control and standard operating procedures, 57–58

Health workers *(Continued)*
interpersonal emotional building mechanisms, 55–56
interpersonal problem solving mechanisms, 53
intrapersonal coping strategies, 57
mental health and psychosocial challenges, 41, 52–53
methods, 40
morale boosting from workmates, 56–57
pandemic response services, 39
patient-centered care, 62
psychosocial factors, 48–51, 64
response strategies, 39
response team, 53
sense of calling to serve patients, 58–59
special contribution, 60
spirituality, 60–62
staying away from family, 58
sub-Saharan Africa, 39
Hepatitis B vaccine (HBV), 188–189
Hierarchical regression analyses, 286–287
High dose of intravenous vitamin C (HIVC), 190
Highly active antiretroviral therapy (HAART), 188–189
Home-based physical exercise, 220
Human motivation, 133–134

I

ICBT. *See* Internet-delivered cognitive behavioral therapy (ICBT)
Imaginal exposure, 307–308
Immune development, 200
Immunity, 188–191, 196–198
In-depth interview techniques, 40
Individualized case formulation, 304–305
Inflammatory bowel disease (IBD), 193–194
Informal market economy, 82
Informal support systems, 32
Intellectual disabilities, 225–226
International College of Obsessive Compulsive Spectrum Disorders (ICOCS), 178–179
Internet-based strategies, 219
Internet-delivered cognitive behavioral therapy (ICBT), 311
Interpersonal coping factors, 52
Interpersonal emotional building mechanisms
hobbies that kill off stress, 55–56
keeping staff together, 56
Interpersonal problem solving mechanisms, 53
Interpersonal theory of suicide, 123
Intrapersonal coping strategies, 57
In vivo exposure, 306–307
Isolation syndrome, 138–139
Isolation treatment unit (ITU), 43

L

Latvian government, 10
Loss of appetite, 52
Low- and middle-income countries (LMICs), 70
Lower respiratory tract infections (LRTI), 193–194

M

Malnutrition, 160, 188, 192, 204–205
Mass sensitization, 85
Mediation analysis, 95–96
Mental health
disaster management plans, 218
high transmission rate, 217–218
impacts, 291, 295–296
nutrition, 202–204
professionals, 284
psychosocial challenges, 41
repercussions, 3
sedentary behavior, 218
Meta-regression analysis, 190
Micronutrients, 188–189, 191, 205–206
Mind-body exercises, 221
Mindfulness-based interventions, 309
Morale boosting from workmates, 56–57
Multiinformant assessment, 302
Multimethod assessment, 302
Multinomial logistics regression analysis, 201–202
Multiorgan dysfunction, 190
Multivitamin supplementation, 193
Musculoskeletal health, 216

N

Negative socioemotional changes, 293
Neuromotor exercise training, 221
Neuroticism, 273
Novel Coronavirus Disease 2019 (COVID-19), 89, 138, 216
Nutraceuticals, 188–189
Nutrition
background, 188
COVID-19
contemporary evidence, 199
immune development, 200

infectivity, 200–201
management, 204–205
optimal mental health, 202–204
recoveries, 201–202
disease recovery, 194–195
immunity, 188–191
infection cycle, 192–193
infectivity, 193–194
respiratory illness, 195–199

O

Obsession with COVID-19 Scale, 302–303
Obsessive-Compulsive and Related Disorders Research Network, 178–179
Obsessive-compulsive disorder (OCD)
bimodal distribution, 171–172
clinical features, 172
compulsions, 172–173
cortico-striato-thalamo-cortical pathways, 173–174
Covid-19 pandemic
effect of, 175–179
excessive behavior, 174
diagnosis, 173
dimensional approach, 172–173
intolerance of uncertainty, 175–176
prevalence, 179–181
symptoms, 171
Older adults
loneliness
mental health impacts during coronavirus pandemic, 120–123
older age and mental health implications, 118–120
online communication
during coronavirus pandemic, 126
social media, 123–126
Ongoing cardiac stress test, 253
Online communication
during coronavirus pandemic, 126
social media, 123–126
technologies, 283–284, 288, 296–297
Orphan and vulnerable children (OVC), 19–20
Orthographic principles, 40
Orthorexia nervosa, 160–161

P

Parallel disaster management interventions, 69–70
Paranoia, 269–270
Parental burnout, 247–250
Parenting
burnout, 247–250
coping strategies, 235, 250–253
landscape
blended and extended family, 236–237
corporate family, 236
financial, social and emotional support, 237
positive reinforcement, 237–238
provision of opportunity, 238
psychological flexibility and adaptability, 236–237
school-type environments, 237–238
multitasking, 235
parent-child dynamic, 238–240
posttraumatic growth, 253–254
stressors, 240–247
Passive engagement, 287–288
Patient Health Questionnaire, 303
Perceived risk, 271–273
Personal protective equipment (PPE), 42–43, 60
Physical activity
chronic diseases, 216
consequences, 217–218
Down syndrome, 224–226
economic impact, 216
musculoskeletal health, 216
national and international public health policies, 216
prevention, COVID-19 spread, 217
psychological well-being, 216
SARS-CoV-2, 216
sedentary behavior, bed rest and physical inactivity, 218–219
sports, 219–226
Physical distancing, 104–105, 118
Physical inactivity, 215, 218–219
Pornography addiction, 12–14
Positive socioemotional changes, 293
Positive thinking, 59
Posttraumatic growth, 253–254
Posttraumatic stress disorders, 301
PPE. *See* Personal protective equipment (PPE)
Probiotics, 188–189
Problematic pornography use (PPU), 12–13
Problem-solving coping strategies, 53, 57–58
Procrastination, 293
Psychoeducation, 181, 305
Psychological distress, 89–96, 106–109, 121
Psychological flexibility, 94–97
Psychological wellbeing, 122, 216, 268
social connectedness, 285, 295
social media and negative impacts, 287

Psychosocial stress, 7
Psychotherapy process, 176–177
Public health agencies, 275–276
Public Health Emergency of International Concern (PHEIC), 103–104
Public health professionals, 263–264
Purposive sampling, 21

Q
Qualitative data analysis, 289–294
Quantitative data analysis, 289
Quarantinos, 49

R
Relationship initiation, 290
Relationship maintenance, 290
Remote cognitive behavioral therapy (CBT), 311–312
Residential care, 20
Resilience, 33, 80–81, 84, 252–253, 285
Respiratory illness
  immunomodulatory effect, 195
  low calcifediol levels, 195
  nutrition
    immunity, 196–198
    recovery, 198–199
    respiratory infectivity, 195–196
Risk allowances, 38
Royal Spanish Football Federation, 224

S
Safety behaviors, 308
SARS-CoV-2. *See* Severe acute respiratory syndrome coronavirus 2 (SARS-CoV-2)
Selective serotonin reuptake inhibitors (SSRI), 173–174
Selenium (Se), 190–191, 202, 205–206
Selenoprotein P (SELENOP), 190–191
Self-care self-efficacy, 92–93
Self-esteem, 297
Self-imposed/voluntary *vs.* enforced isolation, 137–138
Self-perceived pornography addiction (SPPA), 12–13
Semistructured interview, 73
Severe acute respiratory syndrome (SARS), 89–90
Severe acute respiratory syndrome coronavirus 2 (SARS-CoV-2), 106–107, 216
Sex and love addicts anonymous (SLA), 12
Sexual addiction, 10–12
Sexual behaviors, 10–12
Sexually transmitted diseases (STDs), 11–12
Situation selection, 305
Sleep deprivation, 246
Sleep disorders, 77–78, 301
Sleep hygiene, 310
SMF. *See* Social media fatigue (SMF)
SNSs. *See* Social networking sites (SNSs)
Social capital, 125
Social connectedness
  and psychological wellbeing, 285
  social media, 285–287
Social damage, 138–139
Social distancing
  definition, 103–104
  and isolation, 155–156
  measures, 118
  quarantine measures, 89
  restrictions, 3–4
  self-quarantine measures, 159–160
Social exclusion, 63–64
Social isolation, 161–162, 165
  behavioral effects, 138–140
  decreased social support, 165
  definition, 136–137
  depression laboratory model, 133–134
  lockdown, 253–254
  loneliness, 203, 284
  physiological effects, 140–142
  self-imposed/voluntary *vs.* enforced isolation, 137–138
  sociality, 134–136
  staying at home, 225
  stress reaction and hallucinations, 155–156
  task, 273
  uniquely human aspect, 142–143
Sociality, 134–136
Socially assistive robot (SAR), 125–126
Social malfunction, 80
Social media
  defined, 283
  elements, 283
  frequency count, 289, 289*t*
  health-related misinformation, 266–267
  method, 288–289
  methodological limitations, 287–288
  negative impacts, 287
  online communication, 123–126
  overuse, 291
  positive and negative psychological effects, 283–284
  qualitative data analysis, 289–294

quantitative data analysis, 289
rationale, 288
and social connectedness, 285–287
themes
mental health impacts, 291
news/discussion, 294
passive and less connection, 290
relationship maintenance and initiation, 290
relieve boredom, procrastinate/entertain, 293
Social media fatigue (SMF), 267–268
Social networking, 82, 89, 123
Social networking sites (SNSs), 283
Social stress, 135–136
Social support, 79–80, 92–94, 107–108, 165, 251
Socioeconomic status (SES), 244
Socioemotional selectivity theory, 122
SOPs. *See* Standard operating procedures (SOPs)
Spirituality
adequate training and preparedness, 61
emotion coping, 60–61
medical condition, 61
mental health and psychosocial challenges, 60
mild symptoms, 60–61
opportunity to learn, 62
personal protective equipment, 60
Sports
athletes, 223–224
children and adolescents, 222
elderly, 220–222
healthy adults, 219–220
immunological system, 219
monitor exercise, 219
SPPA. *See* Self-perceived pornography addiction (SPPA)
SSRI. *See* Selective serotonin reuptake inhibitors (SSRI)
Standard operating procedures (SOPs), 42–43, 57–58, 62–63
STDs. *See* Sexually transmitted diseases (STDs)
Stereotype embodiment theory, 120–121
Stigmatization, 48–50, 112–113
Stressors
emotional and behavioral sequelae, 241
family separation, 247
financial burden, 246
health anxiety, 241–242
implications, 241
role collision and navigation
guidance counselor, 244–245
teacher, 243–244
worker, 242–243
sleep deprivation, 246
Stress reduction, 309
Structured interview schedules, 302
Structured problem solving, 308–309
Subjective wellbeing, 287–288
Substance use disorders, 301
Suicidal ideation, 119–120
Support services providers, 38
Swallowing training techniques, 205

T

Telehealth, 167–168
Telemedicine, 178–179
Telephone-delivered cognitive behavioral therapy (TCBT), 311–312
Thematic network analysis, 23, 73, 286–287
Transaction stress model, 250
Traumatic event, 240
Tricyclic antidepressant (TCA), 140
Trisomy 21. *See* Down syndrome

U

Uganda, 19, 69, 71, 76
Ugandan government, 69
Unemployment, 20
United Nations Human Development Index, 19
University of Ghana Medical Centre (UGMC), 42–43
Upper respiratory tract (URT), 190
Urban refugees
anger/irritability, 75–76
anxiety, 76–77
design, 71
fear of COVID-19, 75
financial distress, 76
lethal communicability, 70
loss of personal control, 83
loss of social support, 79–80
neighboring countries, 71
procedures, 72–73
psychosocial impact, 70, 73–75, 84–85
public health measures, 69
resilience and coping mechanisms, 80–81, 84
ruptured lives, 83
sample, 71–72
sleep disorders, 77–78
social and physical isolation, 78–79

Urban refugees *(Continued)*
social malfunction, 80
social role limitations and lost identity, 82
sociodemographic characteristics, interviewees, 73, 74*t*
vulnerable groups, 69–70

V

Videoconferencing-delivered cognitive behavioral therapy (VCBT), 311–312
Virtual reality (VR), 125–126
Vitamin C, 202, 205–206
Vitamin D supplements, 192–193, 196

W

Weight management, 219
Wellbeing
emotional, 122
psychological, 122, 216, 268, 285, 287, 295
social connection, 296
subjective, 287–288
Working memory, 139–140, 154–155
Work readiness programs, 20–21
World Health Organization (WHO), 12, 89–90, 103–104, 117–118, 171, 215–216, 220, 222
Worry exposure, 307–308

Y

Yale-Brown Obsessive-Compulsive Scale (YBOCS), 177–178